OXFORD MEDICAL PUBLICATIONS

Post-operative Complications

Oxford Specialist Handbooks

Post-operative complications

Second Edition

Edited by

David Leaper

Visiting Professor
Department of Wound Healing
Cardiff University, UK

Iain Whitaker

Plastic, Reconstructive and Burns Surgery
Welsh Centre for Burns and Plastic Surgery
Morriston Hospital
Swansea, UK

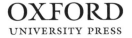

OXFORD
UNIVERSITY PRESS

OXFORD
UNIVERSITY PRESS

Great Clarendon Street, Oxford, OX2 6DP,
United Kingdom

Oxford University Press is a department of the University of Oxford.
It furthers the University's objective of excellence in research, scholarship,
and education by publishing worldwide. Oxford is a registered trade mark of
Oxford University Press in the UK and in certain other countries

Published in the United States of America by Oxford University Press
198 Madison Avenue, New York, NY 10016, United States of America

British Library Cataloguing in Publication Data
Data available

Library of Congress Cataloging in Publication Data
Data available

ISBN 978-0-19-954626-8

Preface

As we started to compile this second edition of *Post-operative Complications* we felt it important to define what a complication is. If you perform a PUBMED search using the phrase 'surgical complication(s)', depending over how long a period you search, over 900 articles will be returned. Despite their importance and prevalence, there seems to be no agreed definition. An appropriate definition has been devised by Adedeji et al., in their article 'Ethics of Surgical Complications', which we felt was appropriate:

A surgical complication is any undesirable, unintended, and direct result of surgery affecting the patient which would not have occurred had the surgery gone as well as reasonably hoped.

Adedeji et al., *World Journal of Surgery*, 2009

Complications following surgical procedures are associated with significant morbidity and mortality, add immensely to the psychological burden of the patient, and are disappointing for the surgical team. Unfortunately they are a fact of life, although we should continue to strive for the lowest incidence. Recent research has led to a greater understanding of the response to surgery and anaesthesia, and great advances have been made in pre-operative preparation with appropriate investigations and pharmacological prophylaxis. These have reduced the incidence of many complications, but the risks are impossible to remove completely.

In addition, patients are increasingly aware of the risks and complications of surgery, and are keen to help to minimize their risk in whatever way they can. Information and 'league tables' regarding surgical success rates are increasingly available in various forms. However, these should be viewed with caution, as they are not always adjusted to allow for patient co-morbidities or the level of surgical difficulty. Things are rarely black and white in surgery.

Regular audits should be undertaken by surgical teams in order to optimize patient care and to learn lessons where possible. Doctors are more aware of the power of EBM (evidence-based medicine) than they may have been some years ago. All surgeons will hopefully be aware of the Cochrane database, which collates best evidence, and adhere to the ever-expanding guidance and protocols emanating from the National Institute for Health and Clinical Excellence (NICE) and the Scottish Intercollegiate Guidelines Network (SIGN). Most surgical expertise is still passed on by apprenticeship, experience, reading peer-reviewed journals and continuing medical education. Although the expectations of surgery by the general public are increasing, surgical trainees are spending less time learning, particularly in the operating theatre, than ever before. The impact of the European Working Time Directive (EWTD) and changes in surgical training will no doubt produce a different type of surgeon. Nevertheless, he or she must not only be aware of all the potential complications for each procedure performed, but also how to minimize the occurrence of such complications.

This handbook is aimed at educating medical undergraduates, surgical trainees, and multi-disciplinary theatre and ward staff with regard to both general complications and those complications associated with specific procedures. We believe it will help medical staff to consent and counsel patients, and care givers to have a greater understanding.

ISW
DJL
2009

Foreword

Complications are an important cause of morbidity and mortality after surgery. They are feared by surgeons and patients alike; surgeons because they feel they have let their patient down, and patients, relatives and carers as they have been let down. In addition there is an extra cost to our health service in terms of the need for additional care, and delayed return to home and work for the patients, which can be devastating and hard to measure. Many complications are avoidable, and the introduction of 'flight lists' as used by the airline industry has been shown to reduce errors and attendant complications. The Safer Surgery Saves Lives campaign, promoted by the World Health Organization, has been tested and proved to be a great advance. Following the use of this checklist there is a consequent reduction in deaths and injuries with less likelihood for system errors and lack of communication, and litigation (outlined in Chapter 24), which may follow complications after surgery. The reduction in complications after surgery and improvement of the quality of care reflects my recommendations in the NHS *High Quality Care for All* report.

The authors have built on the previous handbook from the popular Oxford Specialist Handbook series by combining the complications after surgery in general in the first half of the book, followed by complications after specialty surgery in the latter half. The majority of surgical specialties are represented, including gastrointestinal, cardiothoracic and peripheral vascular surgery, orthopaedic, urological, ENT, and plastic surgery. In using free text and checklists the authors have avoided too much repetition so the reader is able to dip into appropriate sections for rapid answers and advice.

There are few textbooks available to offer information on complications after surgery, how to avoid and recognise them, and how to treat them when they occur. Training and education are essential to ongoing improvements in healthcare and it is encouraging to see the authors focus on this aspect of the surgical pathway. This specialist handbook is comprehensive, up-to-date, logically presented and should be a useful pocket book, with wide appeal, for trainee surgeons, medical students, and allied professions.

Professor the Lord Darzi of Denham KBE

Contents

Contributors

A Ross Anderson
SpR in ENT, Head and Neck
Surgery
Hull Royal Infirmary, UK
(Chapter 19)

M A Benton
Department of Haematology
ABMU Trust and
Welsh Blood Service,
Singleton Hospital Swansea, UK
(Chapter 6)

Scott Cairns
Research Registrar
Department of Wound Healing
Cardiff University, UK
(Chapter 22)

Anwar Chahal
Fellow in Cardiovascular Medicine
Critical Care Unit
St George's Hospital
London, UK
(Chapter 3)

Joanna Chikwe
Consultant Cardiothoracic
Surgeon
Mount Sinai Medical Center
New York, USA
(Chapter 11)

Jonathan Cooke
Director of Research and
Development and Clinical
Director of Pharmacy and
Medicines Management
University Hospital of South
Manchester NHS Foundation
Trust, UK
(Chapter 8)

Renee Debray
Surgical Pharmacist
University Hospital of South
Manchester NHS Foundation
Trust, UK
(Chapter 8)

Andrew Elsmore
Consultant Neurosurgeon
Royal London Hospital, UK
(Chapter 22)

Martin Gardner
Consultant Anaesthetist and Lead
Clinician Acute Pain Service
Epsom and St Helier NHS Trust
Surrey, UK
(Chapter 1)

Alison Gregg
Directorate Pharmacist for
Theatres, General Anaesthetics
and Pain
University Hospital of South
Manchester NHS Foundation
Trust, UK
(Chapter 8)

Dean Harris
Specialist Registrar
Cardiff and Vale NHS Trust, UK
(Chapter 9)

L Y Hiew
Consultant Plastic and Breast
Reconstructive Surgeon
Welsh Centre for Burns and
Plastic Reconstructive Surgery
Morriston Hospital
Swansea, UK
(Chapter 20)

Sam Huddart
Specialist Trainee Registrar in
Anaesthetics & ITU,
St George's School of Anaesthesia,
London, UK
(Chapter 1)

Nicholas Inston
Consultant Surgeon
University Hospitals Birmingham
NHS Foundation Trust, UK
(Chapter 12)

Paul Jones
Consultant Urological Surgeon
Morriston Hospital
Swansea, UK
(Chapter 18)

Amelia Jukes
Nutrition Support Dietitian –
Clinical lead
University Hospital of
Wales, UK
(Chapter 5)

Sairan Koron
ST Trainee in Medicine
Lancashire Teaching Hospitals
Trust, UK
(Chapter 4)

Hamish Laing
Consultant Plastic, Reconstructive
and Hand Surgeon, Welsh
Centre for Burns and Plastic
Surgery Communication Officer,
British Association of Plastic,
Reconstructive and Aesthetic
Surgeons
(Chapter 7)

David Leaper
Visiting Professor
Department of Wound Healing
Cardiff University, UK
(Chapter 2)

Lyndon Mason
Specialist Trainee
University Hospital of Wales, UK
(Chapter 16)

Jonathan Mackay
Consultant Physician
Victoria Hospital,
Blackpool, Fylde and
Wyre Hospitals NHS Trust
(Chapter 4)

James McDaid
Specialist Registrar in Transplant
Surgery
West Midlands Deanery, UK
(Chapter 12)

Ruth Murdoch
Principal Pharmacist for Surgery
and Education/Development
University Hospital of South
Manchester NHS Foundation
Trust, UK
(Chapter 8)

Nagmeh Naderi
Core Surgical Trainee,
Welsh Centre for Burns and
Plastic Surgery,
Swansea, UK
(Chapter 6)

Warren M Rozen
Senior Research Fellow
Jack Brockhoff Reconstructive
Plastic Surgery Research Unit,
University of Melbourne,
Victoria, Australia
(Chapters 7, 21, 23)

Julian Scott
Professor of Vascular Surgery
Leeds Institute of Genetics,
Health and Therapeutics (LIGHT),
University of Leeds and
Leeds Vascular Institute, and
General Infirmary,
Leeds Teaching Hospitals
NHS Trust,
Leeds, UK
(Chapters 10, 13, 14, 15, 17)

Kayvan Shokrollahi
Specialist Registrar
Welsh Centre for Burns and
Plastic Reconstructive Surgery
Morriston Hospital
Swansea, UK
(Chapter 24)

N D Stafford
Professor of Otolaryngology/
Head & Neck Surgery
Postgraduate Medical Institute
University of Hull, UK
(Chapter 19)

Hafiz Syed
Consultant Physician in
Stroke and Internal Medicine,
Department of Geriatric Medicine,
Newham General Hospital,
London, UK
(Chapter 3)

Ian Thomas
Specialist Registrar in General
Surgery
Morriston Hospital
Swansea, UK
(Chapter 18)

Jared Torkington
Consultant Surgeon
Cardiff and Vale NHS Trust, UK
(Chapter 9)

Max Troxler
Specialist Registrar in
Vascular Surgery
Leeds Vascular Institute,
Leeds General Infirmary, Leeds, UK
(Chapters 10, 13, 14, 15, 17)

Iain Whitaker
Plastic, Reconstructive and Burns
Surgery
Welsh Centre for Burns and
Plastic Surgery
Morriston Hospital
Swansea, UK
(Chapters 7, 21, 23)

Jamie Wooton
Consultant Orthopaedic Surgeon
Wrexham Maelor Hospital, UK
(Chapter 16)

Symbols and abbreviations

~	approximately
📖	cross reference
↓	decreased
↑	increased
→	leading to
±	plus/minus
🕮	website

AAA	abdominal aortic aneurysm
ABCDE	airway, breathing, circulation, disability, exposure (in trauma patients)
ABG	arterial blood gases
ABPI	ankle brachial-pressure index
ACA	American College of Cardiology
ACE	angiotensin-converting enzyme
ACL	anterior cruciate ligament
ACS	acute coronary syndrome
ADH	anti-diuretic hormone
ADRs	adverse drug reactions
AF	atrial fibrillation
AGNB	aerobic gram-negative bacilli
AHA	American Heart Association
AIDS	acquired immunodeficiency syndrome
AKA	above knee amputation
ALP	alkaline phosphatase
ALS	advanced life support
AMI	acute myocardial infarction
APACHE	Acute Physiology and Chronic Health Evaluation
APC	argon plasma coagulation
APTR	activated partial thromboplastin time ratio
APTT	activated partial thromboplastin time
ARDS	acute respiratory distress syndrome
AST	aspartate aminotransferase
ATN	acute tubular necrosis
AV	arteriovenous
AVN	avascular necrosis
AVNRT	atrioventricular nodal re-entrant tachycardia

AVR	aortic valve replacement
AVRT	atrioventricular re-entry tachycardia
BAHA	bone-anchored hearing aid
BG	blood glucose
BIPP	bismuth iodoform paraffin paste
BKA	below knee amputation
BMA	British Medical Association
BNF	British National Formulary
BP	blood pressure
BPF	bronchopleural fistula
BPH	benign prostatic hypertrophy
CABG	coronary artery bypass graft
CAM	community acquired meningitis
CARS	compensatory anti-inflammatory response syndrome
CBF	coronary blood flow
CCU	coronary care unit
CDAD	*Clostridium difficile*-associated diarrhoea
CEA	carotid endarterectomy
CFV	common femoral vein
CK	creatine kinase
CK-MB	creatine kinase membrane bound
CMV	cytomegalovirus
CNI	calcineurin inhibitor
CNS	central nervous system
COPD	chronic obstructive pulmonary disease
COX	cyclo-oxygenase
CPAP	continuous positive airway pressure
CPB	cardiopulmonary bypass
CPP	cerebral perfusion pressure
CPR	cardiopulmonary resuscitation
CRP	C-reactive protein
CRPS	complex regional pain syndrome
CSF	cerebrospinal fluid
CSU	catheter-specimen of urine
CSW	cerebral salt wasting
CT	computed tomography
CV	cardiovascular
CVA	cerebrovascular accident
CVP	central venous pressure
CVS	cardiovascular system
CVVHF	continuous veno-veno haemofiltration

CXR	chest X-ray
DGF	delayed graft function
DH	Department of Health
DI	diabetes insipidus
DIC	disseminated intravascular coagulation
DIEP	deep inferior epigastric artery perforator
DIPJ	distal interphalangeal joint
DO_2	oxygen delivery
DS	degree of substitution
DSWI	deep sternal wound infection
DVT	deep vein thrombosis
EBM	evidence-based medicine
ECA	external carotid artery
ECF	extra-cellular fluid
ECG	electrocardiogram
ECHO	echocardiogram
EDH	exradural haematoma
EMD	electromechanical dissociation
EMG	electromyogram
EMLA	eutectic mixture of local anaesthetic
EMRSA	epidemic meticillin resistant *Staphylococcus aureus*
ENT	ear, nose, and throat
EPUAP	European Pressure Ulcer Advisory Panel
ERCP	endoscopic retrograde cholangiopancreatography
ESR	erythrocyte sedimentation rate
ESWL	extracorporeal shockwave lithotripsy
ET	endotracheal
$ETCO_2$	end tidal carbon dioxide
EUA	examination under anaesthetic
EVAR	endovascular aneurysm repair
EVC	external ventricular catheter
EWTD	European Working Time Directive
FAP	familial adenomatous polyposis
FBC	full blood count
FES	fat embolism syndrome
FESS	functional endoscopic sinus surgery
FEV_1	forced expiratory volume in one second
FFP	fresh frozen plasma
FRC	functional residual capacity
FTSG	full-thickness skin graft
GA	general anaesthetic

GABA	gamma-aminobutyric acid
GCS	Glasgow Coma Scale
GFR	glomerular filtration rate
GI	gastrointestinal
GIT	gastrointestinal tract
GMC	General Medical Council
GORD	gastro-oesophageal reflux disease
GRE	glycopeptide-resistant *Enterococci*
G&S	group and save
GSW	gun shot wound
GTN	glyceryl trinitrate
GvHD	graft versus host disease
HAART	highly active anti-retroviral therapy
HAS	human albumin solution
HAT	hepatic artery thrombosis
HBV	hepatitis B virus
HCAI	healthcare associated infection
HCV	hepatitis C virus
HDI	human development index
HDU	high-dependency unit
HES	hydroxyethyl starch
HIT	heparin-induced thrombocytopaenia
HITT	heparin-induced thrombocytopaenia and thrombosis
HIV	human immunodeficiency virus
HLA	human leukocyte antigen
HR	heart rate
HRT	hormone replacement therapy
HT	hypertension
IABP-CP	intra-aortic balloon pump counter-pulsation
iaDSA	intra-arterial digital subtraction arteriography
IAP	intra-abdominal pressure
ICA	internal carotid artery
ICB	intracranial bleeding
ICH	intracranial haematoma
ICP	intracranial pressure
IHD	ischaemic heart disease
IL	interleukin
IM	intramuscular
IMA	inferior mesenteric artery
IMHA	independent mental health advocate

INR	international normalized ratio
ISC	intermittent self-catheterization
ITU	intensive therapy unit
IV	intravenous
IVC	inferior vena cava
ivDSA	intravenous digital subtraction arteriography
JVP	jugular vein pressure
LA	local anaesthetic
LAD	left axis deviation
LBBB	left bundle branch block
LDH	lactic dehydrogenase
LDL	low-density lipoprotein
LFT	liver function test
LiDCO	lithium dilution cardiac output
LIMA	left internal mammary artery
LMWH	low molecular weight heparin
LOC	loss of consciousness
LP	lumbar puncture
LSVG	long saphenous vein graft
LSV	long saphenous vein
LV	left ventricle
LVF	left ventricular failure
MAOI	monoamine oxidase inhibitor
MAP	mean arterial pressure
MCA	Mental Capacity Act
MCP	metacarpophalangeal
MHRA	Medicines and Healthcare products Regulatory Agency
MI	myocardial infarction
MODS	multiple organ dysfunction syndrome
MRCNS	multiply resistant, coagulase-negative *Staphylococcus*
MRI	magnetic resonance imaging
MRSA	meticillin resistant *Staphylococcus aureus*
MS	mitral stenosis
MSA	multiple stab avulsion
MSU	midstream urine
MVR	mitral valve replacement
NBM	nil by mouth
NBTC	National Blood Transfusion Committee
NGT	naso-gastric tube
NICE	National Institute for Health and Clinical Excellence

NMDA	N-methyl-D-Aspartate
NPSA	National Patient Safety Agency
NPT	negative pressure therapy
NPUAP	National Pressure Ulcer Advisory Panel
NSAIDs	non-steroidal anti-inflammatory drugs
NSTEMI	non-ST elevation myocardial infarction
OGD	oesophagogastroduodenoscopy
OM	obtuse marginal
OPSI	overwhelming post-splenectomy infection
ORS	oral rehydration solution
PA	pulmonary artery
PAF	platelet activating factor
PBC	primary biliary cirrhosis
PCA	patient controlled analgesia
PCAS	patient controlled analgesia system
PCEA	patient controlled epidural analgesia
PCNL	percutaneous nephrolithotomy
PDA	posterior descending artery
PE	pulmonary embolism
PEA	pulseless electrical activity
PEEP	positive end-expiratory pressure
PEG	percutaneous endoscopically-placed gastrostomy
PEM	protein-energy malnutrition
PFO	patent foramen ovali
PHTN	pulmonary hypertension
PIC	peripheral inserted catheter
PICC	peripherally inserted central venous catheter
PIPJ	proximal interphalangeal joint
PMH	past medical history
PMN	polymorphonuclear neutrophil
PN	parenteral nutrition
PONV	post-operative nausea and vomiting
PPM	permanent pacemaker
PPN	peripheral parenteral nutrition
PPPD	pylorus-preserving pancreaticoduodenectomy
PR	pulmonary regurgitatio
PRBCs	packed red blood cells
PRN	*pro re nata* (i.e. when required)
PS	pulmonary stenosis
PSA	prostate specific antigen
PSC	primary sclerosing cholangitis

PT	prothrombin time
PTC	percutaneous transhepatic cholangiography
PTDM	post-transplant diabetes mellitus
PTFE	polytetrafluoroethylene
PTLD	post-transplant lymphoproliferative disorders
PVA	polyvinylalcohol
PVD	peripheral vascular disease
PVR	pulmonary vascular resistance
RBC	red blood cell
RCA	right coronary artery
RIMA	reversible inhibitor of monoamine type A
RPG	radiologically-placed gastrostomy tube
RSD	reflex sympathetic dystrophy
RSTL	relaxed skin tension lines
RT	respiratory tract
RTI	respiratory tract infection
rtPA	recombinant tissue plasminogen activator
RV	right ventricle
RWMA	regional wall motion abnormality
SA	sinoatrial
SC	subcutaneous
SDD	selective decontamination of the digestive tract
SDH	subdural haematoma
SFJ	saphenofemoral junction
SG	specific gravity
SHOT	Serious Hazards of Transfusion Report
SIADH	syndrome of inappropriate ADH secretion
SIGN	Scottish Intercollegiate Guidelines Network
SIRS	systemic inflammatory response syndrome
SNHL	sensory neural hearing loss
SPJ	saphenopopliteal junction
SSG	split-thickness skin graft
SSI	surgical site infection
SSRI	selective serotonin re-uptake inhibitors
SSV	short saphenous vein
STEMI	ST elevation myocardial infarction
SVC	superior vena cava
SVR	systemic vascular resistance
SVT	supraventricular tachycardia
TAA	thoracoabdominal aneurysm
TACO	transfusion-associated circulatory overload

TE	thromboembolism
TED	thromboembolism disease
TENS	transcutaneous electrical stimulation
TFT	thyroid function tests
THR	total hip joint replacement
TIA	transient ischaemic attack
TKR	total knee replacement
TLSO	thoracic lumbar sacral orthotic
TNF	tumour necrosis factor
TOE	transoesophageal echocardiogram
TOS	thoracic outlet syndrome
TPN	total parenteral nutrition
TPW	temporary pacing wire
TR	tricuspid regurgitation
TRAM	transrectus abdominus muscle (flap)
TRIM	transfusion-associated immunomodulation
TRISS	Trauma and Injury Severity Score
TRUS	trans-rectal ultrasound
TS	tricuspid stenosis
TTE	transthoracic echocardiography
TURBT	transurethral resection of bladder tumour
TURP	transurethral resection of the prostate
UC	ulcerative colitis
U&Es	urea and electrolytes
UFH	unfractionated heparin
UGT	urogenital tract
UNC	ureteroneocystostomy
USS	ultrasound scan
UTI	urinary tract infection
VAP	ventilator associated pneumonia
VATS	video-assisted thoracic surgery
VF	ventricular fibrillation
VO_2	oxygen uptake (i.e. volume of oxygen utilization)
VRE	vancomycin-resistant *Enterococci*
VSD	ventricular septal defect
VT	ventricular tachycardia
VTE	venous thromboembolism
WBC	white blood cell
WCC	white cell count
WHO	World Health Organization

Section 1

General complications

Post-operative pain

Pain physiology

Pain has been defined as 'an unpleasant sensory and emotional experience associated with actual or potential tissue damage, or described in terms of such damage'. In essence pain is whatever the patient says it is, when they say it is. It is influenced by psychological (attitude, perception, previous experience) and environmental factors. Attention to patient education and psychological factors pre-operatively can improve outcome.

Acute pain is related to actual or perceived tissue damage. Chronic pain is that which is experienced beyond healing of the original insult; often, however, there is no identifiable cause.

Pain is mediated by nociceptive somatic nerve fibres with their cell bodies in the dorsal root ganglion of the spinal cord, or in the case of the head and neck, in the trigeminal ganglia. Tissue damage leads to the direct stimulation of nociceptors and indirect stimulation via the release of mediators. Nociceptive fibres synapse with second order neurons in the dorsal horn of the grey matter of the spinal cord (lamina I-V). With this there is a complex network of interneurons regulating transmission (including stimulatory NMDA receptors, substance P, glutamate, and inhibitory GABA-ergic and glutamine-ergic receptors). From here the second order neurons cross to the contralateral cord and ascend in the lateral spinothalamic tracts to the thalamus and periaqueductal grey matter. Third order neurons project to the sensory cortex. Descending tracts modulate ascending transmission in the posterior horn of the spinal cord.

Management of pain is aimed at modulating the transmission of pain at points along this pathway. Non-steroidal anti-inflammatory drugs and paracetamol prevent the production of prostaglandins, a group of important inflammatory/nociceptive mediators. Local anaesthetics block fast sodium channels preventing the propagation of action potentials along axons, thereby halting neuronal transmission. Ketamine blocks stimulatory NMDA receptors. Opioids and clonidine act on receptors that enhance inhibitory mechanisms.

Why treat pain?

The most obvious reason to treat pain is to relieve patient suffering. Poorly treated acute pain can progress on to chronic pain. Acute pain causes numerous detrimental physiological responses, which can lead to increased morbidity and mortality, delayed recovery, and prolonged hospital stay.

The sympathetic stimulation caused by painful stimuli increases heart rate and myocardial contractility leading to an increase in myocardial oxygen demand, strain on the myocardium, and potentially ischaemia. Diaphragmatic splinting by a painful abdomen and/or pain from chest wounds/fractured ribs lead to an increased incidence of respiratory failure and infections. Effects on the gastrointestinal tract include delayed gastric emptying, bowel transit time, and absorption. Changes in regional blood flow can reduce perfusion to other organs and the operative site itself. These changes can impair renal function, cause delayed repair of tissue damage, and have a detrimental effect on recovery. Pain can also lead to urinary retention. Immobility caused by pain on movement can predispose to pressure sores and thromboembolic complications.

Causes of post-operative pain

Commonly, post-operative pain is caused by **surgical** factors. Post operative patients are also at an increased risk of **non-surgical** complications. Detailed history, examination and investigation are essential in establishing the cause(s) of pain, to exclude complications or life-threatening conditions.

Surgical

- Pain relating to surgery (e.g. wound pain).
- Complications of the surgery itself (e.g. bleeding, infection, perforation, ischaemia, obstruction, ileus, compartment syndrome).
- Nerve palsies secondary to surgery or intra-operative patient positioning.

Non-surgical

- DVT (secondary to immobility and hypercoagulable state).
- Myocardial ischaemia.
- Pleuritic pain (pulmonary embolus, pneumonia).
- Pressure areas (especially in immobile patients).
- Incidental pathology unrelated to surgery (including pre-existing painful conditions).

Assessment

Acute pain management primarily revolves around identifying the cause, treating the underlying condition, and treating the pain. A thorough pain history should include site, onset, duration, character, intensity, associated symptoms, exacerbating/relieving factors (including current and prior treatments), radiation, effect of activity, and effect of pain on sleep pattern. Pain has been termed the fifth vital sign and as such should be assessed and recorded regularly. Severity scores are useful in guiding initial management and the ongoing efficacy of treatment. Scoring systems include numerical scales (0–3 or 0–10), verbal rating scales (mild/moderate/severe), and visual scales. Paediatric pain severity can be estimated using pictorial scales and behavioural assessment scales. Scoring systems are subjective but are useful in assessing and monitoring the response to interventions/treatments. They must be appropriate for the patient's age, development, and mental status. It is probably irrelevant which scale is used but their use must be consistent and regular.

Multimodal analgesia

Multimodal analgesia describes the treatment of pain using different classes of drugs aimed at various points along the pain pathway (e.g. paracetamol, NSAIDs, opioids, local anaesthetics). The aim is to provide adequate analgesia while keeping unwanted side effects to a minimum. Multimodal analgesic regimens have been shown to reduce the need for strong opioids and the incidence of clinically meaningful events (e.g. vomiting associated with opioids). By adequately treating pain and avoiding unnecessary side effects morbidity is reduced, patients are more satisfied, and their length of stay in hospital is shorter.

The analgesic ladder

The World Health Organization (WHO) has a well-established approach to pain management, originally devised as a guide to the management of pain associated with cancer. The analgesic ladder can be used as a framework for the management of acute pain. Treatment can begin at any step depending on severity, moving up the ladder if the pain is not controlled with the intervention.

Step 1 (mild pain):   **non-opioid** (e.g. paracetamol)
↓   ± NSAID

Step 2 (moderate pain):   **addition of mild opioid**
                          (e.g. codeine, tramadol)
↓   + regular paracetamol, ± NSAID

Step 3 (severe pain):   **stronger opioid**
                          (e.g. morphine), dose titrated to analgesia
                          + regular paracetamol, ± NSAID

At any point adjuvant pain relief can be given, e.g. **non-steroidal anti-inflammatory drugs** (**NSAIDs**), if appropriate for the type of pain and the co-morbidities. Multimodal pain relief should be given regularly ('by-the-clock') and in adequate doses. If in doubt call for senior advice; any further queries can be referred to the acute pain service or on-call anaesthetist.

The acute pain team

Most hospitals have an acute pain service, run by the anaesthetic department. It is made up of anaesthetists, specialist nurses, and trainee anaesthetic doctors. Their role in the management of pain is through education of staff and individual patient review (on request by the team, those with known pain problems, and the management of epidural/PCA analgesia). They are an excellent source of information regarding the treatment of pain in difficult patients. Out-of-hours pain management advice can be sought through the on-call anaesthetist. The pain team can be contacted for advice, for example, if pain is poorly controlled on an adequate multi-modal analgesic regime (i.e. regular paracetamol, ± NSAID, with adequate opioid dose). They can also advise on patients with difficult pain issues such as chronic pain and substance misuse. Any issues arising with patient controlled analgesia (PCA) or epidurals are dealt with by the pain team/on-call anaesthetist.

Paracetamol

Paracetamol is a drug with anti-pyretic and analgesic actions. Its mechanism of action is unknown but is thought to involve inhibition of prostaglandin synthesis in the CNS, possibly via inhibition of the cyclo-oxygenase-3 enzyme.

It can be administered orally, rectally, or intravenously. Oral administration is effective in 20–40 minutes and is cheap. Rectal administration has unpredictable bioavailability and is relatively expensive. Intravenous paracetamol has rapid onset of clinical effects, but again is relatively expensive and can lead to hypotension when rapidly infused.

Adult dosage is up to 4g in four divided doses in 24 hours, and paediatric dosage is up to 80mg/kg in four divided doses in 24 hours.

Paracetamol has relatively few side effects. It is metabolized by the cytochrome p450 system in the liver. When taken in overdose this system becomes saturated and a build-up of the substrates of metabolism leads to hepatic and renal toxicity. Care should be taken when using regular paracetamol in patients with impaired hepatic function.

Non-steroidal anti-inflammatory drugs (NSAIDs)

This broad group of drugs have anti-inflammatory, anti-pyrexial, and analgesic actions. They act by inhibiting the enzyme cyclo-oxygenase (COX). COX is responsible for the production of thromboxanes and prostaglandins from arachidonic acid. Inhibition of prostaglandin production accounts for their anti-inflammatory effects peripherally and their anti-pyretic effects centrally. Inhibition of thromboxanes leads to reduced platelet aggregation. Many subtypes of prostaglandins have been identified, accounting for the variation in side effect profiles of different groups of NSAIDs. There are two subtypes of cyclo-oxygenase inhibited by NSAIDs, COX-1 and COX-2. Broadly speaking, inhibition of COX-1 is responsible for the side effects. Inhibition of COX-2 accounts for the anti-inflammatory, anti-pyretic, and analgesic effects. As such NSAIDs can be classed as either non-specific COX inhibitors (e.g. aspirin, ibuprofen, diclofenac, ketorolac) or COX-2 selective inhibitors (e.g. meloxicam, celecoxib, parecoxib).

The use of NSAIDs is limited by their side effect profile:

- *Gastrointestinal effects* – inhibition of gastro-protective prostaglandins leads to gastric irritation, ulceration, and bleeding (acute haemorrhage iron deficiency anaemia). Bleeding is further compounded by the anti-platelet effects of NSAIDs. Preferential COX-2 selection can reduce the incidence of GI effects.
- *Asthma* – inhibition of the COX enzyme leads to a build-up of arachidonic acid and an increase in leukotriene production. This can lead to acute severe bronchospasm in up to 20% of susceptible asthmatic patients. Selective COX-2 inhibition appears not to induce bronchospasm in aspirin-sensitive asthmatics.
- *Renal impairment* – prostaglandins are involved in regulation of renal blood flow, hence reducing their production can reduce renal blood flow leading to acute renal impairment/failure. This can be compounded in the post-operative patient by factors such as hypovolaemia, hypotension, and sepsis. Selective COX-2 inhibition displays the same renal toxicity.
- *Fluid retention* – NSAIDs cause fluid retention, which can lead to heart failure in susceptible patients.
- *Anti-platelet effects* – the anti-platelet effect of NSAIDs, via inhibition of thromboxane production, can lead to increased bleeding post-operatively. COX-2 inhibitors do not display the same anti-platelet effect.
- *Drug interactions* – NSAIDs are highly protein bound in the plasma and as such can displace other highly protein bound drugs, potentiating their effects (e.g. warfarin). Lithium levels can increase with NSAID use.
- *Hepatotoxicity* – NSAIDs have been associated with impaired hepatic function.
- *COX-2 inhibitors and cardiovascular risk* – rofecoxib was withdrawn from the market in 2004 after several studies demonstrated an increased risk of myocardial infarction and cerebrovascular accidents. Similar concerns over the safety of other drugs in this class have been raised.

Cautions:
- post-op bleeding
- avoid in hypotensive/septic patients
- anticoagulation
- non-NSAID-sensitive asthmatics.

Contraindications:
- renal failure
- history of upper GI bleed
- patients on warfarin
- asthmatics with history of NSAID-induced bronchospasm.

Common NSAIDs

Ibuprofen
- non-selective COX inhibitor, only available orally
- adult dose: 400mg 8 hourly with food
- paediatric dose: 5–10mg/kg 8 hourly.

Diclofenac
- non-selective COX inhibitor, available in oral, rectal, and intravenous preparations
- adult oral dose: 50mg 8 hourly.

COX-2 selective inhibitors
- fewer GI side effects, appear safe in aspirin-sensitive asthmatics, no anti-platelet effect
- similar renal toxicity to regular NSAIDs
- questions over cardiovascular safety
- adult dose celecoxib: 100–200mg orally 12 hourly
- adult dose valdecoxib: 10–20mg orally once daily
- adult dose parecoxib: 20–40mg IV 6–12 hourly (max. 80mg/24hrs)
- valdecoxib/parecoxib contraindicated after cardiac surgery due to increased incidence of CV events.

Opioids

Opioids are naturally occurring or synthetic compounds that are agonists at the opioid receptor. Opioid receptors are found throughout the CNS, spinal cord, and peripheral nervous system. Stimulation of the receptors modulates transmission of pain and other signals. There are three classes of opioid receptor: mu, delta, and kappa (the sigma subclass has been shown not to be blocked by naloxone and has therefore been removed from the opioid receptor classification).

Routes of administration

- Oral – dependent on ability to ingest and absorb, limited by nausea and vomiting.
- Intramuscular/subcutaneous – fast and effective, limited by lipid solubility and changes in regional perfusion.
- Intravenous – rapid onset, titrate small boluses up to adequate pain relief, vigilance to ensure early detection of side effects.
- Trans-mucosal – sublingual/buccal/intranasal – fast and effective, limited by lipid solubility.
- Transdermal – limited to lipophilic opioids (e.g. fentanyl).
- Epidural/caudal/intrathecal – possible delayed onset of side effects.

Effects

All opioids display a similar side effect pattern, but to varying degrees:
- analgesia
- nausea and vomiting
- sedation, euphoria, dysphoria
- respiratory depression
- bradycardia, hypotension secondary to histamine release
- reduced bowel mobility, constipation
- urinary retention
- itching.

Common opioids

Morphine
- Naturally occurring opiate, reference opioid to which all others are compared.
- Given IV, IM, SC, orally (as short acting or slow release preparations), intrathecal/epidural (associated with delayed respiratory depression).
- Adult oral dose 10–30mg 4 hourly, IM/SC dose 5–10mg, titrate intravenous dose in small boluses (1–2mg every ~5 minutes) until adequate pain relief (close monitoring for signs of side effects).
- Paediatric oral doses 0.3–0.5mg/kg 4 hourly, titrate IV doses in boluses (50–100µg/kg every ~5 minutes).
- Peak effects IV/SC/IM ~10–30 minutes, duration of action 3–4 hours.
- Metabolized via active metabolites to varying degrees. This may explain inter-patient differences in effect. Metabolites are renally excreted and can accumulate in renal failure.
- More pronounced effect in extremes of age.

Diamorphine

- Naturally occurring pro-drug converted to morphine *in vivo*.
- More lipid soluble than morphine, therefore reaches the effector site in higher concentration, therefore potency is up to two times that of morphine.
- Marked euphoria, hence it has become drug of abuse.
- Used IV, IM, SC, epidural, and intrathecal. High first pass metabolism therefore not used orally.
- Adult dose 2.5–5mg 4 hourly.
- Other uses include respiratory distress associated with acute LVF.

Pethidine

- Synthetic opioid, given IM, SC, or IV.
- Adult dose IM/SC 25–100mg, IV 22–50mg 3 hourly.
- No better than morphine for renal/biliary colic.
- Active metabolites renally excreted and accumulate in renal failure.
- Not reversed by naloxone.
- High doses associated with hallucinations and seizures.
- Interacts with monoamine oxidase inhibitors (MAOIs).
- Side effects and interactions make pethidine less suitable than morphine.

Codeine

- Natural opioid, acts directly as a weak opioid agonist and indirectly ~10% metabolized to morphine.
- Given orally, IM, PR in children. Not given intravenously as associated with histamine release, profound hypotension, and death.
- Adult dose 30–60mg 4–6 hourly.
- Paediatric dose 0.1mg/kg 6 hourly (max. 3mg/kg per 24 hours).
- Genetic variability in the proportion of conversion to morphine; this explains the marked effects in some patients and lack of in others.
- Particular problems with constipation; patients may need laxatives.
- Other uses: cough suppressant, anti-diarrhoeal agent.

Tramadol

- Non-selective synthetic opioid agonist, inhibits noradrenaline re-uptake and enhances serotonin release.
- Used IV, IM, and orally.
- Adult dose 50–100mg 4–6 hourly (max 400mg/24 hours).
- Paediatric dose 1–2mg/kg 6 hourly (not licensed for children under 12 years, max 400mg/24 hours).
- Comparatively favourable side effect profile.
- Side effects include nausea, sedation, dizziness, and dry mouth.
- Caution in epilepsy and concurrent with monoamine oxidase inhibitors (MAOI).
- Not antagonized by naloxone; will precipitate withdrawal in opioid-dependent patients if used alone.
- Metabolized in the liver to active metabolites that are predominantly renally excreted, therefore accumulates in renal failure.

Fentanyl
- Synthetic opioid often used in anaesthesia.
- Used IV, epidural, intrathecal, transdermal, and buccal (due to high lipid solubility).
- Transdermal patches take up to 12 hours to reach equilibrium with plasma levels.
- Post-operatively can be used in a PCA pump intravenously.
- New patient-controlled active transdermal systems are available, though not yet widely used.
- Inactive metabolites excreted in the urine, therefore does not accumulate in renal failure.

Dosages given are intended as a guide only, and for the initial management of acute pain in an average, opioid-naïve patient. Reduce dose for elderly/frail patients; increase dose appropriately for opioid-tolerant patients.

Adult doses

Drug	Dose – IV	Dose – IM/SC	Dose – oral
Morphine	titrate 1–2mg bolus up to 0.1–0.2mg/kg 3–4 hourly	5–10mg/kg 3–4 hourly	10–30mg 4 hourly, increase dose as required
Diamorphine	2.5–5mg 4 hourly	2.5–5mg 4 hourly	–
Pethidine	25–50mg 4 hourly	25–100mg 4 hourly	–
Codeine	–	30–60mg 4–6 hourly	30–60mg 4–6 hourly
Tramadol	50–100mg 4–6 hourly (max 400mg/24 hours)	50–100mg 4–6 hourly (max 400mg/24 hours)	50–100mg 4–8 hourly (max 400mg/24 hours)

Paediatric doses

Drug	Dose – IV	Dose – IM/SC	Dose – oral
Morphine	Titrate IV doses in boluses of 50–100µg/kg	0.1–0.2mg/kg 3–4 hourly	0.3–0.5mg/kg 4 hourly
Pethidine	0.5–1mg/kg 4 hourly	0.5–1mg/kg 4 hourly	–
Codeine	–	0.1mg/kg 6 hourly	0.1mg/kg 6 hourly
Tramadol	1–2 mg/kg 6 hourly	1–2 mg/kg 6 hourly	1–2 mg/kg 6 hourly

Narcosis

Treatment of opioid overdose is initially supportive. Ensure the following:
- Patent airway (give 100% oxygen via high-flow device,
  e.g. non re-breathe mask).
- Adequate respiration (may need to assist with bag-valve-mask
  ventilation – if so call arrest team).
- Call for help early.
- If respiratory arrest, begin bag-valve-mask ventilation and call arrest
  team (2222).
- If cardiac arrest/cardiovascular collapse, begin CPR/resuscitation and
  call arrest team (2222).
- Secure intravenous access; treat bradycardia and hypotension.
- Give naloxone intravenously in small bolus doses. If carefully titrated
  naloxone can reverse the sedative and respiratory depressive effects
  without reversing the analgesic effects.

Naloxone
- Opioid antagonist used in the treatment of the over-opiated patient.
- Competitive antagonist predominantly at the mu receptor.
- Adult dose 200–400µg, paediatric dose 5–10µg/kg. Use small
  intravenous boluses and titrate to effect.
- Duration of action of ~20 minutes so care must be taken as the effects
  of the opioid can outlive the effects of naloxone; repeated doses or an
  infusion may be required.
- Side effects include hypertension, pulmonary oedema, and arrhythmias,
  and it can be antianalgesic or cause withdrawal symptoms in opioid
  users.
- Other uses include treating pruritus, nausea, and respiratory
  depression associated with epidural/spinal opioid administration.

Patient controlled analgesia (PCA)

The term PCA most commonly refers to intravenous opioid administered via a programmed pump on demand by the patient. The pump is
programmed such that demands for doses are only administered at set
intervals (e.g. 1mg morphine bolus with 5 minute lockout). PCA programmed pumps can also be used to administer local anaesthetic/opioid
mix via epidural and opioids intravenously/subcutaneously. The principle
of patient administration relies on just that; only the patient should be
allowed to administer a dose. If the patient begins to become drowsy secondary to the opioid they will not be able to actuate another dose until
they are more alert, thereby, in theory at least, protecting against opioid
side effects. However, as for any opioid administration, patients with a
PCA still require regular assessment and monitoring for signs of narcosis.
PCA pumps are usually controlled by the acute pain service. If there are
any urgent issues with patients receiving PCA opioids, contact the on-call
anaesthetist or the pain team who will assist in troubleshooting problems.

Local anaesthetics

Local anaesthetics act by blocking fast sodium channels, preventing the propagation of the action potential down a nerve. They are non-selective and act on all nerves: sensory, motor and autonomic, central, and peripheral. However, smaller nerves are more readily affected so sensory block will develop at lower doses than the motor effects. They can be administered as a local infiltration (e.g. around a wound), around target nerves (e.g. epidural, caudal, intrathecal, specific nerve block), or topically (e.g. EMLA, Ametop). Lignocaine can be given intravenously (e.g. Biers block) to produce limb anaesthesia, or intravenously as an anti-arrhythmic agent.

Commonly encountered local anaesthetics:

Lignocaine (lidocaine)
- Rapid onset, medium duration of acting, less cardiotoxic than bupivacaine.

Bupivacaine
- Slow onset, long acting, not used intravenously due to its cardiotoxicity.

Levobupivacaine
- Enantiomer of bupivacaine. Effects and dosing as bupivacaine but less cardiotoxicity/neurotoxicity.

Care must be taken when using local anaesthetics that the maximum dose is not exceeded. All local anaesthetics come in a variety of concentrations. It is therefore essential to check the drug carefully and calculate the dose permissible prior to injection.

Drug	Toxic dose (mg/kg) plain	Toxic dose (mg/kg) with adrenaline
Lignocaine	3mg/kg	7mg/kg
Bupivacaine/ levobupivacaine	2mg/kg	2mg/kg

Side effects of local anaesthetics relate to their action on sodium channels. They can be severe and life-threatening.

CNS effects
- Circumoral tingling, metallic taste, seizures, and coma.

CVS effects
- Bradycardia, hypotension, cardiovascular collapse, and cardiac arrest.

Emergency treatment of local anaesthetic toxicity
- Call for help (cardiac arrest call 2222).
- Airway (with 100% O_2), Breathing, and Circulation.
- Treat arrhythmias as appropriate.
- Intralipid is a lipid suspension that can be used in the treatment of cardiac arrest secondary to local anaesthetic toxicity. It binds local anaesthetics in the plasma rendering them inactive. Initial intravenous dose is 100ml stat.

Regional anaesthesia

Regional anaesthesia refers to the targeted use of local anaesthetics to produce analgesia/anaesthesia and includes nerve blocks, peri-neural infusions, wound-catheter infusions, and spinal/epidural anaesthesia. Principles of management and complications are similar to those encountered with epidural analgesia (📖 see section on epidural complications, p.20). If there is uncontrolled pain with continuous local anaesthetic infusions (peri-neural or wound infiltration), instigate additional multimodal pain management regimen, avoiding NSAIDs (anti-platelet effect can lead to bleeding/haematoma), and contact the pain team for further advice.

Epidural analgesia

Epidural analgesia describes the administration of local anaesthetics (and/ or opioids/adjuvant drugs) into the epidural space via a specially placed catheter. Epidural catheters are inserted pre-operatively by the anaesthetist. A lumbar epidural can be used for low abdominal incisions and lower limb surgery. Thoracic epidurals are used for analgesia of pain associated with high abdominal incisions. A mix of local anaesthetic (e.g. bupivacaine 0.1%) with or without opioid (e.g. fentanyl 2µg/ml) is infused into the epidural space. This infusion can be given continuously or as a bolus ± background infusion. Boluses can be doctor, nurse, or patient administered (patient controlled epidural analgesia (PCEA)) depending on specific hospital protocols.

Side effects, complications, and their management

Failure/patchy block

- If the patient has uncontrolled pain, contact the pain team/on-call anaesthetist for review and management.
- Options include: alternate patient positioning, epidural top-up, moving the catheter, or stopping the epidural and instigating alternative pain management plan (e.g. regular paracetamol with PCA or intermittent opioids).
- Avoid NSAIDs – anti-platelet effects can cause bleeding/haematoma and subsequent nerve damage/cord compression.

Shivering and itching

- Related to epidural mix of opioids and local anaesthetics; self-limiting and benign. Reassure patient.
- Contact pain team in severe persistent cases for advice on management. Treatment options include antihistamines and naloxone.

Hypotension

- Establish cause of hypotension (epidural related, sepsis, hypovolaemia).
- Give colloid challenge and observe response in BP and urine output.
- Contact on-call anaesthetist for advice/review.

High block

- A high block can include the sympathetic chain leading to autonomic instability, bradycardia, and hypotension. Inclusion of the cervical nerve roots can lead to respiratory compromise and diaphragmatic paralysis.
- This is an emergency:
  - call for help
  - support Airway (with 100% O_2), Breathing and Circulation
  - stop epidural infusion
  - sit patient up if possible
  - if suspected call the on-call anaesthetist immediately
  - in the case of cardiac collapse or respiratory arrest call cardiac arrest team (2222).

Local anaesthetic toxicity
(📖 See Local anaesthetics, p.18)

Post-dural puncture headache
- Puncturing the dura causes a leak of CSF and the associated drop in pressure and subsequent stretching of the meninges leads to a classical occipital headache that is worse on sitting/standing.
- Treatment includes simple analgesia, bed rest, and if persistent an epidural blood patch.
- If suspected contact the on-call anaesthetist/pain team.

Nerve damage
- Patch of numbness and/or weakness in a group of muscles that continues beyond the expected effect of the epidural. Can be difficult to differentiate between epidural nerve damage and nerve damage secondary to surgery/intra-operative patient positioning. If suspected refer to the anaesthetic department.

Epidural haematoma/abscess
- Symptoms and signs of cord compression.
- Surgical emergency – if suspected refer immediately to on-call anaesthetist. Surgical decompression has a good outcome if performed within 8 hours of the onset of symptoms.

Inhalational analgesia

Nitrous oxide (N_2O) can be used as an effective analgesic agent for relief of pain associated with procedures, labour, or acute pain relief in the emergency department. It is presented as a 50:50 mix of nitrous oxide and oxygen. It is administered via a breath-actuated valve. It has a rapid onset and offset; efficacy relies on patient compliance and good breathing technique. It is eliminated from the body via the lungs and expired. Side effects include euphoria, dysphoria, nausea, dissociative state, and bone marrow suppression. It is a potent greenhouse gas and pollution is inevitable. Has been associated with spontaneous abortion in healthcare staff exposed over time. It causes distension of gas-filled spaces, for example middle ear, bowel. Do not use in patients with a pneumothorax; you may turn a simple pneumothorax into a tension pneumothorax. Useful in episodic and procedural pain (e.g. in the Emergency Department). Unsuitable for ongoing pain relief in the post-operative setting.

Adjuvant drugs

Various classes of drugs are used in addition to the analgesic ladder outlined earlier. They are usually prescribed after consultation with a pain specialist or the pain team.
- Gabapentin, tricyclic antidepressants, and anticonvulsants are used in the treatment of neuropathic pain, but there is limited evidence for their use in acute or post-operative pain.
- NMDA antagonists – ketamine is an anaesthetic agent. When used peri-operatively, morphine-sparing has been demonstrated. They are limited by side effects, which include hallucination, disorientation, and agitation.
- Alpha-2 agonists – clonidine, but use is limited by hypotension and sedation.

Non-pharmacological methods

TENS (transcutaneous electrical stimulation) stimulates cutaneous sensory nerves. This modulates pain transmission in the dorsal horn of the spinal cord. It is ineffective and impractical in the post-operative period. Acupuncture can be used in the treatment of acute and chronic pain, but it is of little relevance post-operatively. Psychological techniques (e.g. combined sensory procedural information, training in coping methods, hypnosis) have been shown to be effective in reducing post-operative pain.

Specific patient groups

Certain groups of patients present specific difficulties in acute pain management. The general approach involves using multimodal analgesics, and tailoring doses according to the patients' condition and co-morbidities. The pain team are an approachable source of advice and, if appropriate, will review the patient on request.

Chronic pain

If possible, continue regular medication plus additional analgesia to treat acute episode pain. Chronic pain patients are often taking long-term opioids and as such may show significant tolerance. If you are changing the analgesic regimen be sure to account for their pre-admission opioid intake and the additional opioid requirements to treat the acute post-operative pain.

Substance abuse

Treatment of acute pain in drug-dependent patients requires an understanding of dependence and tolerance. Chronic misuse leads to physical dependence; stopping acutely leads to physical symptoms of withdrawal. Use over time leads to tolerance – increasing doses required to induce the same effect. Tolerance and dependence are part of a disease process. Inadequate doses of opioid or sole use of tramadol will not treat their pain and may lead to withdrawal. Patients with chronic opioid misuse must be treated for the acute episodic pain associated with their procedure, often requiring higher doses than otherwise expected (to account for regular intake of opioid, associated low pain threshold, and that needed to provide pain relief). Continue pre-admission replacement regimens (e.g. methadone) at the regular dose if possible and give additional pain relief to cover the acute pain from the procedure itself. There are often concerns over drug seeking and misappropriation; this is less likely post-operatively with a genuine reason for pain. Patients recovering from previous substance abuse should be reassured that relapse is unlikely with opioid treatment for acute pain.

Hepatic and renal impairment

Hepatic and renal disease often cause anxiety when prescribing analgesics. Paracetamol should be avoided in liver disease. NSAIDs should not be given to patients with acute or chronic renal failure, and used with caution in hepatic disease. Opioids should be used cautiously as their active metabolites may accumulate in renal failure. If in doubt seek senior advice.

Elderly patients

As patients get older there are changes in physiology and an increased incidence of co-morbidities. In addition, elderly patients can often have a stoical attitude and a high pain threshold. This must be taken into account when assessing and treating pain in this group of patients. Avoid NSAIDs and employ cautious dosing of opioids.

Paediatric patients

Paediatric patients in acute pain are often frightened and confused. It is important to treat pain appropriately, with as little distress as possible. Memories of a distressing hospital stay have marked effects on the child's attitude towards future healthcare interactions. Children often require higher doses of pain relief; pain scores should be assessed regularly (pictorial scale) and the pain regimen altered accordingly. Be sure to observe recommended maximum doses and monitor regularly for signs of side effects. Paracetamol, ibuprofen, and opioids are all considered safe to use in children, provided there are no contraindications. Aspirin should be avoided in children. However, NSAIDs are considered safe over the age of 6 months. Avoid needles if at all possible, but in severe pain use the intravenous route if available. If intravenous access or venepuncture is necessary, ensure a topical local anaesthetic agent (e.g. EMLA) is applied and given adequate time to work. Use distraction techniques during any procedure and keep parents informed at all stages. Patient controlled analgesia (PCA) is very effective in children who have the capacity to use it correctly. The paediatric team are a useful source of help and advice in this group of patients.

Pregnancy and breastfeeding

Opioids and paracetamol are considered safe for short periods of treatment in a healthy pregnancy. If ongoing treatment is required consult the obstetric team. Avoid NSAIDs in the first and third trimesters (as they can cause an increased incidence of miscarriage and premature closure of the patent ductus arteriosus).

All analgesic drugs pass into breast milk to a certain degree, but do not cause any ill effects in the child. Local anaesthetics, paracetamol, some NSAIDs (e.g. ibuprofen), and morphine are all considered safe in lactating women. If high dose opioids are used then the child may become drowsy. If pain relief is required then it should not be withheld; careful explanation and discussion with the mother is essential. If possible, try to time breastfeeding before doses of strong analgesia.

Pain management in the Emergency Department

Pain is a very common presenting feature of acute surgical conditions. It has been shown that treating pain does not mask the symptoms and signs of the underlying pathology. Give adequate doses of multimodal pain relief appropriate to the presenting condition and severity of pain. In the treatment of renal colic, NSAIDs (IV over parenteral) are equally as effective as opioids, and pethidine is no better than morphine. In the Emergency Department it is essential not to delay analgesia for any reason and regularly assess the patient as presenting conditions and symptomatology can change rapidly.

Post-operative nausea and vomiting

Post-operative nausea and vomiting (PONV) is a major cause of morbidity, including patient suffering, prolonged hospital stay, dehydration, electrolyte disturbances, increased bleeding, wound dehiscence, graft failure, aspiration, and oesophageal rupture. The aims are to ensure a balanced approach to PONV so that appropriate anti-emetic medication is administered regularly. There should also be a prescribed 'as necessary' alternative on. When assessing the nauseated/vomiting patient, careful history and examination are essential to establish probable cause(s). Ensure adequate hydration, analgesia, and oxygenation.

Aetiology

Patient factors

- Increased risk of PONV in:
  - females
  - young patients
  - non-smokers
  - those with history of travel sickness/PONV.
- Post-op hypoxia, hypotension, electrolyte disturbances, uncontrolled pain.

Surgical factors

- Various types of surgery are associated with an increased risk – ENT, laparoscopic, laparotomy, gynaecological.
- Gastric stasis secondary to ileus/obstruction.
- NG tube irritation, early resumption of oral intake.

Drug factors

- Anaesthetic agents (except propofol, which has anti-emetic properties), opioids, and antibiotics are all associated with PONV.
- Opioid drugs are potent emetics; management must be aimed at maintaining the target site concentration of opioid within the analgesic corridor between too low a concentration, which will be ineffective, and too high, which will increase PONV.

Treatment

It is important to use anti-emetics that work in different ways with first-line (regular) and second-line (PRN) prescriptions; remember regular prescriptions can be omitted if not necessary. PRN drugs are often given more on the feelings of the staff that they are necessary rather than those of the patient, especially if the ward is busy.

Routes available are:

- IV – suitable if there is a cannula *in situ*
- IM – will take longer to work, painful
- oral – problematic if the patient is actively vomiting
- buccal
- subcutaneous – not generally used in the management of PONV.

Commonly used anti-emetics:

Cyclizine
- Piperazine-derived, antihistamine antagonist at the H1 receptor.
- Effective in the treatment of nausea/vomiting associated with opioids, motion sickness.
- Available as IV, IM, and oral formulations.
- Adult dose: 50mg PO/IM/slow IV 8 hourly.
- Paediatric dose: 1mg/kg (up to 50mg) 8 hourly.
- Central anti-muscarinic effects of sedation, may worsen prostatic hypertrophy and glaucoma.
- Causes tachycardia, which may increase myocardial oxygen demand and exacerbate ischaemic heart disease.

Ondansetron
- 5HT3 antagonist.
- Now available in generic form.
- Usable routes: IV, IM, oral, rectal.
- Adult dose: 4mg 6 hourly.
- Paediatric dose: 0.1mg/kg 6 hourly.
- Hepatically metabolized, renally excreted, half life 5–6 hours.

Prochlorperazine
- Phenothiazine.
- Little evidence to support its use as an anti-emetic; however, it is frequently used to treat PONV.
- Adult dose: IM 12.5mg, buccal 3mg, PO 20mg initially then 5–10mg 8 hourly.
- Side effects include sedation, extrapyramidal effects, jaundice, skin sensitization, and blood dyscrasias.

Metoclopramide
- Dopamine receptor antagonist.
- Adult dose: PO/IV 10mg 8 hourly.
- Pro-kinetic action.
- Side effects include extrapyramidal reactions, dystonias, agitation, hypotension, and arrhythmias.

Dexamethasone
- Particularly helpful in Day Surgery Unit setting as an adjunct to 5HT3 antagonists.
- Usually given as one-off dose intra-operatively.
- Steroid side effect profile; can cause distressing perineal burning sensation when given IV.
- Also used in control of chemotherapy (N/V) and cerebral oedema due to altitude sickness/intracranial masses.

Infection

Infection

Infection is a major complication of operative surgery and surgical management. It is associated with appreciable morbidity and mortality, and no field of surgery is exempt. Post-discharge and inpatient surveillance need to be in place for accurate data collection, which is increasingly being used for inter-hospital and inter-surgeon comparisons. Definitions also need to be understood, as without them meaningful measurements cannot be made.

The Egyptians, Greeks, and Romans described infections, antiseptic salves, and how to drain pus, but the advent of antiseptic technique and modern antiseptics, aseptic technique, and the development of antibiotics are relatively recent advances. However, the 'wash your hands' campaign to prevent cross infection, on surgical wards in particular, is not a new concept but is still widely ignored.

The advent of antibiotic therapy has been associated with the associated risks of microbial resistance, for example meticillin resistant *Staphylococcus aureus* (MRSA), and microbial emergence, for example *Clostridium difficile* enteritis. It is probable that the greatest single cause of these complications follows antibiotic overuse. There are relatively few new antibiotics becoming available and the use of antibiotics will have to be far more rational if these complications are to be avoided; for example antibiotics should not be used to treat an undiagnosed cause of post-operative pyrexia, nor should a course of them be unnecessarily prolonged. Production of new antibiotics is a lengthy and expensive cost to industry and we may be in danger of running out of antibiotics to treat these infections caused by resistant organisms.

In the United Kingdom the 'search and destroy' tactics, in force in many hospitals in Northern Europe, cannot always be fully enacted because of bed pressures and lack of isolation facilities, waiting list targets, and inadequate numbers of infection control staff. However, in the background of operative surgery and surgical practice the importance of environmentally acceptable operating theatres and wards (for example the laminar, microbiologically filtered air in orthopaedic theatres), sterilization of re-useable instruments, and assurance of sterility of disposable materials is easy to overlook. These time-honoured rituals do not need randomized controlled trials to prove their worth.

Surgeons in training need to combine their knowledge of the pathophysiology of infection with these changing trends in infection observed in surgical practice, and its management. In this chapter the healthcare associated infections (HCAIs) with relevance to surgical practice in general will be described, with sections on pyrexia, systemic inflammatory response syndrome (SIRS), sepsis, multiple organ dysfunction syndrome (MODS), and organ failure.

Healthcare associated infection (HCAI)

Infection still poses a huge and continuing threat worldwide. Infectious diseases account for about a third of deaths, almost half in developing countries. Despite huge advances in antimicrobial therapy and vaccines there is global concern about the rise of microbial resistance. It seems almost paradoxical that treatment in primary care, or a hospital admission, could end in the acquisition of a new infection but this has become a major healthcare issue with political overtones. The single most likely cause of this rise in healthcare associated infection (HCAI) is the inappropriate, prolonged, or excessive use of antibiotics. The problems that come with HCAIs are around the development of resistance (the classic example being meticillin resistant *Staphylococcus aureus* (MRSA), which leads to complications of hard-to-treat SSIs, particularly when a hip or knee prosthesis is involved) and emergence (of organisms such as *Clostridium difficile*, which cause life-threatening colitis that can be of almost epidemic proportions).

The HCAIs that are relevant to surgical practice are:
- surgical site infection (SSI)
- urinary tract infection (UTI)
- respiratory tract infection (RTI), particularly ventilator associated pneumonia (VAP)
- vascular line infection and bacteraemia
- *Clostridium difficile* enteritis.

The political overtones have been translated into close surveillance of these infections and MRSA and *C. difficile* have led to huge campaigns to 'search and destroy' these unwanted pathogens. We have seen the 'clean your hands' campaign, which has led to alcoholic gels being widely distributed around the hospitals of the UK, but they are only effective against MRSA. To eradicate *C. difficile*, hand-washing with soap and water is necessary. There has been a similar campaign to encourage deep cleaning of hospitals, but systems to disinfect spores need time to work as it is not just a case of routine cleansing between patients. All this is difficult if there are not the facilities to isolate infected patients, and there are targets to be met and rapid bed turnover.

The monitoring of antibiotic use is clearly important and we should be grateful to our infection control teams and pharmacists in this regard. Intensive surveillance and isolation with adequate cleaning do come at a substantial cost.

We have been in a strong position with the introduction of many new antibiotics with good performance against these organisms. As resistance climbs we may run out as the cost of producing and introducing new antibiotics spirals and is delayed by clinical trial methodology. We need to respect and optimally use the antibiotics we have.

Surgical site infection (SSI)

Surgical site infection is a common complication of surgery. With the increasing trend to day-case or short-stay surgical it is unusual to see it in hospital practice as patients are discharged to primary care before it becomes manifest. Careful definition, assessed by a blinded trained observer with an adequate follow-up period (e.g. 6 weeks) is the only way to be sure of infection rates. The median time to a wound infection is 8–10 days; spreading cellulitis caused by β-haemolytic *Streptococci* may be seen 3–4 days after surgery, whereas some superficial and deep *Staphylococcal* infections may manifest themselves 5–6 weeks post-operatively. In the case of orthopaedic, prosthetic hip and knee surgery, SSIs can present up to and even beyond a year after surgery.

Recognition and treatment of superficial surgical site infections is often transferred to primary healthcare, where recognition may be delayed and inappropriate treatment given (antibiotics instead of removal of a suture to release pus, for example). SSIs can be expensive to healthcare services, particularly when complex procedures have to be used for their management or when there is a delay in return home. Post-discharge surveillance of SSI rates is clearly important and the following definitions and classification should be used for this purpose.

Definition of surgical site infection

For audit purposes it is critical that wounds are assessed by a trained unbiased observer using adequate definitions. A wound infection may be described as the discharge of pus or fluid from which a pathogen can be cultured, sometimes with spreading erythema. A 30-day surveillance should be used for best accuracy, a period advocated by the American Centers for Disease Control. Most SSIs are superficial, involving the skin or subcutaneous layers. Deep incisional SSIs involve the musculofascial layers, and organ or cavity SSIs might present as a liver abscess after hepatobiliary surgery or an empyema after a lung operation.

A minor wound infection should not delay the planned date of return home, but a major one may do so with systemic complications of pyrexia and SIRS (see later) and with wound disruption. The grading of wound infection is usually reserved for research purposes, a useful scheme being the ASEPSIS score based on **A**dditional treatment, the presence of **S**erous discharge, **E**rythema, **P**urulent exudate, **S**eparation of deep tissues, **I**solation of bacteria, and the duration of inpatient **S**tay. In research the interval data given by a scoring system are more useful than categorical present or absent data.

The cause of infection can be related to the time of bacterial exposure. Exogenous SSIs arise from an external source (e.g. poor theatre environment with inadequate laminar flow or air filtration, or poor ward discipline of contaminated hands at dressing change). Endogenous SSIs arise from patients' own bacterial flora (e.g. organisms from their own skin or bowel) during surgery.

Classification of SSI

This has been traditionally related to the theoretical risk of contamination (📖 see Table 2.1), and there is evidence that these classes do work. It has been estimated that contamination with 10^6 potential pathogens/gram of tissue is required to lead to a wound infection, but this is exponentially lower, as few as 100–1000 organisms, in the presence of ischaemia or foreign bodies (such as silk sutures or prosthetic grafts). Antibiotic prophylaxis is given empirically to cover the spectrum of anticipated organisms (e.g. flucloxacillin in clean prosthetic surgery against *Staphylococci*; or cefuroxime and metronidazole in elective colonic surgery to cover aerobes such as *Escherichia coli* and anaerobes such as *Bacteroides* spp.).

Rational antibiotic prophylaxis has been associated with falls in wound infection from 20–30% to <10% in clean contaminated operations; 60% to 15–20% in contaminated surgery, and over 60% to <40% in dirty surgery. There is currently some controversy surrounding wound infection rates after non-prosthetic, clean-wound surgery, particularly for breast surgery, where rates of >15% have been reported when in-depth post-discharge surveillance has been used. The use of prophylactic antibiotics is also controversial but the evidence of their value in clean, prosthetic surgery is not contested. In vascular graft surgery and orthopaedic joint surgery, infection rates should be less than 5% and 1%, respectively; antibiotic prophylaxis is extended for 24 hours in such surgery. However, there is no substitute for aseptic technique (together with ultraclean air in orthopaedics), as infection in these fields of surgery can be disastrous with high rates of mortality and morbidity and revision surgery.

In dirty surgery, the rate of wound infection is so high with its attendant risks of superficial and deep wound disruption that a case for leaving the wound open can be made. Infection is thereby minimized and once there is a clean granulating wound it can be closed by delayed primary (within five days) or secondary closure. Antibiotic prophylaxis in such cases should be extended as treatment for five days. There are many other risk factors than operative site contamination (📖 see Table 2.2).

Table 2.1 Categories of wound contamination

Ia	clean (e.g. hernia, varicose veins, breast)	hollow viscus not opened
		no inflammatory process encountered
Ib	clean prosthetic surgery (e.g. vascular grafts, joint prosthesis)	no break in aseptic ritual
II	clean-contaminated (e.g. elective open cholecystectomy)	GIT, RT, or UGT opened without significant spillage
III	contaminated (e.g. appendicectomy or elective colorectal surgery)	acute inflammation encountered without pus
		gross spillage from an open viscus or major break in asepsis
IV	dirty (e.g. abscess or faecal peritonitis)	pus or perforated viscus encountered

GIT – gastrointestinal tract; RT – respiratory tract; UGT – urogenital tract.

Table 2.2 Risk factors for wound infection (few have a level one evidence base)

Local	operative technique (haematoma or roughly handled tissues)
	thin devascularized skin flaps (local hypoxia)
	inflammatory disease (without infection being present)
	previous surgery (breast biopsy)
Systemic	malnutrition
	blood transfusion
	age
	immunosuppression of any cause
	chemotherapy or radiotherapy
	medical complications (diabetes, renal or liver failure, vascular disease)
	shock of any cause (haemorrhagic, septic, myocardial infarction)
	cancer
	remote infections
General factors	long pre-operative hospital stay
	long operations
	shaving (which ought to be immediately pre-operatively, if undertaken at all)
	use of pre-operative antiseptic showers
	operating theatre and ward rituals

Management of wound abscess/infection

- Release pus, remove any retaining sutures, and ensure adequate drainage.
- Debride necrotic non-viable tissue; this may need several sessions, including general anaesthetic in the operating theatre.
- Antibiotic empirical therapy (or based on microbiological analyses) for associated cellulitis, lymphangitis, or systemic complications of sepsis or bacteraemia.
- Topical antimicrobials (such as povidone iodine – which is useful against meticillin resistant *Staphylococcus aureus* (MRSA) – or chlorhexidine).
- Keep wound moist with appropriate surgical dressings.
- In the presence of clean granulations consider grafting or secondary suture.

When taking pus from an infected wound, fresh specimens (large volumes of pus preferably in a sterile pot rather than on a swab) need to be sent for microbiological identification and sensitivities. Communication with a microbiologist gives the best results and the best choice of an antibiotic if needed.

Urinary and respiratory infections and post-operative peritonitis

Urinary tract infection

This is a common and costly HCAI just as SSI is. The risk factors for post-operative urinary infections are:

- presence of neoplasm
- urinary obstruction/urinary stasis
- presence of urinary catheter
- presence of urinary stent
- urinary calculi and other underlying disease.

The definition of a lower urinary tract infection (UTI) depends on symptoms (not present with a urethral catheter in place) of 'cystitis' – i.e. frequency, dysuria, haematuria. An MSU may show sterile pyuria but it needs a bacteriuria of 10^5 organisms/ml to be diagnostic. Lower numbers of bacteria may represent commensals. In the presence of significant UTI, bacteraemia may follow instrumentation and antibiotics should be given prophylactically and as treatment, particularly when patients have a prosthesis or replaced heart valve. All Trusts have antibiotic protocols for this, which are based on current national guidelines and local bacterial sensitivity patterns, and should be followed. Upper urinary tract infection can follow ascending infection or bacteraemia. It is more likely to present with high pyrexia (~40°C) and rigors.

The organisms causing UTIs are mostly aerobic Gram-negative bacilli: principally *E. coli*, but also *Proteus* and *Pseudomonas* spp. (the latter can be an unwanted colonizing organism prevalent on urology wards and ITUs). *Staphylococci* may colonize the lower urinary tract when there is a catheter and *Candida* spp. may appear after prolonged catheterization, particularly after prolonged antibiotic use. Urinary tract infections are a common cause of post-operative pyrexia.

Treatment involves the use of large-volume fluid therapy to ensure an adequate diuresis and appropriate antibiotics, preferably chosen from the results of culture and sensitivities. Underlying obstructive and other disease should be attended to, with early removal of catheters and stents when possible.

Resistance is another growing problem with the rise of extended spectrum β lactamases arising in many of the coliform organisms that cause UTIs, particularly in secondary care (Ⓛ see Chapter 18, Complications of urological surgery, p.347).

Respiratory tract infection

The alveolar–capillary interface, and ventilation–perfusion balance, is a delicate one. Post-operative respiratory tract infections (RTIs) can be anticipated in patients with restricted airways: where lung volumes are reduced but patients have a reasonable one-second forced expiratory volume – FEV_1 (such as fibrosing alveolitis, chest wall disease, after pneumonectomy, and pneumoconiosis); and in obstructive airways disease with a reduced FEV_1 of <70% (those patients with chronic bronchitis, smokers, and asthmatics). These patients can be accurately identified using spirometry – an FEV_1 of <1 litre is particularly poor. Arterial blood gases identify the 'pink puffer' with a low $PaCO_2$ and the 'blue bloater' with a high $PaCO_2$ (cor pulmonale and right ventricular failure). Pre-operative physiotherapy and choice of the time for surgery when respiratory function is optimized may reduce post-operative respiratory tract infection. Cessation of smoking at least 4–6 weeks prior to surgery results in an improvement in respiratory function and less viscid bronchial secretions.

Atelectasis during the first 24–48 hours is recognized as poor basal air entry, dullness to percussion, and extra sounds. It is a common cause of early post-operative pyrexia and responds to good pain relief and physiotherapy. Chronic obstructive pulmonary disease may become acute, with an increase of pathogens such as *Haemophilus* spp. and Pneumococci. Progression to bronchopneumonia can be prevented with physiotherapy and appropriate antibiotics. Aspiration leads to profound pneumonitis, which may progress to lobar pneumonia or lung abscess without bronchial lavage and respiratory support. Pneumonias involving aerobic Gram-negative bacilli are common after prolonged ventilation on ITU and are related to sepsis and MODS, including ARDS. Ventilation may be required if physiotherapy, antibiotics, and aids to breathing fail.

Resistance is being seen in the *Enterococci* (vancomycin resistance, VRE, and other glycopeptide resistance, GRE), which are causes of ventilator associated pneumonia (VAP). This is in addition to increasing resistance being seen in 'conventional' respiratory pathogens such as *Streptococcus pneumoniae*. (📖 Also see Post-operative pyrexia, p.40 and Respiratory compromise in sepsis, p.49, and Chapter 11, Complications after cardiothoracic surgery, p.231.)

Post-operative peritonitis

Post-operative peritonitis may follow an anastomotic leak after oesophageal, rectal, colonic, pancreatic, or biliary surgery; or it may follow inadequate source control at emergency operations for community-acquired peritonitis (perforated peptic ulcer, pancreatitis, perforated appendix, gallbladder, or colonic pathology).

Post-operative ileus associated with peritonitis may be difficult to differentiate from obstruction during the early post-operative days. There is now evidence that giving early enteral feeding helps to prevent intestinal mucosal atrophy with resulting intestinal colonization and translocation to mesenteric lymph nodes and the promotion of sepsis. Certainly, attention should be given to nutrition whilst determining the cause of an ileus/obstruction and assessing whether re-laparotomy is necessary. Gastric and small bowel ileus is treated with decompression. Enteral nutrition can be provided by nasojejunal feeding or direct jejunal feeding using a jejunostomy that has been placed at the primary operation.

Enteral feeding is always preferable to total intravenous parenteral nutrition, which carries the risk of complications of insertion as well as a major risk of infection and further sepsis. Water, electrolyte, and acid–base balance can usually be managed using a peripheral IV line (📖 see Chapter 5, Complications of nutrition, p.99).

Signs of SIRS and MODS need to be monitored and early appropriate organ support instituted if necessary; in particular, signs of acute tubular necrosis associated with hypovolaemia, ARDS, and the need for cardiovascular support with fluids and inotropic support. (📖 See SIRS, sepsis, MODS, and organ failure, p.46.)

Antibiotics need to be considered, but complications of resistance (MRSA, multiple-resistant coagulase-negative *Staphylococci*, and vancomycin-resistant *Enterococci*), emergence (fungal infection, *Clostridium difficile* enteritis), toxicity, and allergy need to be taken into account. A second line of antibiotics, agreed by protocol, should be used to empirically cover the spectrum of likely organisms. This may either be monotherapy (using, for example, a carbapenem such as imipenem or meropenem) or combination therapy (such as piperaeillin-tazobactam and metronidazole), but not with the same antibiotics used to treat the peritonitis that led to the first operation.

Second look operations to exclude an abdominal cause of sepsis, such as a pelvic or subphrenic abscess or a suspected anastomotic leak, should be made on demand rather than on a routine basis. Although percutaneous drainage using imaging control may be appropriate, it cannot substitute peritoneal lavage with exteriorization of bowel ends after an anastomotic leak. The development of abdominal compartment syndrome should always be considered with the need for laparostomy (📖 see Chapter 9, Complications of gastrointestinal surgery, p.159).

Post-operative pyrexia

Patients who have a post-operative pyrexia will be seen on every ward round on a surgical ward; it is a common complication that should neither be ignored nor treated blindly with antibiotics. The most likely cause can be considered by reference to the post-operative time-scale (📖 see Table 2.3 below).

Table 2.3 Likely causes of post-operative pyrexia

Days 1–3	metabolic response to trauma
	atelectasis
	systemic or local inflammatory response
	pre-existing disease
	SIRS or extensive local dissection/haematoma
	drug reactions
	IV fluids (pyrogens; incompatibility)
	IV-line infection
	instrumentation of urinary tract
	endoscopy (ERCP)
Days 4–6	spreading wound infection (*Strep. pyogenes*)
	chest infection (early)
	urinary infection
	IV-line (peripheral and central) infection
Days 7–10	suppurative wound infection
	chest infection
	urinary infection (if catheter still in place)
	deep venous thrombosis
	deep abscess

ERCP – endoscopic retrograde cholangiopancreatography

Early (days 1–3)

As part of the metabolic response to trauma and systemic inflammatory response, the release of cytokines, and other mediators, may cause a low-grade early pyrexia (📖 see Fig. 2.1). Atelectasis is a more common cause of pyrexia, particularly when there is inadequate pulmonary effort related to inadequately controlled post-operative pain or pre-existing pulmonary disease. Atelectasis means there is an absence of gas in the alveoli – examination of the lungs may reveal poor basal air entry with retained secretion and dullness to percussion. Poor gas exchange may lead to hypoxia and poor saturation on oximetry. Treatment is adequate physiotherapy, with pain control involving the pain team if necessary, with humidified oxygen to prevent secondary infection. Antibiotics are usually unnecessary at this stage.

Local inflammation, related to extensive dissection or haematoma, may also add to the metabolic response. Systemic inflammation, expressed as systemic inflammatory response syndrome (SIRS), may relate to pre-existing disease. For example, a patient who had an appendicectomy for a gangrenous perforated appendix the day or night previously may well still have a persisting pre-operative temperature, although hopefully settling following successful surgery.

Drugs may cause a pyrexia, as may any IV fluids that are not pyrogen-free or are contaminated. Remember that blood or blood products may also cause pyrexia and need to be discontinued to avoid incompatibility complications.

Peripheral IV lines may also cause a local inflammatory reaction, particularly if the same line is being used 2–3 days after surgery. Central lines put in as an emergency for therapy or monitoring may also be a source of pyrexia. All intravascular lines need to be removed as soon as they are no longer needed and should never be used for dual function because of the risk of contamination; for example taking blood for laboratory analysis from a feeding central line is risking superadded infection and bacteraemia. Treatment is removal or replacement and, in the case of central catheters, culture of the catheter tip and antibiotic therapy if there is proven bacteraemia or sepsis.

Instrumentation or endoscopy of a viscus may cause a marked pyrexia, also relating to a transient bacteraemia. Cystoscopy in an infected urinary tract is an example. Persisting pyrexia should not be ignored – antibiotics alone may not be sufficient, particularly if there is a perforation. Always seek an underlying cause that can be corrected.

Intermediate (days 4–6)

Spreading surgical site infection caused by β-haemolytic *Streptococci*, or one of the synergistic gangrenous infections (or very rarely *Clostridium perfringens*) may be seen as early as this. There are often systemic signs of infection (hyperdynamic circulation, with hypotension and SIRS) as well as local signs of crepitus, cellulitis, or lymphangitis. In subdermal gangrene diagnosis may not be so obvious.

By this post-operative time specific chest infections (other than atelectasis) may be apparent. Patients with pre-existing pulmonary disease are most at risk: chronic bronchitis and emphysema, chronic obstructive pulmonary disease, reduced respiratory reserve, and of course smokers. Specific pathogens such as *Haemophilus influenzae* or *Streptococcus pneumoniae* may be the cause in pneumonias. Aerobic Gram-negative bacilli are usually the cause of pneumonias in surgical patients being ventilated on intensive care units (ventilator associated pneumonia). After aspiration with pneumonitis patients may develop pneumonia, usually of lobar type, and patients with small-bowel intestinal obstruction are particularly at risk of this unless they are decompressed by adequate nasogastric aspiration. A 'soup' of organisms may be expected in this situation, but *Staphylococcus aureus* is a common offender and may lead to a lung abscess.

Clinical features of dullness to percussion and inadequate ventilation follow with hypoxia and SIRS, together with cough, sputum, and occasionally haemoptysis. Chest X-ray may show diffuse changes (in aspiration) or bilateral basal bronchopneumonia or a lobar pneumonia with a pleural effusion. Progression to empyema or lung abscess occurs later but respiratory failure may supervene early.

Treatment is urgent with humidified oxygen, physiotherapy, and monitoring on a high dependency unit, or an intensive care unit if ventilation is required. Although sputum (from expectoration or aspiration) needs to be sent for microbiology, the empirical use of antibiotics should be considered. If aspiration has occurred, early bronchoscopy and lavage may be life-saving.

Urinary tract infections are common if a urinary catheter has been in place for more than a few hours, particularly in female patients. Catheter care is an important aspect of prevention. Symptomatic patients, once a catheter is removed, justify treatment with fluids and urinary antiseptics. Antibiotic therapy should be reserved for those patients who have a midstream urine/catheter-specimen urine (MSU/CSU) report that shows $>10^5$ bacteria/ml or a white cell count of >50 or red cell count (in the absence of surgery or trauma) of >100 cells/high-power field on microscopy. Culture and sensitivities may confirm that an empirical choice of antibiotic was justified or indicate that a change is needed if the clinical response is unsatisfactory. The treatment of sterile pyuria is controversial. The removal of a urinary catheter should be undertaken as soon as possible with promotion of urinary output (📖 see Fig. 2.2).

Later (days 7–10+)

Surgical site infections (SSIs) are more likely in this later period and are of suppurative, rather than spreading, type. The commonest pathogen overall is *Staphylococcus aureus* (but especially after clean surgery); other offending organisms usually relate to contaminated surgery (e.g. the synergy of a coliform with *Bacteroides* spp. after colorectal surgery). The median time to presentation of this type of wound infection is 8–10 days, and it is less likely to be associated with systemic signs, such as SIRS, unless it is an organ space SSI.

Organ space abscesses usually have a predisposing cause such as peritonitis or occur after an anastomotic leak. They are associated with the classical 'church spire' swinging temperature (📖 see Fig. 2.3). These abscesses can be imaged using ultrasound, computed tomography (CT), magnetic resonance imaging (MRI), or occasionally isotope scans. Because such abscesses tend to 'point' they may be safely drained by interventional techniques without the need for open surgery.

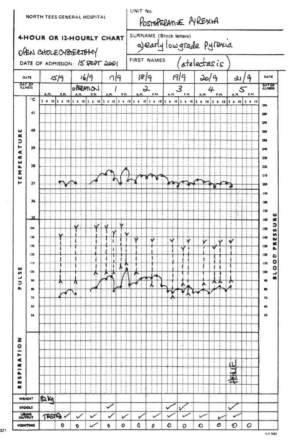

Fig. 2.1 Post-operative patterns of pyrexia. (a) Early low-grade pyrexia (e.g. atelectasis).

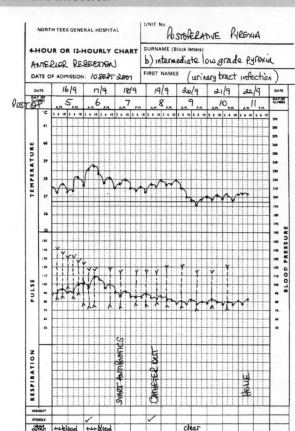

Fig. 2.2 Post-operative patterns of pyrexia. (b) Intermediate low-grade pyrexia (e.g. wound infection, UTI, RTI).

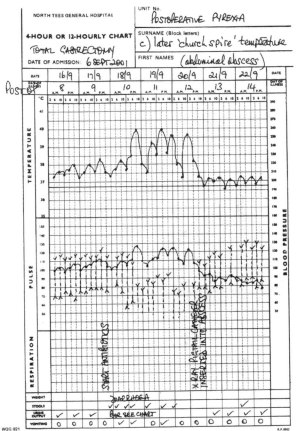

Fig. 2.3 Post-operative patterns of pyrexia. (c) Later 'church spire' temperature of abdominal abscess.

SIRS, sepsis, MODS, and organ failure

Many meanings have been ascribed to the term 'sepsis'. It should not be used as an expression of infection, but should specifically relate to the systemic inflammatory response syndrome (SIRS) that is triggered by infection. Similarly, terms such as 'Gram-negative sepsis', 'septic shock', and 'multiple organ failure' can be confusing.

SIRS may be regarded as an excessive systemic or hyperinflammatory response associated with vasodilatation and capillary leakage. It is an expected, pathophysiological, and complex response to injury or infection and there are compensatory regulatory mechanisms that, if interfered with, may worsen SIRS. This feedback mechanism has been termed 'compensatory anti-inflammatory response syndrome' (CARS). Unchecked systemic inflammation may progress to multiple organ dysfunction syndrome (MODS), multiple organ failure, and death. These definitions are summarized below.

Systemic inflammatory response syndrome (SIRS)
- Pyrexia (>38°C) or hypothermia (<36°C).
- Tachycardia (>90 beats/min in absence of β-adrenergic blockade).
- Tachypnoea (>20 breaths/min).
- Raised WBC count (>12 × 10⁹/l) or low WBC (<4 × 10⁹/l).

Any two of the above four criteria confirms SIRS.

Sepsis
SIRS with a documented focus of infection (can be of chest, wound, peritoneal, urinary, or bloodstream origin).

Sepsis syndrome (or severe sepsis)
Sepsis with evidence of organ failure.

Initiation of SIRS and MODS
Several sources that can lead to these syndromes are initiated and promoted by a complex pattern of mediators (see the following list).

Initiating 'Is' of SIRS and MODS
- INJURY
- INFLAMMATION
- INFECTION
- ISCHAEMIA
- iatrogenic
- intoxication
- immune
- idiopathic.

A simple mnemonic is to consider the 'Is', with some examples:
- *injury* – multiple trauma or extensive burns
- *inflammation* – severe acute pancreatitis
- *infection* – faecal peritonitis
- *ischaemia* – following shock of any cause or tissue ischaemia – reperfusion.

Less important (in surgery) are iatrogenic, intoxication, immune, and idiopathic causes.

Infection is the most important cause in general surgical practice and may involve Gram-negative organisms (principally *E. coli* and its lipopolysaccharide endotoxin, which stimulates macrophages to release mediators); but superantigens related to *Staphylococcus aureus*, and fungi are also important organisms (📖 see Fig. 2.4).

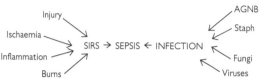

Fig. 2.4 Initiating factors in sepsis.

Although non-infectious causes exist (e.g. multiple trauma or acute pancreatitis), blood cultures should be taken as part of the investigation of patients with SIRS and MODS.

Table 2.4 Mediators involved in SIRS and MODS

cytokines	complement
nitric oxide	proteases
prostaglandins	kinins
leukotrienes	histamine
platelet activating factor (PAF)	oxygen free radicals

The mediators involved in SIRS (📖 see Table 2.4) lead to the activation of complement with stimulation of macrophages and polymorphonuclear neutrophils (PMNs). Activated PMNs are involved in systemic inflammation and their interaction with endothelium leads to changes in coagulation with the release of platelet activating factor (PAF). Increased margination and white cell diapedesis can be measured as the expression of adherence molecules (selectins and integrins). PMNs release oxygen free radicals (superoxide O_2^-, hydrogen peroxide H_2O_2, and hydroxyl radicals OH^-) with proteases, and together with other molecules (when in excess) go beyond physiological protective mechanisms and lead to tissue damage. With macrophages there is release of proinflammatory cytokines (principally interleukin-6 (IL-6), tumour necrosis factor (TNF), and IL-1), prostaglandins from the arachidonic acid cascade, leukotrienes through eicosopentanoic acid, the potent vasodilator nitric oxide, kinins, and histamine. Lymphocytes are also involved and there may be anergy. In untreated SIRS, CARS and other compensatory feedback mechanisms may be overwhelmed leading to organ failure.

Definition of MODS (📖 see Table 2.5)

Organ failure follows SIRS and sepsis, and several organs are involved. Various scoring systems have been devised to recognize early organ dysfunction; some are based on trauma (TRISS, Trauma and Injury Severity Score), others on physiological variables (APACHE, Acute Physiology and Chronic Health Evaluation (severity of illness score)) or the extent of organ failure (Goris). They may be an adjuvant to therapy, and sequential scoring may anticipate the need for surgery or higher planes of monitoring or additional therapy (HDU and ITU).

Table 2.5 Definitions of multiple organ dysfunction (MODS)

Pulmonary	ARDS	PaO_2 <9.3kPa PaO_2/FiO_2 <30 (reduced compliance, increased PEEP, CXR appearance)
Renal	ATN	<120ml urine/4h (raised urea, creatinine, K^+)
Cardiovascular		lactate >1.2mmol/l SVR <800dynes/s/cm³ (cardiac depression, lowered CO_2, arrhythmias)
Coagulation	DIC	decreased platelets, increased D-dimers (bleeding tendency)
CNS		GCS <15 (in absence of head injury)
Hepatic		(increased bilirubin, AST, reduced albumin)
Intestinal		(gastric stress ulceration, ileus)

Brackets indicate associated but non-definitive variables.

ARDS – acute respiratory distress syndrome; PEEP – positive end-expiratory pressure; CXR – chest X-ray; ATN – acute tubular necrosis; SVR – systemic vascular resistance; DIC – disseminated intravascular coagulation; GCS – Glasgow Coma Score; AST – aspartate aminotransferase.

Management of SIRS and MODS

- anticipate/predict complications
- resuscitate (fluids and oxygen)
- investigate
- remove precipitating cause
- treat with antibiotics (based on empirical therapy)
- give nutritional support and vaso-active drugs.

SIRS and MODS are more likely in some presenting surgical illnesses and after specific types of surgery; they can be anticipated and avoided or, at the earliest sign, recognized and prevented quickly. Resuscitation is based on ABCDE (airway, breathing, circulation, disability, exposure, as in trauma patients). A rapid response to high-flow oxygen (the re-breathing Hudson mask can give an FiO_2 of 60%) and a rapid intravenous infusion

(0.5 to 1.0l in adults) of colloid or crystalloid (not 5% dextrose) fluid challenge should be given. Systems scoring may be helpful and encouraging. Once organ failure is established (APACHE >20, Goris 2+ systems failure) mortality can reach 80–100%. Inotropes may be considered once the fluid deficit is corrected (based on pulse, BP, CVP, urine output, and markers of cardiopulmonary performance such as blood gases, oximetry, and transoesophageal-measured cardiac variables, which have replaced the Swan Ganz catheter technique). Fluid and oxygen therapy is as important in early hyperdynamic circulatory states, when oxygen consumption (VO_2) is high and oxygen delivery (DO_2) falls behind. The development of late 'cold' hypotensive shock is an ominous sign of myocardial and peripheral circulatory failure.

Investigation needs to identify the cause, particularly a focus of infection. Interventional radiology now has an important role; not only can collections of pus be accurately imaged (using ultrasound, CT, radionuclide scans, and MRI), but guided drainage is successful and may avoid the need for open or even minimally invasive surgery. Occasionally, surgery is necessary for the evacuation of pus and has a place in excluding ischaemia, particularly in second-look operations or when there is an abdominal compartment syndrome (which may require bowel exteriorization-resection, or laparostomy). Catheter-related infections (central venous catheters (CVCs) and urinary catheters) usually require removal of the catheter before sepsis can be controlled.

Antibiotics are given on a considered, empirical basis. This can involve combination chemotherapy or monotherapy to cover the likely organisms. Most Hospital Trusts and ITUs have strict protocols for antibiotic use. As an example, first-line combination antibiotic therapy for faecal peritonitis following a perforated sigmoid diverticulum should cover aerobes and anaerobes (a wide-spectrum penicillin or second- or third-generation cephalosporin together with an imidazole, such as metronidazole, would suffice); whereas for a nosocomial infection, for example a post-operative pneumonia, a second-line monotherapy drug might be used (such as a carbapenem, like meropenem or imipenem). Samples should always be sent for microbiological culture whenever possible (blood, sputum, urine, pus) and sensitivities may justify a change in antibiotic therapy if the clinical response is unsatisfactory.

Specific treatments involving monoclonal antibodies to endotoxin or cytokines such as TNF have been disappointing. The cause of sepsis may initially be unclear, and interference with the complex septic process may upset the feedback mechanisms of SIRS and CARS. Nevertheless, the search to modulate mediators continues.

Respiratory compromise in sepsis

The most common cause of poor conscious levels in post-operative surgical patients relates to cardiopulmonary performance. Respiratory failure may be of type I (when there is failure of oxygen uptake) or type II (when, in addition, there is failure of carbon dioxide removal). Blood gas levels in failure include a PaO_2 of <8kPa and a $PaCO_2$ >7kPa; oxygen levels in this low range relate to the steep part of the dissociation curve when saturation can rapidly fall under 90%. There may be pre-existing COPD in a surgical patient with airflow obstruction, but in septic conditions there may be an acute fall in functional residual capacity (FRC), for example in pneumonia, or increased pulmonary vascular dysfunction, as in ARDS.

ARDS is recognized when the PaO_2/FiO_2 ratio is <30 and the PaO_2 falls under 9.3kPa. The high FiO_2 (0.6) of a re-breathing mask may be inadequate and as compliance falls there is a need for CPAP or ventilation with increasing PEEP.

Cardiovascular compromise in sepsis

In sepsis there is a need for oxygen supplementation and an assurance that adequate fluid has been given before inotropes are considered. The fluid loss to the 'third space' may be large in septic states. Myocardial depression may occur with arrhythmias; but when cardiac preload and myocardial performance have been corrected, a fall in systemic vascular resistance (SVR <800dynes/s per cm^3) may need inotrope support. Dobutamine can improve myocardial contractility and heart rate by stimulating β_1-adrenergic receptors, but if there is hypotension this may be worsened (through β_2-adrenergic receptor stimulation, although there is some α-adrenergic receptor effect). Dopamine is similar, but is not as effective. The use of small 'renal' doses of dopamine is controversial. Noradrenaline (norepinephrine) is an effective α-adrenoreceptor stimulant and raises SVR but with some degree of renal vessel constriction. The titration of optimal fluid input, myocardial support, and inotropes may be complex. Cardiac performance variables, measured using transoesophageal ultrasound, are used to measure cardiac pressures and aid in the measurement of preload and afterload and myocardial performance – particularly in sepsis and MODS, ARDS, and monitoring of inotropes.

Renal compromise in sepsis

Loss of fluid to third-space compartments must also be corrected for optimal renal function. If, despite this and with the appropriate cardiopulmonary support, there is evidence of renal failure (oliguria, rising potassium concentration, rising urea and creatinine levels with sodium and water overload) renal replacement therapy may be required. Peritoneal dialysis is rarely appropriate and haemofiltration or dialysis is required.

The acid-base balance will also need to be addressed. In sepsis, there may be a renal failure to excrete hydrogen ions, and a respiratory compromise (e.g. ARDS) when there is a failure to remove CO_2. In sepsis, there is also an added metabolic acidosis.

Gastrointestinal compromise in sepsis

In sepsis, many gastrointestinal protective mechanisms are lost. With starvation and increased metabolic rate there is a rapid atrophy of enterocyte function with falls in IgG in gastric mucus and gut-associated lymphoid tissue function. This may be severe in shock states, particularly after ischaemia-reperfusion injury. In jaundice, there is also a loss of protective enteral bile salts.

The normally sterile upper gastrointestinal tract becomes colonized, principally with aerobic Gram-negative bacilli in sepsis, and this can also occur where there is a risk of sepsis development, such as a multiply injured patient being ventilated on ITU. There is translocation of bacteria to the mesenteric lymph nodes, and following macrophage stimulation the release of proinflammatory cytokines and other mediators that cause sepsis add to the development of ileus. The colonization of the gut has been termed the 'motor' of sepsis and multiple organ failure. Translocation and sepsis has been convincingly proven in animal models but is still controversial clinically. Nevertheless, efforts to selectively decontaminate the digestive tract (SDD) have been made using topical, poorly absorbed antimicrobials (amphotericin B, tobramycin, polymyxin E) with parenteral cephalosporins to reduce HCAIs on ITUs, particularly ventilator associated pneumonia (VAP). The effect on mortality is less clear. Other methods to decontaminate the GI tract, including the use of probiotic bacteria and early enteral nutrition with immunostimulating diets (containing nucleic acids, arginine, and polyunsaturated fatty acids), need further proof before being widely used.

The stomach is at risk of acute stress gastritis in sepsis with the risk of significant bleeding manifested as bloody naso-gastric aspirates or haematemesis, and melaena. The use of antacids (proton pump inhibitors or H2-receptor antagonists) reduces gastric acidity and further increases the risk of gastrointestinal microbial colonization. Gastric cyto-protective agents, such as sucralfate, should be considered as an alternative.

Bacterial resistance and emergence

'Superbugs'

The β-haemolytic organisms can cause rapidly spreading cellulitis and lymphangitis after surgery. Some carry superantigens and may relate to high mortality (referred to in 'outbreaks' a few years ago as the 'Gloucester flesh-eating virus'). They may be associated with the similar organism 'soups' seen in synergistic gangrene and need to be treated with the same aggression and urgency. Animal and human bites may result in these infections but they are rare after elective surgery.

MRSA was reported as being an important pathogen in 1961 and has since been implicated in several surgical ward epidemics. There are now epidemic strains (EMRSA). This epidemic potential is clearly a concern in surgery, particularly when a prosthesis has been implanted. MRSA is an opportunistic pathogen that colonizes theatre and ward environments as well as open wounds (such as chronic ulcers, pressure sores, and incised wounds that have broken down). It can be difficult to eradicate, and controversy over the need to attempt this escalates. In some hospitals, colonization may reach >40% of surgical patients and infection control can be a costly business. Containment involves ward and theatre closure, isolation of patients with full barrier nursing, identification of carriers, and the use of mupirocin and topical antiseptics in all those so infected.

Multiply resistant, coagulase-negative *Staphylococcus* (MRCNS) is another colonizing opportunistic pathogen and the principal cause of infected intravascular devices, vascular grafts, and orthopaedic prostheses. Short pre-operative stays reduce the risk of colonization before surgery.

Intravascular lines, even peripheral intravenous cannulas, are a major source of MRSA and MRCNS bacteraemia. They need to be removed as soon as they are not needed. Strict aseptic precautions are needed for all manipulations of intravascular devices; if these precautions are used then the catheters can last for months without infection. This is seen in long-term chemotherapy and feeding central venous catheters, even on intensive care and renal units where super-added infection with these resistant organisms is more likely. Always consider an intravascular line as a cause of post-operative prexia; remove it if it is not required and if suspicious send the tip for microbiological culture.

If antibiotic use is not controlled then the incidence of MRSA and MRCNS (and other organisms such as glycopeptide-resistant *Enterococci*, those organisms expressing extended spectrum β lactamases, and *C. difficile*) will increase with a corresponding decrease in the numbers of effective antibiotics. Vancomycin is still usually effective in the treatment of MRSA, although resistance is increasingly being seen, and even the new effective agents such as linezolid are having reports made of resistance.

Other relevant surgical infections, including HIV and hepatitis

Synergistic gangrene

This is caused by a mixed pattern of organisms and often a 'soup' of opportunistic pathogens is responsible – coliforms, *Staphylococci*, *Bacteroides* spp, anaerobic *Streptococci*, and *Peptostreptococci* have been implicated. It is more commonly seen in patients who are immunocompromised and even more unusual bacteria may be seen.

Risk factors for immunocompromise and synergistic wound infection include:

- malnutrition
- cancer
- diabetes
- anti-cancer therapies – chemo- and radiotherapy
- steroids and other drugs
- immunosuppressing diseases, e.g. acquired immunodeficiency deficiency syndrome (AIDS).

These infections can, in susceptible patients, follow even clean wound operations such as herniorrhaphy with several related eponyms – Meleney synergistic hospital gangrene (abdominal wall); Fourniér's gangrene (scrotum). This may be overlooked in the early stages as the infection is subdermal, but it is soon clear that the patient is profoundly unwell with SIRS and the risk of a multiple organ dysfunction syndrome (MODS). There may soon be obvious non-viable changes in dermal tissues with severe pain; and crepitus may be felt or gas seen on imaging (X-ray or ultrasound). Gas is not confined to *Clostridium perfringens* infection.

Therapy includes:

- IV fluids
- systemic organ support
- antibiotics
- early, aggressive, widespread debridement of non-viable tissue with laying open of wound
- hyperbaric oxygen (controversial)
- skin grafting once debrided areas are clean.

Clostridial gas gangrene

The spores of *Clostridium perfringens* are widely distributed, being present in soil and normal human faeces. Again, immunocompromised patients are more at risk and gas gangrene can follow surgery or a needle-stick injury when contaminated instruments are used, or when bacteria or spores are not cleaned from the incision site. Patients most susceptible are those with contaminated anaerobic tissues, particularly muscle, and those in whom foreign bodies are present. These are the typical conditions after military injuries, particularly high-velocity missile injuries where the kinetic energy ($\frac{1}{2}mv^2$) is high and dissipates into widespread soft-tissue injury and cavitation. There is also a 'sucking' action at the entry wound that promotes the entry of foreign bodies such as clothing and soil. The exotoxins and proteases released by *Clostridia* spp. cause widely spreading gangrene with crepitus (and gas seen on X-ray) and severe septicaemia. Wide debridement is necessary with organ support, antibiotics, and hyperbaric oxygen.

Tetanus

This is a very rare complication of surgery. After implantation of spores there is a long prodromal period (a shorter period of a few days indicates a poor prognosis) while the neurotoxin is taken up by the anterior horn cells of the spinal cord. The local inflammatory reaction at the implantation site or wound may be trivial or often resolved before the patient presents with painful spasms, respiratory failure, and aspiration pneumonia in the most severe form. Tracheostomy and prolonged drug-induced paralysis and ventilation may be needed. The rarity of this infection may relate to the widely accepted programme of immunization with tetanus toxoid and, of course, the excellence of operating theatre environments.

Clostridium difficile enteritis (CDAD)

Antibiotic-related colitis is common, but *Clostridium difficile* enteritis can be profound with blood loss and dehydration shock. Although the organism can be cultured from normal stools, the diagnosis is made by assay of toxin. The disease can be of epidemic proportions locally and is spread by poor ward hygiene. Older patients are particularly susceptible, and they may suffer relapses.

The antibiotics most commonly associated with the syndrome are broad-spectrum penicillins or cephalosporins, particularly when they are prolonged in use or changed over, but most antibiotics have been implicated. Treatment is usually effective using metronidazole or vancomycin with removal of existing antibiotic therapy.

Recognition follows suspicion and assay of the toxin. Sigmoidoscopy, which is not recommended for diagnosis because of the risk of perforation, shows the classical pseudomembrane of fibrin and sloughed mucosa (hence its alternative name). If the colitis becomes fulminant it may lead to a toxic megacolon with the risk of life-threatening bleeding or perforation. Colectomy may be life-saving; however, aggressive IV replacement therapy is usually successful, although often needing high-dependency unit (HDU) monitoring and isolation barrier nursing.

Fungal infections

These can occur as complications of prolonged broad-spectrum antibiotic therapy, again particularly in immunosuppressed patients. *Candida* is a yeast that may result in infection of the gastrointestinal tract, mostly mouth and oesophagus, and respiratory tract. Rarely, there may be systemic candidiasis often related to intravascular catheter infection, which may require therapy with fluconazole or ketoconazole. Nystatin is only useful in managing oral thrush. The filamentous organisms of the *Aspergillus* genus may be seen in patients who have prolonged stays on ITUs; amphotericin is the antibiotic of choice.

Fungal infections are often missed or the diagnosis is delayed. The usual help can be gained by communication with a microbiologist when there is suspicion of a fungal infection, and appropriate recognition methods can be used.

HIV, AIDS, and hepatitis

The type I immunodeficiency retrovirus (HIV) can be transmitted by body fluids, particularly blood, and is a complication to the operating team when known infected or high risk patients are being operated on. The virus is transmitted through homosexual and heterosexual contact, intravenous drug addiction, and transfusion with infected blood, and is prevalent in sub-Saharan Africans. The risk by 'needle-stick' injury to healthcare staff and in the operating room is small but very important. In the early weeks after infection, when there may be a flu-like illness, and during seroconversion there is the greatest risk of transmission through exposure to body fluids. Untreated HIV progresses to AIDS with opportunistic infections and neoplasms with a high fatality. It is in the early phases that highly active anti-retroviral therapy (HAART) is most effective. If a sharp injury occurs during surgery then the injured part should be washed under running water. Local occupational health policies are needed to determine the use of HAART or HIV testing.

Viral hepatitis is another major world health problem. There are well recognized acute and chronic liver diseases caused by hepatitis A, B, and C, and now D and E. Hepatitis B (HBV) and C (HCV) are transmissable by blood and body fluids.

The operative team need to take universal precautions when a known infected or at risk patient presents for necessary surgery. These involve:

- wearing of full face mask or protective spectacles when there is a high risk from splashing, for example with power tools in orthopaedics
- use of fully waterproof, disposable gowns and drapes
- wearing of boots, not clogs, to avoid injury from dropped sharps
- double gloving with the larger size glove on the outside
- avoidance of excessive movement or unnecessary people in the operating theatre
- respect and eye contact for passing of sharps (in a dish, not hand-to-hand)
- slow meticulous operative technique with minimal bleeding.

Chapter 3

Cardiovascular complications after surgery in general

Introduction

Cardiovascular (CV) disease remains the largest cause of disease burden in the developed world and is now the largest killer worldwide. With an increasingly ageing population, most of us will encounter patients with CV disease. Complications after anaesthesia and surgery are a major cause of morbidity and mortality. Identifying patients most at risk pre-operatively, and the use of invasive monitoring in the peri-operative period, have increased the safety of surgery. Nevertheless, myocardial infarction, dysrhythmias, cardiac failure, and stroke occur relatively frequently, reflecting the need for better understanding of the basic pathophysiology, diagnosis, and management of cardiovascular complications. It must be noted that rapidly evolving advances in cardiovascular diagnostics and therapeutics have resulted in an increasing dependence on technology. There is no substitute for excellent clinical skills – a few minutes of carefully invested time can pay huge dividends. This chapter is divided into three sections: a brief refresher section on physiology and pharmacology; the clinical skills; and the commonest conditions, in context with the latest guidelines for surgical patients. This does *not* include management of cardiac surgery patients (refer to Chapter 11, Complications after cardiothoracic surgery, p.231).

Cardiovascular history and examination

This should include the past and present history of cardiovascular disease; is there a history of chest pain, dyspnoea, paroxysmal nocturnal dyspnoea, orthopnoea, pre-syncope, syncope, palpitations, limb weakness, dysarthria, changes in vision?

A general examination should involve checking:

- Pulse – rate, rhythm, character; collapsing, parvus, alternans, bisferiens, slow-rising.
- Capillary refill time and temperature of peripheries.
- BP – systolic is peak, diastolic is trough, and the difference gives the pulse pressure; mean arterial pressure (MAP) is the average pressure during the cardiac cycle which equates to ~1/3 pulse pressure + diastolic. Check for pulsus paradoxus (note that this is not a paradoxical fall in pulse rate but an exaggeration of the normal physiological response of decreased BP with inspiration, a fall of >20mmHg is considered significant).
- Heart sounds 1 and 2 (S3 and S4 are both diastolic sounds suggestive of heart failure) (📖 see Fig. 3.1).
- Murmurs – location, timing, nature, intensity, radiation, other features (📖 see Fig. 3.2) – *the key question is: are they new or changing?*
- Signs of congestive heart failure: basal crepitations, peripheral oedema, hepatomegaly, raised JVP.
- Urine output.
- Radial, brachial, carotid, femoral, popliteal, posterior tibial, and dorsalis pedis pulses.

Timing of murmurs

- Right-sided murmurs i.e. TS/TR/PS/PR occur at the same points in the cardiac cycle as their left-sided equivalents.
- Tricuspid valve pathology will cause same timing of murmurs as MV pathology and PV as AV.
- Example TR has the same PSM as MR, PS has same ESM as AS.
- Similarly MS and TS are similar as is AR and PR.
- Right sided murmurs become louder on inspiration.
- Left-sided murmurs become louder on expiration.

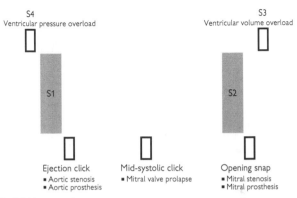

Fig. 3.1 Heart sounds.

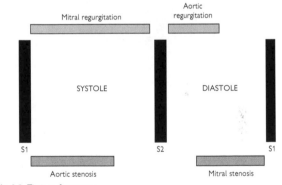

Fig. 3.2 Timing of murmurs.

Cardiovascular physiology

Understanding CV physiology and haemodynamics can be very confusing. However, mastering CV physiology can be easily achieved by thinking of the system as having two components: a pump (the heart) and plumbing (arteries and veins). Their regulation is complex with the ultimate homeostatic aim of maintaining adequate organ perfusion. The body endeavours to survive above all odds and has to be able to respond to constantly changing factors. In times of 'shock' the body prioritizes limited blood and oxygen supplies by maintaining perfusion to the brain and then the kidneys above other organs.

There are two main equations concerning cardiac output and blood pressure:

- Cardiac output (CO), which is the amount of blood pumped out of each ventricle per minute:
  CO (ml/min) = stroke volume (ml) × heart rate (bpm)
- BP = cardiac output × total peripheral resistance.

Blood pressure (BP) refers to the force exerted by blood on vessel walls and, used in the commonest context, refers to systemic arterial pressure. Occasionally clinicians flip between referring to venous, portal, and pulmonary pressures, but in reality all vessels have a pressure within them. Mean aortic pressure is determined by cardiac output and total systemic resistance. Cardiac output is influenced by those factors listed in the first equation above.

Peripheral arterial resistance is determined by vessel stiffness, length, and lumen size. Blood pressure is maintained by these factors interacting with neurohormonal components such as adrenaline production.

Determinants of cardiac output

Preload – the degree to which the myocardium is stretched before it contracts. Mainly determined by circulating blood volume. This is also affected by: atrial contraction, venous tone, intrathoracic pressure, intrapericardial pressure, and posture.

Afterload – the resistance against which the heart has to eject blood. It is determined mainly by peripheral vascular resistance and arterial vasoconstriction/dilatation. This is also affected by viscosity of blood, compliance and inertia of large arteries, and the radius of the ventricular cavity.

Myocardial contractility – the intrinsic inotropic state of the heart muscle is affected by the autonomic impulses, circulating catecholamines, hypoxia, acidosis, hypercapnia, ischaemia, and drugs.

The Frank Starling principle describes the length–tension relationship in cardiac muscle, where the more the muscle is stretched, the greater the tension developed in the muscle, and hence the greater the force of contraction. As the stretch becomes more extreme, no further tension is developed, and eventually the force of contraction declines. The curve is moved up and to the left with increased contractility, but shifts downwards and to the right in heart failure (see Fig. 3.3).

The Frank Starling curve illustrates the relationship between the end-diastolic volume and the stroke volume, or, in a clinical context, the relationship between atrial pressure and cardiac output.

Note that all of the above factors interact to maintain cardiac output and blood pressure, and cannot be thought of in isolation. In disease states compensatory mechanisms may not function or maladaptive responses occur.

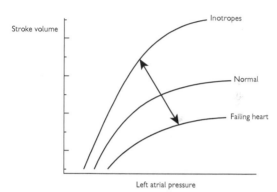

Fig. 3.3 The Frank Starling curve.

Coronary blood flow (CBF)

- Is normally about 225ml/min at rest.
- The heart has a very high (70–80%) oxygen extraction ratio, even at rest.
- Increased delivery of oxygen to the myocardium at times of increased need can therefore only be achieved by increasing the blood flow.
- The major determinants of myocardial oxygen consumption are myocardial contractility, heart rate, and intramyocardial tension.
- CBF to the left ventricle mainly occurs during diastole.
- Increasing heart rates lead to a shortening of diastole, and a reduction in CBF.

Cardiac disease can be due to:

- ischaemia
- valvular disease
- dysrhythmias
- cardiomyopathies
- pericardial disease
- infective causes

When assessing cardiac disease it is useful to think of the primary problem and complications that occur. For example, a primary issue may be valvular heart disease leading to cardiac failure and/or secondary dysrhythmias.

It is useful to think about effects on the heart chambers secondary to valvular problems as:
• stenoses causing pressure overload and usually hypertrophy
• regurgitation as causing volume overload and thereby dilatation.

With major vessels disease may present as:
• dissections
• embolus
• aneurysm
• inflammation, as in the vasculitides.

These complications can occur in **any** part of the vasculature.

Investigations

General
- venous blood for FBC, U&Es, coagulation profile, cardiac enzymes, lipid profile, glucose
- arterial blood gases (ABG)
- ECG
- CXR.

Specialized

Table 3.1 Summary of specialized cardiac investigations and their uses in surgical patients

Type	Investigation	Post-operative uses and indications
Non-invasive	Trans-thoracic echo	Regional wall motion abnormalities that occur in ischaemia.
		Valvular incompetence.
		Diastolic function and physiological determinants of cardiac output.
		Pericardial disease.
		LV and RV systolic function.
	Carotid and vertebral artery 2D US and Doppler	For stenosis, aneurysms, and pseudo-aneurysms.
	CT head	CVA – embolic or haemorrhagic intracranial bleeds.
	Cardiac CT and cardiac MRI	Useful for imaging heart for looking at coronary arteries if unable to perform cardiac catheterization (requested on advice of specialist).
		Cardiac MRI is sensitive for cardiomyopathies.
	Myocardial perfusion scans (functional assessment)	These scans are used to identify areas of inducible ischaemia. • the heart is stressed either through exercise or usually via chemical stimulation (dobutamine, adenosine) • can be done as dobutamine-stress echocardiography, myocardial perfusion scintigraphy with SPECT, perfusion cardiac MRI.

Table 3.1 Summary of specialized cardiac investigations and their uses in surgical patients (*continued*)

Type	Investigation	Post-operative uses and indications
		Used to stress the heart for troponin-negative acute coronary syndromes in patients who are unable to undertake exercise tolerance testing.
Invasive	Trans-oesophageal echo	Can do above and in aortic dissection – can rapidly help differentiate Stamford type A, B, and C.
	Cardiac catheterization	'Left heart cath.' – coronary angiography for IHD.
		Can also perform left ventriculo-gram to assess function and mitral and aortic valve disease.
		'Right heart cath.' – for VSD, PFO, TR, pulmonary artery hypertension, MS.
Haemodynamic monitoring (useful in cardiogenic shock)	Pulmonary artery catheterization (Swan-Ganz) LiDCO Trans-oesophageal Doppler PiCCO	Cardiac output, systemic vascular resistance – main use is in guiding IV filling and use of inotropes. Use thermodilution or the Fick principle in determining physiological state.

General management principles

Checklist for patents who have cardiovascular complications includes:
- resuscitation (ABCDE)
- history and examination
- review of notes and charts
- management plan
- appropriate investigations
- specific treatment
- consideration of transfer to higher level of care and senior consultation.

Optimization of cardiac output involves:
- giving oxygen with spontaneous or assisted ventilation
- cardiac preload can be optimized by giving fluids (crystalloid, colloid, blood, or diuretics or nitrates)
- cardiac afterload may be adjusted with vasodilators and adequate pain control
- contractility can be improved by giving inotropes, restoring coronary blood flow
- heart rate and rhythm can be optimized using anti-arrhythmic agents, chronotropic drugs, and transvenous pacing
- mechanical support: intra-aortic balloon pump counter-pulsation, ventricular assist devices.

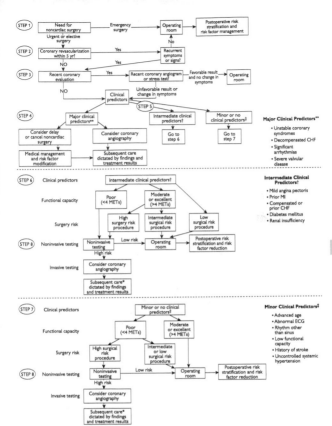

Fig. 3.4 Stepwise approach to preoperative cardiac assessment. Steps are discussed in text. *Subsequent care may include cancellation or delay of surgery, coronary revascularization followed by noncardiac surgery, or intensified care. Reproduced from Eagle, KA, Berger, PB, Clakins H et al. (2002) ACC/AHA guideline update for perioperative cardiovascular evaluation for non-cardiac surgery – executive summary: a report of the American College of Cardiology/American Heart Association Task Force on Practice Guidelines *JACC* **39**: 542–53, with permission from Elsevier.

Acute coronary syndromes

The risk of peri-operative MI in the general surgical population is 0.07%. If surgery is performed within 3 months of an MI, the risk of reinfarction may be as high as 25% and it is important to identify the high-risk group and take precautions to reduce the incidence of MI and subsequent mortality (📖 see Table 3.2). Peri-operative MI is often asymptomatic because of anaesthesia and analgesia. Precipitants can include increasing cardiac workload and hypercoagulability. ECGs often do not show the classic ST elevation of an MI, and cardiac enzymes can be difficult to interpret because of co-existing renal failure, sepsis, pulmonary emboli, and skeletal muscle damage.

Acute coronary syndrome (ACS) is an umbrella term that covers all types of unstable angina and myocardial infarction. Traditionally, a diagnosis of myocardial infarction was made if two out of three positive findings from history, ECG, and cardiac enzymes were found. Many people have been mislabelled as having an MI – it is common to meet those who claim to have had seven heart attacks! The term myocardial infarction should be used when there is evidence of myocardial necrosis in a clinical setting consistent with myocardial ischaemia. The new definiton of MI (agreed by Joint Task Force ESC/AHA/WHF) requires:
1) a rise in a biomarker;
2) any of the following: symptoms, ECG changes, imaging evidence of new loss of myocardium or new wall motion defect.

Troponins are the most sensitive biochemical markers of acute myocardial injury. MI is extremely unlikely in the presence of a normal troponin (excellent negative predictive value). The different subtypes of myocardial infarction are important as they guide the immediate and medium-term management and reflect injury and prognosis. ST elevation MIs (STEMIs) require primary angioplasty. The thrombolysis criteria (ST elevation 1mm or more in one or more chest leads and 2mm or more in any other lead, new left bundle branch block, and prolonged cardiac chest pain) are the same criteria for primary angioplasty. This is now the first-line treatment for the ST elevation ACSs. If your patient fulfils these criteria seek an urgent cardiology referral.

Unstable angina refers to angina at rest, that of abrupt onset, rapid deterioration of previously stable angina, or prolonged chest pain not relieved with anti-anginals, but without ST elevation/bundle branch block changes. These so-called non-ST elevation ACS patients must be anti-coagulated to *prevent* an infarction. If they have a positive troponin rise they are defined as non-ST elevation MIs (NSTEMI). These patients should have cardiac catheterization performed within 48–72 hours as an inpatient provided they are able to tolerate the procedure. 📖 Figure 3.4 stratifies those non-ST elevation ACSs and shows who should receive coronary angiography and when.

Q-wave MI and non-Q wave MI are terms used to describe those infarctions that have pathological Q-waves (normally more than two small squares) and those that do not, since they are prognostically important. Q-wave MIs suggest a fully completed infarction and one that has involved a full segment of myocardium, sometimes called transmural or 'full thickness infarct'. Non-Q wave MIs suggest sub-myocardial damage and carry a better prognosis.

Table 3.2 Clinical predictors of increased peri-operative cardiovascular risk (myocardial infarction, heart failure, death) – taken from ACC/AHA *Guideline Update for Peri-operative Cardiovascular Evaluation for Non-cardiac Surgery*

Major

Unstable coronary syndromes:

Acute or recent myocardial infarction with evidence of important ischemic risk by clinical symptoms or non-invasive study.

Unstable or severe angina (Canadian class III or IV).

Decompensated heart failure.

Significant arrhythmias.

High-grade atrioventricular block.

Symptomatic ventricular arrhythmias in the presence of underlying heart disease.

Supraventricular arrhythmias with uncontrolled ventricular rate.

Severe valvular disease.

Intermediate

Mild angina pectoris (Canadian class I or II).

Previous myocardial infarction by history or pathological Q waves.

Compensated or prior heart failure.

Diabetes mellitus (particularly insulin-dependent).

Renal insufficiency.

Minor

Advanced age.

Abnormal ECG (left ventricular hypertrophy, left bundle branch block, ST-T abnormalities).

Rhythm other than sinus (e.g. atrial fibrillation).

Low functional capacity (e.g. inability to climb one flight of stairs with a bag of groceries).

History of stroke.

Uncontrolled systemic hypertension.

Classification of MI

Type 1: spontaneous MI related to ischaemia due to a primary coronary event such as plaque erosion and/or rupture, fissuring or dissection.

Type 2: MI secondary to ischaemia due to either increased oxygen demand or decreased supply, such as coronary spasm, coronary embolism, anaemia, arrhythmias, hypertension, or hypotension.

Type 3: MI in sudden cardiac death

Type 4: after PCI

Type 5: after CABG

Pathophysiology

Ischaemic necrosis results from an imbalance in the supply and demand of oxygen in the myocardium. Haemodynamic alterations occurring peri-operatively influence the development of MI. Tachycardia results in increased oxygen demand and reduced supply because of shortened diastole. Hypotension results in reduced coronary perfusion pressure, thereby reducing oxygen supply, and hypertension results in increased oxygen demand. Left ventricular overfilling results in increased oxygen demand and reduced supply secondary to augmented tissue pressure.

Clinical features

Chest pain, crushing or constricting in nature, retrosternal, radiating to the jaws or both arms and wrists (NB chest pain radiating to the jaw is almost always from the heart). There may be an atypical presentation (painless heart failure or gastrointestinal symptoms), which is common in the elderly, diabetics, or peri-operatively. Nausea, vomiting, dyspnoea, and autonomic disturbances occur. The physical examination is often negative, unless there is a complication or overt cardiac failure.

Investigations

Bloods

FBC, U&E, blood glucose, lipids, coagulation screen, G&S.

Electrocardiography

Typical changes accompanying acute MI are:
- ST segment elevation 1mm in precordial leads or 2mm in limb leads
- reciprocal ST depression in the opposite leads
- development of new Q waves if they are wide (above 0.04s) or deep (more than one-third of the height of the following R wave)
- T-wave inversion (not diagnostic by itself)
- location of these changes on the ECG identify the region of the infarction:
  - inferior: II, III aVF
  - antero-septal: V3–V4
  - antero-lateral: V5–V6
  - posterior: V1 + V2.

(Note that results **must** be compared with old ECGs – new or dynamic changes are high-risk patients.)

Enzyme changes

Troponin and CK. Serial cardiac enzymes are rarely performed now.

Echocardiography

This is helpful in equivocal cases and may reveal immobility of a discrete area of ventricular wall and help to titrate the dose of angiotensin-converting enzyme (ACE) inhibitors. RWMA is a very sensitive marker of ischaemia. This will also help detect post-MI complications and guide management in cardiogenic shock.

Treatment of myocardial infarction

Immediate for ALL types of MI

- Transfer to coronary care unit (CCU).
- Oxygen as needed.
- Nitrates – sublingual glyceryl trinitrate (GTN) or buccal suscard. If this is ineffective give IV GTN at a dose of 1–10mg per hour for continuing chest pain or pulmonary oedema if the systolic blood pressure is >90mmHg and the patient has not received a phosphodi-esterase inhibitor (ie. sildenafil) within 24 hours. (Prescribe GTN 50mg in 50 ml 0.9% normal saline).
- Analgesia with morphine and anti-emetics – morphine also helps as a vasodilator.
- Aspirin 300mg (even if on 75mg) PO (if allergic seek advice).
- Clopidogrel 600mg or 300mg (depending on your local guidelines).
- Statin (beneficial in an acute setting as helps in acute plaque stabilization). All patients should have a lipid profile performed with baseline bloods, and then be started on a statin **before** the result. For patients with an LDL <4.5mmol/l give simvastatin 40mg od; for patients with an LDL >4.5mmol/l give atorvastatin 40mg od.
- Beta blockers are recommended for all patients except those with:
  - a history of bronchospasm
  - heart failure requiring therapy
  - bradycardia of less than 50bpm
  - second or third degree AV node block
  - cardiogenic shock
  - allergy or hypersensitivity to beta blockers.
  A reasonable choice is metoprolol, which should be given as an initial oral dose of 12.5mg tds. If there is persistent tachycardia or hyperten-sion metoprolol can be given IV at a dose of 5mg. A reasonable oral maintenance dose of metoprolol is 25mg tds.
- Glucose control – all patients with STEMI and a known history of diabetes mellitus or a blood glucose (BG) >11.0mmol/l should be managed with tight glycaemic control. Stop all existing oral hypoglycaemic therapy before, and for 48 hours after, coronary intervention. Refer newly diagnosed diabetic patients to a diabetes specialist. If BG is >11.0mmol, use a background infusion of 5% glucose at 50–100ml/hr. Additionally, use a solution of 50 units Actrapid in 50ml 0.9% sodium chloride (1 unit/ml), titrate on a sliding scale as follows:

Blood glucose	Actrapid infusion rate (1 unit/ml)
BM >17	5ml/hr
BM 13–16	4ml/hr
BM 8–12	2ml/hr
BM 4-7	1ml/hr
BM <4	0ml/hr

After 24 hours convert to SC insulin or oral anti-diabetic medication as appropriate.

Subsequent treatment

For STEMI or new LBBB then primary angioplasty

- This needs the cardiology team or medical registrar for appropriate urgent transfer to a primary angioplasty centre.

For all other acute coronary syndromes

- Heparin, either unfractioned or low molecular weight (MW) heparins (enoxaparin, dalteparin).
- The decision to anti-coagulate is always based on risk-benefit. Patients who are immediately post-op (within hours) are at the highest risk of haemorrhage compared with those who are several days post-op. However, a myocardial infarction may result in major complications and death.
- Caution should be taken with low MW heparins and renal failure as they accumulate and are not excreted. See local guidelines for dose adjustment or unfractioned heparin.

12 hour troponin – if elevated this suggests an NSTEMI. These patients should have angiography performed within 48 hours. Benefits include early revascularization, which has lower risk of death and allows risk-stratification for further events.

Complications post-MI

- Cardiac arrest (due to ventricular fibrillation, VF) – the commonest cause of death.
- Pump failure, i.e. cardiogenic shock.
- Arrhythmias – may require temporary pacing wires.
- Acquired ventricular septal defect (VSD).
- Cardiac rupture.
- Pericardial tamponade.
- Ventricular aneurysm.
- Mitral regurgitation.

Seek specialist advice for management of the above complications.

Prevention

To be forewarned is to be forearmed and a delay of elective surgery for 3–6 months after an MI makes obvious sense. Extended monitoring in the intensive care unit of high-risk patients may be planned after assessment with echocardiography, radionuclide cardiac imaging, or angiography. The treatment of ischaemic heart disease (IHD) can be optimized pre-operatively, including coronary revascularization strategies. If the patient has had revascularization via angioplasty and stent insertion, they may be on dual anti-platelet therapy, i.e. aspirin and clopidogrel. Discuss with the patient's cardiologist or your local cardiology team **before** stopping these. This is a common cause of peri-operative myocardial infarction.

A rise in troponins can occur for a number of reasons, not just infarction (📖 Table 3.3). Any inflammatory process (e.g. myocarditis, sepsis) can cause a release in troponin. However, MI is extremely unlikely in the presence of a normal troponin. They are released within 4–6 hours and peak at 12 hours. They can remain elevated for at least 7 days and up to 10–14 days. Renal failure gives many falsely elevated troponin levels as they are renally cleared. It should be noted that the value of the troponin rise does not reflect the size of an infarction (i.e. mass of necrosed myocardium). For this reason a CK-MB (requested with a troponin) can be very useful as this is a better reflector of infarct size.

Table 3.3 Elevations of troponin in the absence of overt ischaemic heart disease (from 'Universal definition of myocardial infarction', *European Heart Journal*, 2007)

Cardiac contusion or other trauma including surgery, ablation, pacing, etc.

Congestive heart failure – acute and chronic

Aortic dissection

Aortic valve disease

Hypertrophic cardiomyopathy

Tachy- or bradyarrhythmias, or heart block

Apical ballooning syndrome

Rhabdomyolysis with cardiac injusry

Pulmonary embolism, severe pulmonary hypertension

Renal failure

Acute neurological disease, including stroke or subarachnoid haemorrhage

Infiltrative diseases, e.g. amyloidosis, haemochromatosis, sarcoidosis, and scleroderma

Inflammatory diseases, e.g. myocarditis or myocardial extension of endo-/pericarditis

Drug toxicity or toxins

Critically ill patients, especially with respiratory failure or sepsis

Burns, especially if affecting >30% of body surface area

Extreme exertion

Cardiac failure

(📖 See Fig. 3.5.)

Cardiac failure is common after myocardial infarction. It can also be due to valvular dysfunction or diastolic failure and is worsened by dysrhythmias. Diastolic dysfunction refers to impaired ventricular filling due to inability of the myocardium to relax. These patients are highly dependent on active atrial filling. Many surgical patients develop atrial fibrillation, albeit transient, and this can result in cardiac failure, which may be rapidly reversible with adequate control/cardioversion.

Cardiogenic shock refers to inadequate organ perfusion due to primary cardiac 'pump' failure. This is very difficult to manage and is associated with a poor prognosis. Seek specialist input early and consider referral to a tertiary centre. An acutely damaged heart needs to rest in order to facilitate recovery. However, a satisfactory systemic arterial pressure needs to be generated, at the very least, to perfuse the brain and kidneys. These patients usually require inotropic and/or vasoconstrictor support. This conversely, may contrict the coronary arteries or make the patient tachycardic, all of which reduce perfusion on to the starving myocardium. Add to this the increased workload in generating larger cardiac outputs and it is easy to see why cardiogenic shock carries such a poor prognosis. Many develop renal failure, usually secondary to acute tubular necrosis due to hypoperfusion. These patients may require renal replacement therapy in the form of continuous veno-veno haemofiltration (CVVHF). Interestingly, if patients survive the episode of cardiogenic shock, their long-term prognosis can improve. Better adjuncts include mechanical support with intra-aortic balloon pump counter-pulsation (IABP-CP).

Acute LVF

Acute LVF can occur as a new finding or following a background of chronic cardiac failure. It is important to determine this from the history. A thorough past medical history (PMH), drug history (DH), and previous transthoracic echocardiography (TTE) data can provide helpful data on the baseline state. Management in the initial phase is similar; however, subsequent management differs depending on the aetiology. In a new case of acute LVF an aetiology must be sought. It is important to remember that pulmonary oedema has many causes, of which LVF is one cause (📖 see Tables 3.4 and 3.5).

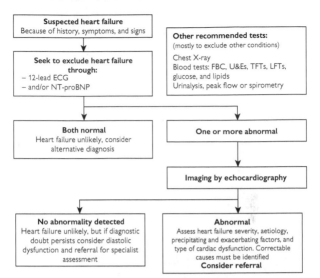

Fig. 3.5 Cardiac failure management steps.

NT-proBNP and acute heart failure

This is a very useful test in heart failure. If your lab offers this test, use it.
- If level <35pmol/l, acute failure is extremely unlikely.
- If aged 50–75, a level >50 pmol/l is compatible with acute decompensation of chronic heart failure.
- If aged >75, a level >212pmol/l is compatible with acute decompensation of chronic heart failure.

Table 3.4 Cardiac causes of pulmonary oedema (in addition to LVF)

Cardiac	
Pulmonary	arterio-venous fistula
	veno-occlusive disease
	ARDS
Renal	reno-vascular disease
Neurogenic	intracranial haemorrhage
	cerebral oedema
	post-ictal
Hypoalbuminaemia	nephrotic syndrome
	liver failure
	sepsis
	dilution

Table 3.5 Causes of heart failure

IHD

Arrhythmia

Valvular or congenital heart disease

Drugs: negatively inotropic and those with fluid-retaining properties (steroids, NSAIDs)

Myocarditis or pericarditis

Cardiomyopathy

Increased metabolic demand:
   pregnancy
   hyperthyroidism
   anaemia

Pulmonary embolus

Inappropriate reduction of therapy (e.g. pre-op anti-heart failure medications stopped)

Concomitant illness

Acute management

Initial steps in management:
- Transfer to CCU or HDU or, if the airway is compromised, ITU.
- High-flow O_2 via mask (unless history of hypercapnic respiratory failure in COPD) and if in Type I RF (pO_2 <7kPa) CPAP.
- Fluid restrict and measure weight daily.
- Nitrates – GTN buccal or IV (50mg GTN in 50ml 0.9% normal saline, titrate to systolic BP of 110mmHg). Aids in redistribution of fluid into capacitance vessels and acutely reduces left atrial pressure.
- Loop diuretic: furosemide (acutely venodilates, and later gives a diuresis causing intravascular volume reduction).

- Digoxin – useful for rate control in AF and has positive inotropic effects.
- Treat underlying cause, e.g. ACS or dysrhythmia.
- If there is renal impairment/hypotensive, start fluid input and output charts.

If the patient fails to respond they may require inotropic support with haemodynamic monitoring, urgent TTE, and mechanical support. If the patient remains dyspnoeic and in respiratory failure, they may require intubation and mechanical ventilation.

IABP-CP

Inserted via the femoral artery and seated with the tip in the arch of the aorta. It consists of a wire with a large 30–50ml helium-filled balloon and is attached to a pneumatic pump. Counter-pulsation means the balloon is inflated during diastole and deflated during systole.

It is a very useful bridge to definitive treatment. It benefits patients by augmenting diastolic pressure (and hence coronary artery perfusion) and decreasing afterload.

Seek specialist input for insertion. Patients with IABPs should be managed on CCU or ITU by appropriately trained staff. NB: IABP-CP contra-indicated if aortic aneurysm/dissection and AR.

Dysrhythmia

Dysrhythmias occurring during the post-operative period are a significant cause of cardiovascular morbidity and mortality. Of the dysrhythmias, AF remains the commonest and may occur in 50% of surgical patients, albeit transiently.

When approaching the management of dysrhythmias it is important to follow a step-wise approach and ask yourself the following questions:

- What are the symptoms? E.g. palpitations, chest pain/tightness, sweating, dyspnoea, pre-syncope, and syncope.
- Are there precipitants? (📖 See Table 3.6.)
- Is there haemodynamic compromise? Assess the patient's peripheral pulses and record blood pressure, and compare with apical rate.
- Does the patient have a structurally normal heart? Look for previous echo data; is there any evidence of valvular abnormalities or cardiomyopathy?
- Thyroid status – which can be erroneous in the post-operative state.

Table 3.6 Precipitating factors for arrhythmia

Precipitating factors	
Age >70 years	Pain and anxiety
Increased catecholamine production	Hypoxia
Ischaemia	Hypercarbia
Electrolyte disturbance	Hypovolaemia
Sepsis	Drugs
Caffeine	

It is useful to classify dysrhythmias as brady- and tachy-arrhythmias. The flow diagram in 📖 Fig. 3.6 will help you to determine a list of differentials.

For management, refer to 📖 Fig. 3.7 for broad-complex tachycardia and 📖 Fig. 3.8 for narrow-complex tachycardia.

General measures for managing dysrhythmias

- History and examination
- O$_2$
- IV access
- Cardiac monitoring
- Attach defibrillator
- 12-lead ECG tracings regularly
- Bloods: FBC, U&E, CRP, TFTs, (calcium, magnesium)
- If there is haemodynamic compromise then DC cardiovert under sedation.

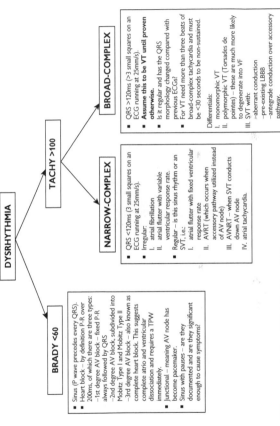

DYSRHYTHMIA

BRADY <60

- Sinus (P wave precedes every QRS).
- Heart block – by definition P-R over 200ms, of which there are three types:
  - –1st degree AV block – fixed P-R always followed by QRS
  - –2nd degree AV block, subdivided into Mobitz Type I and Mobitz Type II
  - –3rd degree AV block – also known as complete heart block. This suggests complete atrio and ventricular dissociation and requires a TPW immediately.
- Junctional – meaning AV node has become pacemaker.
- Sinus with pauses – are they significant and are they documented and are they significant enough to cause symptoms?

TACHY >100

NARROW-COMPLEX

- QRS <120ms (3 small squares on an ECG running at 25mm/s).
- Irregular:
  - I. atrial fibrillation
  - II. atrial flutter with variable ventricular response rate.
- Regular – is this sinus rhythm or an SVT, i.e.:
  - I. atrial flutter with fixed ventricular response rate
  - II. AVRT (which occurs when accessory pathway utilized instead of AV node)
  - III. AVNRT – when SVT conducts down AV node
  - IV. atrial tachycardia.

BROAD-COMPLEX

- QRS >120ms (>3 small squares on an ECG running at 25mm/s).
- **Assume this to be VT until proven otherwise.**
- Is it regular and has the QRS morphology changed compared with previous ECGs?
- For VT need more than three beats of broad-complex tachycardia and must be <30 seconds to be non-sustained.

Differentials:
- I. monomorphic VT
- II. polymorphic VT (Torsades de pointes) – these are much more likely to degenerate into VF
- III. SVT with:
  - –aberrant conduction
  - –pre-existing LBBB
  - –antegrade conduction over accessory pathway.

TPW = temporary pacing wire   LBBB = left bundle branch block

Fig. 3.6 Diagnosing dysrythmia.

Management of atrial fibrillation

This is the commonest dysrhythmia and occurs in 1% of the general population, 10% of those over the age of 70, and may occur in up to 50% of surgical patients, especially if there are precipitants such as infection.

Atrial fibrillation is classified as being:

- paroxysmal or persistent (paroxysmal=going to SR and AF in under 7 days, however many times that may occur)
- acute or chronic
- 'lone' (idiopathic) or secondary.

When managing AF it is important to think about four aspects:

1. Symptoms

Patients may complain of palpitations (be clear in defining this from history and take ECG during episode). AF may occur in a surgical patient with known IHD and make their angina worse (so called rate-related angina). The patient may have diastolic dysfunction and loss of the atrial contribution to ventricular filling, which may lead to pulmonary oedema.

2. Rate control

Beta-blockade is the first-line treatment provided there is no contra-indication. Beta blockers act more quickly than digoxin (which can take at least 6 hours to work). A reasonable choice is metoprolol (12.5mg test dose PO, or 5mg IV, then if tolerated regular dose 12.5mg TDS increased to 25mg or 50mg TDS PO), which is the shortest-acting should there be any concern over intolerance, and will be eliminated more rapidly. If a beta blocker is contraindicated use a calcium-channel antagonist such as diltiazem or verapamil. If these are contraindicated then use digoxin.

3. Rhythm control

Most surgical patients spontaneously cardiovert, in which case consider arrhythmia prophylaxis. Discuss with your cardiology department for suitable drugs. If your patient does not spontaneously cardiovert and is symptomatic in terms of ischaemia or heart failure then consider cardioverting. There are two options available: DC cardioversion and chemical cardioversion with flecainide or amiodarone. Do this with specialist supervision and review. Flecainide in the context of acute ischaemia is contraindicated.

> It is essential to examine for a structurally normal heart, i.e. a recent echo or an urgent echo.
> Do not electively cardiovert patients who have been in AF for >48 hours as this indicates a high probability of the presence of thrombus. These patients have a high chance of stroke if SR is restored.

4. Anticoagulation

Cover acutely with therapeutic doses of low-molecular weight heparin, or unfractioned heparin if GFR <20ml/hour. Discuss with a specialist for long-term anticoagulation. 'CHADS2' scoring system is used for long-term anti-coagulation. Liaise with specialists before doing this.

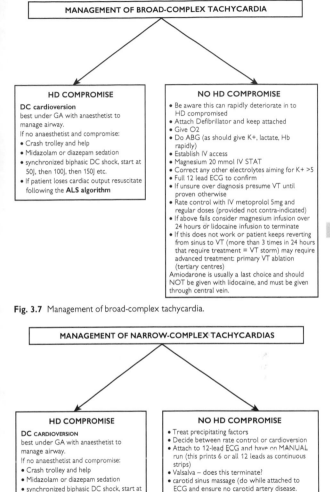

MANAGEMENT OF BROAD-COMPLEX TACHYCARDIA

HD COMPROMISE

DC cardioversion
best under GA with anaesthetist to
manage airway.
If no anaesthetist and compromise:
• Crash trolley and help
• Midazolam or diazepam sedation
• synchronized biphasic DC shock, start at
  50J, then 100J, then 150J etc.
• If patient loses cardiac output resuscitate
  following the **ALS algorithm**

NO HD COMPROMISE
• Be aware this can rapidly deteriorate in to
  HD compromised
• Attach Defibrillator and keep attached
• Give O2
• Do ABG (as should give K+, lactate, Hb
  rapidly)
• Establish IV access
• Magnesium 20 mmol IV STAT
• Correct any other electrolytes aiming for K+ >5
• Full 12 lead ECG to confirm
• If unsure over diagnosis presume VT until
  proven otherwise
• Rate control with IV metoprolol 5mg and
  regular doses (provided not contra-indicated)
• If above fails consider magnesium infusion over
  24 hours or lidocaine infusion to terminate
• If this does not work or patient keeps reverting
  from sinus to VT (more than 3 times in 24 hours
  that require treatment = VT storm) may require
  advanced treatment: primary VT ablation
  (tertiary centres)
Amiodarone is usually a last choice and should
NOT be given with lidocaine, and must be given
through central vein.

Fig. 3.7 Management of broad-complex tachycardia.

MANAGEMENT OF NARROW-COMPLEX TACHYCARDIAS

HD COMPROMISE

DC CARDIOVERSION
best under GA with anaesthetist to
manage airway.
If no anaesthetist and compromise:
• Crash trolley and help
• Midazolam or diazepam sedation
• synchronized biphasic DC shock, start at
  50J, then 100J, then 150J etc.

NO HD COMPROMISE
• Treat precipitating factors
• Decide between rate control or cardioversion
• Attach to 12-lead ECG and have on MANUAL
  run (this prints 6 or all 12 leads as continuous
  strips)
• Valsalva – does this terminate?
• carotid sinus massage (do while attached to
  ECG and ensure no carotid artery disease.
  Slowing the arrhythmia may reveal type
• Adenosine (provided not asthmatic) may
  terminate arrhythmia and will slow down enough
  to reveal underlying rhythm
• If adenosine contra-indicated consider IV
  verapamil 5mg repeat x 3 5 mins apart
• If above fails consider chemical cardioversion
  or electrical cardioversion (SEEK specialist input)

Fig. 3.8 Management of narrow-complex tachycardias.

Stroke

Stroke remains a major health problem, accounting for 11% of all deaths in the UK and results in significant morbidity. It is defined as a focal neurological deficit persisting for more than 24 hours and as such the diagnosis remains clinical. Symptoms include numbness, weakness or paralysis, slurred speech, blurred vision, confusion, and severe headache. A transient ischaemic attack (TIA) is defined as symptoms and signs of stroke that resolve within 24 hours, meaning a TIA is reversible. It is analogous to angina pectoris. The term cerebrovascular accident is avoided.

NICE has recently published guidelines on the diagnosis and initial management of acute stroke and TIA. The key emphasis is on rapid diagnosis with immediate imaging followed by admission to a specialist stroke unit (Ⓠ Fig. 3.9). Acute strokes presenting within 3 hours should be thrombolysed – however, surgery is a relative contraindication to thrombolysis, especially if stroke has occurred within 1 month of surgery. If you suspect your patient has had a stroke, refer for urgent CT imaging and ask for specialist in-put.

For TIAs the mainstay of treatment is to prevent a full infarction. These patients should not be considered lower priority compared with those likely to be strokes. Rather, there should be an aggressive approach to minimize this from occurring. Arrange all investigations and review preventative medications.

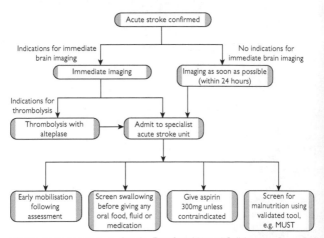

Fig. 3.9 Acute management of stroke. Data from National Collaborating Centre for Chronic Conditions. *Stroke: National clinical guideline for diagnosis and initial management of acute stroke and transient ischaemic attack (TIA).* London: Royal College of Physicians, 2008.

Chapter 4

Complications related to fluid and electrolyte management in surgical patients

Salt and water

Water homeostasis

The water content of the body is controlled by changes in water intake and water excretion. Thirst is a powerful stimulus for increasing water intake. There are obligatory losses of water in the urine and stool, and from the skin and respiratory tract; but water excretion is controlled primarily by the action of antidiuretic hormone (ADH) on the kidneys. Both thirst and ADH secretion are controlled by hypothalamic osmoreceptors which respond to small changes in extracellular fluid (ECF) osmolality so that, in health, plasma osmolality is maintained within narrow limits. ADH release is also affected by volume receptors in the atria and by higher brain centres (responding to stress and pain), both of which can override osmotic control in the context of illness.

Sodium homeostasis

Sodium is mainly an extracellular ion and the normal serum sodium concentration is in the range 135–145mmol/l. The extracellular volume is determined by the sodium content. The renin–angiotensin–aldosterone axis and possibly atrial natriuretic peptide (ANP) modulate sodium excretion by the kidneys. Sodium excretion can be minimal (<10mmol/l) in the context of hypovolaemia. The normal sodium requirement is 1mmol/kg per day, i.e. 70mmol for a 70-kg man.

It is important to stress that plasma sodium does not reflect total body sodium, only the ratio of sodium to water in the ECF. Most acute changes in sodium concentration represent changes in water balance rather than changes in total body sodium. Sodium levels are an important determinant of ECF osmolality. Osmolalities must be the same inside and outside cells, and adjustments occur automatically to preserve this. Thus cells will swell if the ECF osmolality is low and shrink if it is high.

The initial assessment of abnormalities of salt and water balance is clinical. This includes a judgement as to whether the patient is euvolaemic, hypovolaemic, or hypervolaemic. Euvolaemia is typically found in states of water overload; hypovolaemia when there are combined salt and water deficits; and hypervolaemia in oedematous states, as seen in congestive cardiac failure, cirrhosis, and the nephrotic syndrome.

Water deficit

A pure water deficit results in hypernatraemia (with ECF volume depletion only in severe cases because the loss is spread evenly among all compartments of body water).

Situations where this might arise are as follows:

- Inadequate water intake in patients who are acutely confused or demented.
- Inadequate supplements of water in patients fed a high protein intake. Non-utilized protein is broken down to urea which will increase free water clearance by the kidneys.
- Inadequate fluid intake in head injury patients who have developed diabetes insipidus.

Hypernatraemia is associated with an increased plasma osmolality and a raised urine urea. Urine osmolality is inappropriately low in cases with diabetes insipidus due to pituitary disease.

The symptoms of hypernatraemia include thirst, nausea, vomiting, lethargy, weakness, fever, confusion, and even fits. Although the kidney can minimize water excretion via the effect of ADH, a water deficit can be corrected only by an increased intake. Whenever possible, water should be given orally. Failing this, water can be given enterally via a nasogastric or a fine-bore feeding tube, provided the enteral route is accessible and functioning. Parenteral water administration has to be by means of 5% dextrose. Desmopressin will be needed as well for acquired diabetes insipidus in neurological/neurosurgical cases.

Water excess (euvolaemic or dilutional hyponatraemia)

A pure excess of body water results in dilutional hyponatraemia. It results from an intake of water in excess of the kidney's ability to excrete it.

Elevated levels of ADH may persist for several days after surgery and are part of a normal stress response thought to be related to pain afferents and nausea. Falling urine output may prompt excess administration of fluids containing a high proportion of free water, with consequent water retention, hyponatraemia, and the risk of an irreversible neurological deficit. Children and pre-menopausal women are particularly at risk as they are very sensitive to ADH.

The bladder is irrigated with 1.5% glycine or sorbitol solutions during urological procedures such as transurethral resection of the prostate (TURP). This may lead to the rapid and excessive absorption of water into the circulation, with acute onset hyponatremia—the so called TURP syndrome.

The syndrome of inappropriate ADH secretion (SIADH) is an important but probably overdiagnosed cause of hyponatraemia. SIADH may be seen in malignancy (especially lung, pancreas, and prostate), following head injury and may be associated with pneumonia. It is also seen as a result of drug treatment (e.g. carbamazepine, SSRIs, opiates, and some cytotoxics). SIADH is characterized by dilutional hyponatraemia in a patient who is:

- Not clinically hypovolaemic, hypotensive, hypokalaemic, or on diuretics.
- With low plasma osmolality (<280mosmol/l).
- With a urine osmolality that is 'inappropriate', i.e. higher than the plasma osmolality, coupled with a natriuresis (urine sodium >30mmol/l).
- Has normal renal, adrenal, and thyroid function.

Some chronically hyponatraemic elderly patients can fulfil these criteria and have idiopathic SIADH.

Diagnosis of dilutional hyponatraemia

Symptoms from acute onset hyponatraemia indicate encephalopathy: they include headache, nausea, irritability, and confusion, progressing to drowsiness, myoclonic jerks, generalized convulsions, and coma. Hypoxia is often evident, from non-cardiac pulmonary oedema or associated respiratory depression. Examination of the fluid-balance charts may show an excessive administration of intravenous (IV) fluids containing free water.

There is a reduction in the serum sodium and serum osmolality. (Beware a falsely low one-off serum sodium as a result of blood taken from an arm with IV dextrose running!).

Chronic hyponatraemia is less likely to induce neurological symptoms.

Treatment of dilutional hyponatraemia

Rapid correction of electrolyte imbalance should be avoided if possible. Water retention due to increased ADH secretion following surgery usually corrects spontaneously. Established water retention from iatrogenic IV free water is treated by restricting water intake to 500–1000ml per day. Water excess due to the TURP syndrome is normally corrected with restriction of water intake, but in severe forms it may require the use of loop diuretics ± the cautious infusion of 0.9% saline. Cases with severe neurological symptoms, such as fits or coma, may need the cautious infusion of hypertonic saline (3%, 513mmol/l), but at a slow rate of 100–125ml per hour, aiming to increase the serum sodium by no more than 8–10mmol/l in the first 4 hours and by no more than 15–20mmol/l over 48 hours. Hypoxia must be corrected to avoid potentiating cerebral damage.

Treatment of SIADH is with fluid restriction or, if necessary, oral demeclocycline.

Deficits of salt and water (dehydration)

Combined body deficits of sodium and water are more commonly encountered in clinical practice. They result in the signs of dehydration from loss of interstitial fluid (reduced skin turgor) and loss of circulating volume (hypotension, postural hypotension, peripheral vasoconstriction, reduced urine output).

The relative proportion of the deficits of sodium and water are reflected in the plasma sodium. The serum sodium can be normal or raised; but hyponatraemia is often found as volume receptors override hypothalamic osmoreceptors and stimulate ADH release, with consequent thirst and water retention by the kidneys. The body is defending circulating volume at the expense of osmolality.

Volume depletion primarily results from sodium and/or water loss from the following anatomic sites:

- GI losses, e.g. vomiting, diarrhoea, bleeding, and patients with ileostomies are particularly at risk.
- Renal losses and polyuria, e.g. inappropriate diuretics, osmotic diuresis from hyperglycaemia, salt-losing nephropathies, and in the cerebral salt wasting syndrome.
- Skin losses from burns or excessive sweating.
- Third-space sequestration, including intestinal obstruction, crush injury, fracture, peritonitis, and acute pancreatitis.
- Surgical drains.

Cerebral salt-wasting is characterized by hyponatraemia and ECF depletion due to inappropriate sodium loss in the urine. It is seen in some patients after subarachnoid haemorrhage, head injury, or neurosurgery. Treatment is with IV 0.9% saline (in contrast to fluid restriction in superficially similar hyponatraemic cases with SIADH).

Diagnosis of dehydration

The diagnosis of dehydration (combined salt and water deficiency) is primarily clinical. Symptoms from dehydration include fatigue, thirst, muscle cramps, postural dizziness, weakness, and confusion. Clinical and laboratory parameters can be used to assess severity of volume depletion. Dry mucous membranes and decreased skin turgor reflect a decrease in the interstitial fluid, while a decrease in the plasma volume leads to a low systemic blood pressure and jugular venous pressure, as well as postural hypotension. Oliguria, a high urine osmolarity, and a low urine sodium concentration (<20mmol/l) are likely. Serum sodium concentrations may be normal, raised, or low (see 'Sodium homeostasis') but haemoglobin, blood urea, and creatinine levels rise.

Treatment of dehydration

Severe dehydration with hypotension and oliguria may be treated initially with IV colloid, but usually crystalloid infusions of 0.9% saline or Hartmann's solution will suffice. The aim is to administer 50–100ml per hour in excess of continued losses (equal to the sum of the urine output, estimated insensible losses [approximately 30–50ml per hour], and any other losses that may be present). Dextrose or 0.45% saline can be used if hypernatraemia is present or develops with isotonic crystalloid replacement.

Sodium excess

Hypernatraemia is usually due to a water deficit, as outlined in a previous section. However, excessive reliance on 0.9% (150mmol/l) saline or Hartmann's solution for volume replacement; high-dose parenteral penicillin therapy; and the use of 8.4% sodium bicarbonate after a cardiac arrest, all result in a high sodium load and can cause hypernatraemia. In addition, patients with heart disease and the elderly are at risk of being precipitated into heart failure.

The symptoms of hypernatraemia have been outlined previously. With excess sodium there may be signs of fluid overload, with oedema and/or signs of heart failure.

The cause of hypernatraemia can be diagnosed by attention to the history, fluid-balance charts, and electrolyte results. A history of restricted water intake or excessive urine output point to a problem with water balance. A history of positive fluid balance and the application of excessive sodium in IV fluid suggest sodium excess.

Additional free water orally or as 5% dextrose will permit the kidneys to excrete this solute load.

Rapid correction of hypernatraemia should be avoided, particularly if the sodium is >160mmol/l, as rapid movements of fluid can cause cerebral oedema; and the use of 0.45% saline rather than 5% dextrose may be safer.

Patients with heart failure will need loop diuretic therapy.

Potassium

Potassium is the main intracellular ion (~3000mmol), with only 50–60mmol in the ECF. The serum concentration of potassium is 3.5–5.0mmol/l compared with an intracellular concentration of 140mmol/l. Serum potassium levels are not a good indicator of overall potassium balance as losses from the extracellular space are corrected by the migration of potassium from the intracellular space. The serum potassium concentration only shows a significant fall when there are substantial intracellular losses; and in acute illness particularly, serum potassium does not necessarily relate to total body potassium.

Potassium concentration is controlled by the kidney in response to mineralocorticoids—particularly aldosterone—but there is an obligatory loss of 10–20mmol/l of urine. There is a close reciprocal relationship between potassium, hydrogen, and sodium excretion. Potassium excretion falls if there is an intracellular acidosis and rises with an intracellular alkalosis. Also, a plasma pH fall of 0.1 leads to a plasma potassium rise of 1mmol/l (and vice versa). The normal daily requirement of potassium is 1–1.5mmol/kg.

Hypokalaemia

The causes of hypokalaemia in surgical patients include:
- Reduced intake due to dietary deficiency or inadequate potassium replacement with IV fluids.
- Increased GI losses, due to vomiting, nasogastric aspiration, severe diarrhoea, excessive ileostomy output, and fistulae. Hypokalaemia from gastric fluid loss is a particularly potent cause of hypokalaemia because of renal compensation for the associated metabolic alkalosis (with potassium loss in exchange for hydrogen absorption).
- GI fluid sequestration in bowel obstruction and post-operative ileus.
- Increased renal excretion from concomitant diuretic use.
- Hypomagnesaemia.
- Elderly patients and females seem particularly at risk of developing hypokalaemia.

Diagnosis of hypokalaemia

A serum potassium concentration <3.5mmol/l indicates hypokalaemia, but it does not give a good indication of the total potassium deficit, which is usually substantial. The ECG changes of hypokalaemia are flattening of the T wave, ST depression, and a prominent U wave. Severe hypokalaemia (<2mmol/l) may result in cardiac arrhythmias such as supraventricular and ventricular extrasystoles, as well as atrial and ventricular fibrillation.

Treatment of hypokalaemia

Hypokalaemia can often be treated by oral supplementation or by the addition of extra potassium into enteral feeds. IV replacement is with crystalloid fluid (0.9% saline or 5% dextrose) containing 20mmol/l or 40mmol/l of potassium chloride (KCl). Replacement rates of 5–10mmol KCl per hour are usually adequate. Rates should not exceed 20mmol KCl per hour without intensive, hourly monitoring of the serum potassium and ECG, particularly in the context of poor renal function. Up to 200–300mmol of KCl may have to be replaced in severe cases of hypokalaemia.

Hyperkalaemia

A potassium level >5.0mmol/l is abnormal; >6.0mmol/l usually an indication for review of management; and >7.0mmol/l a medical emergency. Severe hyperkalaemia (7–13mmol/l) can be described as the deadly killer, as it leads to depolarization of cell membranes by inactivating sodium channels. This results in skeletal muscle paralysis, initially affecting the limbs, but then respiration. Bradycardia, hypotension, ventricular arrest or fibrillation can follow. A rapid increase in potassium is more dangerous than a slow rise, as some adaptation occurs in a chronic state.

Common causes of hyperkalaemia in surgical patients are:

- Pre-existing renal impairment: more likely to develop hyperkalaemia perioperatively as the initial response to the tissue damage from surgery is a release of potassium from damaged cells.
- Sepsis: leading to renal impairment.
- Increased protein load: e.g. GI haemorrhage; burns and muscle injury with potassium release from damaged tissues (6.25 g protein [1 g nitrogen] releases 2.7mmol potassium).
- Rapid blood transfusion: may elevate the serum potassium, as stored blood contains high levels of potassium.
- Iatrogenic: following inappropriately extended potassium replacement.
- Iatrogenic: from drugs that interfere with potassium excretion, such as potassium-sparing diuretics, angiotensin-converting enzyme inhibitors, angiotensin receptor blockers, and non-steroidal anti-inflammatory drugs.
- Older patients, particularly men with genitourinary disease, seem at greatest risk of developing hyperkalaemia.

Diagnosis of hyperkalaemia

The finding of severe hyperkalaemia (>6.0mmol/l) necessitates an ECG to check for the characteristic changes: tented T waves; then reduced P wave with widening of the QRS complex; then loss of the P wave; and a 'sine wave' pattern as the hyperkalaemia worsens. Also, consider repeating the serum potassium if it is >6.0mmol/l, as a haemolysed blood sample may produce a falsely elevated potassium.

Treatment of hyperkalaemia

Potassium intake should be restricted in high-risk patients, e.g. patients with renal failure. It is important to involve the dietician in cases of persistent hyperkalaemia for advice on low potassium diet. Hyperkalaemic patients receiving enteral and total parenteral feeding should have adjustments made to a low potassium feed.

Severe hyperkalaemia, associated with characteristic ECG changes, requires urgent treatment:

1. IV 10% calcium gluconate 10–20ml over 5 minutes, to prevent fatal arrhythmias.
2. Sodium bicarbonate 1.26% 500ml (75mmol), to correct acidosis.

3. IV insulin and glucose, to drive potassium (temporarily) into cells: 50ml of 50% glucose containing 10 units of soluble insulin is infused over 10–15 minutes. Serum potassium is lowered by about 1mmol/l for about 3 hours.
4. Cation-exchange resins. Calcium Resonium® 15g orally every 6 hours or 30g rectally can be administered, which starts to reduce serum potassium within 4 hours and lasts for 12 hours. There is a risk of calcium overload.
5. Haemofiltration or haemodialysis, if the measures (1) to (3) fail.

Other electrolytes

The other electrolytes – calcium, magnesium, and phosphate – can usually be ignored in the short term as the body contains large pools of these electrolytes. Patients who are unable to eat normally for long periods should have these electrolytes measured weekly and deficits corrected by the administration of supplements.

Hypocalcaemia can occur acutely after parathyroidectomy or parathyroid damage after head and neck surgery, large volume blood transfusions, and sepsis. Manifestations include muscle weakness and tetany, paraesthesia, and cardiac depression. It is treated by infusion of 10–20ml 10% calcium chloride. Regular oral calcium supplements and oral vitamin D (calcitriol or alfacalcidol) may be needed as well.

Hypercalcaemia may occur in association with metastatic malignancy, causing nausea, vomiting, polyuria, and confusion, with dehydration. The patient must be adequately rehydrated with 0.9% saline. Treatment with parenteral bisphosphonates (pamidronate 30–60mg; zolendronic acid 4mg) can help to maintain normocalcaemia.

Hypomagnesaemia may be seen in patients with GI losses or those receiving parenteral nutrition. Hypocalcaemia occurs as well because hypomagnesaemia causes functional hypoparathyroidism. Symptoms include paraesthesiae, cramps, muscle weakness, tetany and fits. Treatment is with 5g (20mmol) magnesium sulphate intravenously, repeated as necessary.

Fluid resuscitation

There is no convincing data to show a difference in survival when using colloid or crystalloid to provide initial resuscitation in major blood loss. The aim of perfusing organs in the short term is met by either of these fluids. However, it has been suggested that there may be a difference between the different formulations of colloid used although this has not yet been investigated.

Crystalloids

These are cheap, effective, and the preferred choice for fluid boluses when administering a dynamic fluid challenge (usually 200-ml boluses of crystalloid with monitoring of urine output, blood pressure, and pulse to assess response). The crystalloids have relatively few adverse effects when compared with colloid.

Balanced salt solutions (e.g. Hartmann's solution)
This is physiologically similar to ECF and is the fluid of choice for restoring ECF volume. It is often administered in the perioperative period by anaesthetists.

Normal saline 0.9%
This can be the fluid of choice for resuscitation of the hypovolaemic patient, although the intravascular half-life is short. It is also useful when replacing electrolyte-rich GI losses. Excessive amounts produce a hyperchloraemic metabolic acidosis.

Glucose (dextrose) solutions
These are usually given in concentrations of 5%, or a dextrose/saline solution of 4% and 0.18% respectively. Dextrose is an appropriate way of treating dehydration and replacing lost water but has no role in plasma expansion/resuscitation. Higher solutions of 10–50% may be used in the treatment of hypoglycaemia but can damage the veins.

Colloids

Colloids are solutions containing substances of large molecular weight that are mainly retained in the intravascular compartment after infusion. Colloids expand the functional plasma volume three times faster than crystalloid solutions and are sometimes referred to as 'plasma expanders'. There are four main colloids: albumin; dextrans; gelatins; and starches. Rapid infusion of colloids can lead to circulatory overload and heart failure. This is a particular risk in the elderly and patients with pre-existing heart failure.

Albumin
Albumin is a natural protein in the circulation and plays an important role in oncotic balance. Human albumin solution (HAS) is derived from pooled human serum and has a molecular weight of 69 000. The use of HAS is expensive and controversial and there is probably no place for its routine use on surgical wards. It is available as a 4.5% solution for the treatment of hypovolaemia and a 20% solution for hypoalbuminaemia. There is concern over the transmission of infection as it is a human blood product.

Albumin should not be used as a replacement for acute blood loss as it has no advantage in this role over synthetic colloid solutions.

Dextrans

Dextrans are solutions containing branched polysaccharides. There are two solutions; dextran 70 (6%) with molecular weight 70kDa, and dextran 40 (10%) with molecular weight 40kDa. Dextrans interfere with blood clotting by reducing factor VIII activity and impairing platelet function. These solutions are little used since the introduction of the gelatins and starches and they will not be discussed in detail. There may be difficulty in blood grouping after a patient has received a dextran solution so it is prudent to discuss this with the laboratory.

Gelatins

Gelatins are short-acting colloid solutions derived from bovine collagen. The molecular weight of these solutions is around 30 000. There are two types of gelatin solutions: succinylated gelatins (e.g. Gelofusine®), and polygelines (e.g. Haemaccel®), which have recently ceased to be manufactured in the UK. Gelatins induce short-term expansion of fluid volume (1–4 hours) after blood loss, in sepsis, and during anaesthesia due to a powerful osmotic effect. Both types of gelatin are provided in solutions of sodium chloride. Anaphylaxis is a rare complication of the use of gelatins.

Starches (molecular weight 70 000–450 000)

A range of starch-based colloids are produced based on hydroxyethyl starch (HES). The molecular weight, concentration, and degree of substitution or DS (number of hydroxyethyl groups per 10 glucose molecules) determines the duration of persistence in the plasma. Starches with a molecular weight <70kDa are excreted by the kidney. Starches with a molecular weight >70kDa are metabolized by α-amylase, and the chains broken down and then excreted by the kidney.

There are hetastarches (DS 0.6–0.7), pentastarches (DS 0.5), and tetrastarches (DS 0.4). The greater the DS, the greater the resistance to degradation which results in an increased duration of action. A recommended maximum dose is provided by the manufacturer which varies with the different formulations. First-generation starches were associated with a number of unwanted effects from pruritus to more serious effects on renal function and clotting. Such side effects are much less common with the newer, lower molecular weight formulations.

Selecting an appropriate intravenous fluid*

When prescribing intravenous fluids, the following should be considered:
• Carefully assess 24-hour fluid balance.
• Clinically assess fluid status.
• Is there a fluid deficit or does the patient require maintenance fluids only?
• If a deficit is identified, what is the nature of the fluid lost?
• Consider insensible losses which will not be represented on the fluid charts.

* Based on recommendations from British Consensus Guidelines on Intravenous Fluid Therapy for Adult Surgical Patients, GIFTASUP ℘ www.ics.ac.uk

- Identify the most appropriate IV fluid.
- Monitor serum electrolytes regularly, particularly sodium and potassium.
- The type of fluid given largely depends on the type of fluid lost and any accompanying electrolyte disturbances. It is important to distinguish between fluid and electrolytes required for maintenance, and those required for resuscitation or replacement of abnormal losses.
- Solutions such as dextrose/saline (4% dextrose plus 0.18% saline) and 5% dextrose are important sources of free water for maintenance, but should be used with caution as excessive amounts may result in hyponatraemia. These solutions are not appropriate for resuscitation or replacement therapy except in conditions of significant free water deficit, e.g. diabetes insipidus.
- Significant losses from gastric aspiration and vomiting should be treated preoperatively with an appropriate crystalloid. Hypochloraemia is an indication for the use of 0.9% saline, with appropriate additions of potassium and care not to produce sodium overload.
- Losses from diarrhoea/ileostomy/small bowel fistula/ileus/obstruction should be replaced volume for volume with a balanced crystalloid solution (e.g. Hartmann's or Ringer's lactate/acetate type solutions).
- Hypovolaemia due predominantly to blood loss should be treated with either a balanced crystalloid solution or a suitable colloid until packed red cells are available.
- Hypovolaemia due to severe inflammation such as infection, peritonitis, pancreatitis, or burns should be treated with either a suitable colloid or a balanced crystalloid.

Complications of nutrition

Malnutrition

Malnutrition results from an imbalance between nutritional intake and requirements over a period of time. The primary feature is depletion of body fat and muscle resulting in weight loss and is often referred to as protein-energy malnutrition (PEM). Malnutrition is common in surgical patients. A number of studies over the last 70 years have shown that 20–40% of patients admitted to hospital are undernourished, and two-thirds of patients lose weight following admission. It has also been clearly shown that malnutrition significantly increases the morbidity and mortality associated with surgery, especially with regard to wound healing and resistance to infection. Awareness of the importance of nutrition is therefore important when planning surgical treatment. Post-operative complications have a significant effect on nutritional requirements. Nutritional support is of even greater importance in patients who may already have had a prolonged period of fasting and may be under considerable stress. Poorly planned or executed nutritional support may itself give rise to potentially life-threatening complications.

Cause of malnutrition

The cause of malnutrition is usually multi-factorial, particularly in the surgical patient, and often develops peri-operatively as a result of a combination of factors including the following examples.

Reduced dietary intake

Poor appetite and intake as a result of illness, anxiety, or depression; symptoms such as swallowing disorders, nausea, vomiting, and pain related to disease or treatment; and prolonged periods of nil by mouth for investigations, procedures, and surgery.

Increased nutritional needs

In contrast to simple starvation, metabolic rate is generally increased during periods of stress and as a consequence of disease such as cancer and treatment such as surgery, particularly if the patient is septic or critically ill.

Impaired absorption or utilization of nutrients

Malabsorption due to diseases such as enteropathies or chronic pancreatitis; surgery including massive intestinal resections; and complications such as fistula, chylothorax, infections, and poor metabolic control including hyperglycaemia.

Consequence of malnutrition

The consequence of malnutrition for the patient and hospital are numerous and can significantly affect morbidity and mortality, increasing patient length of stay and therefore costs to the health service. Malnutrition results in:

- Impaired immune function, predisposing patient to increased risk of infection.
- Delayed post-operative wound healing and increased risk of wound dehiscence and surgical site infection.

- Increased risk of developing pressure sores and delayed healing of pressure sores.
- Reduced respiratory function predisposing patient to increased risk of chest infections.
- Reduced mobility resulting in increased risk of DVT/PE and development of pressure sores.
- Reduced cognitive function resulting in apathy, depression, and self-neglect.
- Reduced cardiac function resulting in heart failure.
- Reduced gastrointestinal function resulting in altered bowel habit.

Nutritional assessment

Nutritional assessment is used to both quantify a patient's nutritional status and identify patients likely to benefit from nutritional support, and to assess the efficacy of nutritional support. There is no one single parameter that can be used to classify malnutrition and a combination of parameters is usually used. This should be undertaken routinely as part of taking a medical history and performing a physical examination on admission, and regularly until discharge home.

Clinical history

General physical appearance including evidence of weight loss, ill-fitting clothes, muscle wasting, hair loss, peripheral oedema, ascites, hydration status, history of swallowing problems, indigestion, nausea, vomiting, change in bowel habit (colour, consistency, frequency), previous medical and surgical history, alcohol intake, and jaundice.

Dietary intake

Recent changes in appetite and food intake and presence of factors affecting intake or therapeutic diets, e.g. diabetic, gluten free, use of nutritional supplements. A dietitian can undertake a more complex dietary assessment.

Anthropometric

Weight and height are the most useful and accessible and in the absence of oedema or ascites, measurement of body weight is a useful tool to quantify nutritional status.

Weight loss as a percentage of pre-illness weight and interpretation

$$\% \text{ weight loss} = \frac{\text{usual weight (kg)} - \text{actual weight (kg)}}{\text{usual weight (kg)}} \times 100$$

- <5%: not significant if intentional or unlikely to continue.
- 5–10%: weight loss not serious unless rapid/already malnourished.
- 10–20%: clinically significant and nutritional support usually indicated.
- >20%: severe and likely to need medium/long-term nutritional support.

NB The more rapid the weight loss the greater the proportion of muscle mass compared to adipose tissue lost, which is of more clinical significance. Very rapid loss (i.e. days rather than weeks) is likely to reflect hydration status.

Body mass index

$$\text{BMI} = \frac{\text{weight (kg)}}{\text{height (m}^2)}$$

Interpretation of BMI:
<16kg/m^2: severely malnourished
16–19kg/m^2: underweight
20–25kg/m^2: normal or ideal range
26–30kg/m^2: mild obesity
31–40kg/m^2: moderate obesity
>40kg/m^2: morbid obesity

NB: BMI measurement in the very elderly is not as accurate as it does not take into account loss of height or muscle mass with age. Gross oedema and ascites also affect accuracy.

Additional anthropometric measurements such as skin fold thickness (measures fat stores), muscle circumference (measures protein stores), and functional measurements such as grip strength are usually undertaken for research purposes and are rarely used in the clinical situation.

Laboratory measurements

These are less useful markers of nutritional status as they are more likely to reflect the disease process. In the absence of renal or liver disease and with normal hydration, low serum levels of urea may reflect short-term inadequate protein intake, and low serum creatinine may reflect reduction in muscle mass. Serum proteins such as albumin and pre-albumin are commonly used as markers but are all affected by disease and hydration. Serum albumin, in conjunction with C-reactive protein, can be used as a general tool. If CRP is normal and albumin low, in conjunction with other nutrition assessment parameters it is likely to reflect poor nutrition; if CRP is high and albumin is low it is usually reflecting an inflammatory or infective process rather than nutrition.

Nutritional requirements

The principle sources of dietary energy are carbohydrates (4kcal/g) and lipids (9kcal/g). Nitrogen or protein is needed to maintain structural and functional proteins in the body (6.25g protein = 1g nitrogen) and may also contribute to energy intake (4kcal/g protein). The body has stores of carbohydrate (liver and muscle glycogen), lipid (adipose tissue), and protein (muscle). When determining the amount and type of nutrition support required, it is important to take into account the normal requirements of the patient and the effect of the disease or its treatment upon them. During simple starvation, the metabolic rate falls to enable the body stores to last as long as possible, so protecting the patient. Eventually, when the carbohydrate and lipid stores are depleted, the body's protein reserves start to become depleted and are broken down to provide energy. Even small amounts of carbohydrate can prevent this.

In contrast, stress or injury, including surgery and infection, result in catabolism where not only carbohydrate and lipid stores but also protein stores are mobilized to provide energy. In patients with sepsis, improvements in nutritional status will not occur in response to nutrition alone – treating the cause of sepsis is essential to achieve effective nutritional support.

There are a number of formulas available to estimate energy requirements, e.g. Schofield and Harris-Benedict equations. The following can be used as a general guide:

• Energy   25–35kcal/kg
• Protein   1–1.5g/kg
• Fluid   30–35ml/kg *
• Sodium   1–2mmol/kg*
• Potassium   1–2mmol/kg*

*Needs may be higher in patients with excessive losses such as gastric fistulas or drain losses.

Nutritional support

The objectives of nutritional support are to provide adequate nutrition (energy, protein, micronutrients, fluid) to either:
• maintain nutritional status in well nourished patients, or
• prevent further deterioration and/or improve nutritional status in malnourished patients.

Additional objectives of nutritional support are:
• to ensure it is administered by the most the appropriate route for the patient and clinical condition
• to minimize the side effects and potential complications of nutrition support.

Methods of nutritional support

NICE (2005) recommend that nutrition support should be considered in people who are malnourished or at risk of malnutrition, as defined by any of the following:
• BMI <18.5kg/m^2 **or** unintentional weight loss >10% in the last 3–6 months
• BMI <20kg/m^2 **and** unintentional weight loss >5% in the last 3–6 months
• patients who have eaten little or nothing for >5 days or are likely to eat little or nothing for the next 5 days or longer
• patients with poor absorptive capacity and/or high nutrient losses and/ or increased nutritional need.

Nutritional support can be provided by the enteral or parenteral route. In general, the gut should be used if it is working. Enteral feeding is less expensive and, in units without special expertise in parenteral nutrition (nutrition support teams), enteral is usually safer. It may also reduce morbidity in critically ill patients by preserving gut epithelial integrity, although this is controversial.

One of the most important aspects of nutritional assessment for the patient anticipating major surgery is to plan the method by which enteral access is to be secured for post-operative nutritional support, i.e. to identify those at risk of post-operative complications.

Enteral feeding tube placement can be undertaken electively pre-operatively without interfering with surgery or it can be undertaken at the time of surgery. This avoids the need for endoscopic and radiological procedures on a patient with poor post-operative intestinal motility or resorting to parenteral nutrition.

Oral feeding

Oral nutrition support is the cheapest, safest, and most physiological method of providing nutritional support, and should be used wherever possible in the conscious patient with an intact gut and normal swallowing mechanism. Patients who are able to take food and fluid orally should receive food fortification advice, and additional snacks and meals. Dietetic input is usually necessary to ensure nutritional adequacy.

Nutritional supplements or sip feeds should be considered if food fortification or additional food intake is not sufficient. These are available as liquids (milk and juice-based, sweet and savoury), which are the most commonly used type. They should be given between meals to maximize intake. Semi-solid or pudding-type supplements are also particularly useful, especially for those requiring altered consistency or who are fluid restricted. Calorie supplements are also available but generally contain few or no proteins or micronutrients.

Enteral tube feeding

Enteral tube feeding is used for patients who are unable to meet their nutritional requirements with food and supplements but who have a functioning and accessible gut. Enteral nutrition is more physiological, safer, and more cost-effective than parenteral nutrition and there are more access routes available.

Enteral tube feeding routes

Naso-gastric (NG) feeding

This is the most commonly used method of providing nutritional support in hospitalized patients. NG tubes can be placed by suitably trained nurses or doctors at the bedside following local policies and procedures. NG tubes are generally a short-term method of feeding (weeks) for patients who are unable to eat due to impaired swallow or altered level of consciousness, or to supplement an inadequate oral intake. Occasionally they may be used for long-term feeding if alternative methods are either unsafe or against patient preference. NG tube placement is contraindicated if there is an obstructive pathology in the oropharynx or oesophagus preventing passage of the tube, facial fractures, basal skull fracture, gastric outflow obstruction, or mechanical bowel obstruction.

Nasojejunal (NJ) feeding

This is used for short-term access for patients with a functioning lower gastrointestinal tract but where the stomach is not emptying as well as it should, for example when there is post-operative ileus, pancreatitis, or where there is a risk of aspiration with gastric feeding. Patients undergoing surgery for emergency repair of aortic aneurysm, or bowel perforation with faecal peritonitis, are at particular risk of gastric paresis. NJ tubes are usually single or double lumen tubes and can be placed at the bedside or at the time of surgery, or more reliably using endoscopic or radiological assistance.

The main problems or complications of NG and NJ tubes include occlusion as a result of feed or medication and displacement (either accidental or intentional), although these can be overcome to a degree by general care such as regular flushing, confirmation of position prior to use, and additional securing devices such as nasal bridles.

Gastrostomy tube feeding

This is a longer-term method of feeding for patients with a functioning gastrointestinal tract who are unable to eat or eat sufficiently, and are particularly useful if placed pre-operatively in patients undergoing surgery or radiotherapy for head and neck cancer. There are a variety of different tubes available and they can be placed using a variety of methods. The most common is a percutaneous endoscopically-placed gastrostomy (PEG), as these tubes can last for a number of years. Contraindications to PEG placement include obstruction of the oropharynx and oesophagus and stomach. Relative contraindications include previous gastric surgery, ascites, portal hypertension, gastric ulceration, bleeding, malignancy, and obesity. The main problems associated with PEG tubes relate to the stoma itself, such as leakage, infection, over-granulation, and buried bumper syndrome. These are generally the result of poor care of the tube and stoma and inadequate fixation, and are therefore avoidable.

Radiologically-placed gastrostomy tubes (RPG or RIG) are usually used in patients where an endoscope is unable to pass through the oesophagus. These tubes are generally more prone to displacement and require replacement every 6–12 months depending on the tube used.

Surgical jejunostomy feeding tubes

These are placed during surgery and are often used routinely in the management of upper GI resections for cancer to enable enteral nutrition post-operatively. Contraindications include jejunal disease such as Crohn's disease or radiation enteritis, or obstructing distal pathology. Relative contraindications include ascites, portal hypertension, and peritoneal dialysis. The main problems associated with jejunostomy tubes include occlusion, infection, and displacement, and can be avoided or minimized with local protocols.

Complications of enteral tube feeding

Enteral feeding is generally safe. Complications or side effects can be divided into the following categories.

Tube related

These depend on the tube used, e.g. occlusion is more commonly associated with NG, NJ, and jejunal feeding tubes as they are usually less than 10Fr in diameter. Displacement is more commonly associated with naso-enteral feeding tubes. Gastrostomy tubes are more prone to stoma site problems due to inadequate fixation and general care.

Gastrointestinal

Vomiting/aspiration/reflux

Gastric feeding can increase the risk of aspiration.

Strategies to prevent or treat should include:
- Patients should be fed in an upright position wherever possible.
- Use of anti-emetics and prokinetics such as metoclopramide or erythromycin.
- Pump feeding rather than bolus feeding.

Post-pyloric feeding such as NJ or jejunal extension to PEG should be considered for those with a non-resolving problem.

Diarrhoea

This is usually multi-factorial, and contributing factors include antibiotic use, prokinetics, liquid medication (often contains sorbitol), low serum albumin, infection such as *C. difficile* enteritis (CDAD), feed formula (low residue or high fibre), or an underlying disease, e.g. malabsorption or colitis.

Treatment should include:
- Exclusion of disease-related pathology, e.g. malabsorption, or infection, e.g. *C. difficile toxin*.
- Medication review, e.g. laxatives, elixirs, antibiotics.
- Review of feeding regimen, e.g. rate/volume/formulae.
- Consider anti-diarrhoeal agents, e.g. loperamide/codeine phosphate.

Constipation

This is usually due to a combination of inadequate fluid intake, reduced mobility, drug therapy, and low residue feeding formulas. Treatment should include exclusion of GI pathology, use of laxatives/suppositories/ enemas, and adequate fluid intake, as well as inclusion of fibre-containing feeds.

Metabolic

📖 See the section on Metabolic complications, p.111.

Parenteral nutrition

Parenteral nutrition (PN) is the administration of nutrition intravenously. It is less physiological, more costly, and is associated with more serious complications compared with enteral tube feeding, and therefore should be reserved for patients in whom:

- the GIT is inaccessible, e.g. oesophageal stricture, severe mucositis
- the GIT is not functioning, e.g. obstruction, motility disorders
- it is not possible to meet nutrition needs using the enteral route, e.g. short bowel syndrome, radiation enteritis.

Factors affecting route/access device include:

- diagnosis and anticipated duration of PN
- clinical issues and potential complications
- availability of suitable access
- method of insertion
- expertise of inserter
- type of catheter available.

Peripheral parenteral nutrition

Peripheral parenteral nutrition (PPN) is generally suitable for those patients who are anticipated to require feeding for less than 14 days and have good peripheral venous access. Nutrition is limited by the osmolarity and pH of the solution and therefore it is generally unsuitable for patients who have high calorie/electrolyte requirements or who are fluid restricted. Peripheral inserted catheter (PIC or midline) should be used in preference to a cannula/venflon.

PIC/midlines

These are usually 15–20cm long, made of polyurethane, and can be inserted at the bedside into the basilic or cephalic vein via the anti-cubita fossa. As they do not enter the central veins there is much less risk associated when compared with central line insertion, and an X-ray is not required for correct positioning. Best results are obtained by a suitably trained person using strict aseptic technique. The main complication associated with PIC lines is thrombophlebitis, which requires the removal of the line.

Central parenteral nutrition

This can include PICC, multi-lumen lines, and tunnelled lines, and generally enables unlimited provision of calories, fluid, and electrolytes.

Peripherally inserted central venous catheters (PICC)

These are made from silicone or polyurethane, 50–60cm long, inserted via the basilica or cephalic vein of the anti-cubital fossa with the tip lying in the superior vena cava. There is a reduced risk of insertion-related complications compared with CVC insertion but placement by a trained person and good venous access are required, and an X-ray to confirm the correct position. Thrombophlebitis can be a limiting factor with PN infusions.

Central venous catheters (CVCs)

Ideally a single-lumen line should be used for PN but more commonly multi-lumen lines (internal jugular/subclavian) are used for short-term PN, and are often placed at the time of surgery. An X-ray is required to confirm the correct position. One lumen should be dedicated to PN infusion and strict aseptic technique used whenever the line is accessed. Femoral vein lines should be avoided wherever possible due to the increased risk of infection and throboembolism. Tunnelled central lines – either single or double-lumen – should be used for patients requiring long-term PN.

Complications of PN

- *Line insertion related* – particularly related to central lines, including pneumothorax, air embolism, haemothorax, arrhythmias, thrombosis, etc.
- *Line related/mechanical* – occlusion results from kinking, lipid deposits, catheter damage, extravasation, displacement, thrombophlebitis (local tenderness, erythema, tracking).
- *Infection* – exit site infection: exudate, inflammation (erythema, tenderness, and induration), or pus.
- *Catheter-related sepsis* – can be serious and life-threatening – pyrexia, increased inflammatory markers (WCC, CRP), rigors, tachycardia, and hypotension.
- *Fluid/biochemical* – fluid overload, electrolyte imbalance, re-feeding syndrome.

Monitoring for parenteral nutrition

Monitoring of patients receiving PN is essential and ideally undertaken by a specialized multi-disciplinary nutrition support team to reduce the complications of PN. The following should be included:

- Line site – should be reviewed at least daily for signs of infection, leakage, etc.
- Clinical condition – daily fluid balance, temperature, pulse, respiratory rate.
- Nutrition – weight, nutritional intake, GI function, oral intake.
- Metabolic/biochemical – strict biochemical protocols should be in place to monitor PN.

Metabolic complications

Metabolic complications may be associated with both enteral and parenteral nutrition and include:

- Re-feeding syndrome – this is the metabolic complication that may arise when re-feeding a very malnourished patient. Signs include hypophosphataemia, hypokalaemia, hypomagnesaemia, altered glucose metabolism, fluid balance abnormalities, and vitamin deficiency. Treatment includes a gradual introduction of nutritional support, supplementation with water-soluble vitamins, close biochemical monitoring, and correction of biochemical abnormalities.
- Over- and under-hydration – all fluids administered should be accounted for, including oral, enteral feed, IV fluids, IV medication, and parenteral nutrition, and fluid balance monitored.

- Hyperglycaemia – elevated glucose levels may be due to insulin-resistance in sepsis or poorly controlled diabetes, and insulin may be required if consistently above 10mmol/l.
- Overfeeding – may be associated with hypercapnoea, azotazaemia, and hyperglycaemia.
- Hepatobiliary and bone – cholestasis, cholelithiasis, liver steatosis, and cirrhosis can all result from PN, but generally occur in patients receiving long-term PN.

Biochemical monitoring of enteral and parenteral nutrition support

The frequency of biochemical tests (☐ see Table 5.1) depends upon the route of feeding, the risk of re-feeding syndrome, as well as the duration of nutrition support. The following should be used as a general guide. Local policy and protocols should be followed if available.

Table 5.1 Frequency of biochemical tests

Parameter	Enteral nutrition	Parenteral nutrition
Sodium, potassium	Baseline then daily until stable, then once or twice weekly	Baseline then daily until stable, then twice weekly
Urea, creatinine	Baseline then daily until stable, then once or twice weekly	Baseline then daily until stable, then twice weekly
Glucose	Baseline then daily until stable, then once or twice weekly in non-diabetic patients	Baseline then 6 hourly for first 24–48hrs, if stable twice weekly
Liver function tests, albumin	Baseline then twice weekly, reduce to once weekly if stable	Baseline, then twice weekly
Calcium, phosphate	Baseline then daily if re-feeding risk, or twice weekly if not, reduce to weekly when stable	Baseline then daily if re-feeding risk, or twice weekly when stable
Magnesium	Baseline then daily if re-feeding risk, or twice weekly if not, reduce to weekly when stable	Baseline then daily if re-feeding risk, or twice weekly when stable
Full blood count	Baseline then once weekly	Baseline, twice weekly
CRP	Baseline then once weekly	Baseline, twice weekly
Trace elements (Zn, Cu, Se, Mn)	If deficiency suspected	After 2–4 weeks PN, then every 2–4 weeks

Complications of blood transfusion and coagulation

Appropriate blood management

Among surgical patients, optimization of pre-operative haemoglobin and assessment of bleeding risk, minimizing blood loss peri-operatively, and critical appraisal of clinical symptoms and haemoglobin level post-operatively, are all key aspects in the prevention and management of anaemia. Surgical blood loss and trauma are major indications for allogeneic blood transfusion as no viable alternatives to red cells currently exist for use in the acute situation. However, identified transfusion risks, reduced supply, increasing costs, and questionable efficacy demand more precise decision-making to ensure that the benefits of blood transfusion balance the risks.

Under physiological conditions, oxygen delivery exceeds oxygen consumption by a factor of up to four. This ensures a sufficient oxygen supply to meet tissue oxygen needs even when there is marked anaemia. Other adaptive responses include blood flow alterations resulting in increased cardiac output, redistribution of blood flow from non-vital to vital organs, and an increase in oxygen extraction ratio. Stored packed red blood cells (PRBCs) undergo a variety of morphological and biochemical changes that adversely affect their ability to deliver oxygen to tissue. Biochemical changes include a low P50 and the loss of 2-3-diphosphoglycerate, both of which result in enhanced haemoglobin affinity for oxygen and, consequently, an impaired ability to offload oxygen at the cellular level. Haemolysis of a proportion of transfused PRBCs is common and results in the release of free haemoglobin along with a variety of other biologically active substances into the circulation. These may trigger an inflammatory response and induce vasoconstriction, exacerbating any reduction in microvascular perfusion. The majority of available data indicate that although global oxygen delivery is increased following transfusion, the cellular uptake of oxygen is relatively unaffected, bringing into question the actual impact of transfused red cells on tissue oxygen delivery.

The Serious Hazards of Transfusion (SHOT) report for 2007 suggests that mortality associated with blood component transfusion is at an all-time low in the UK. A total of 2 914 228 blood components were issued by blood banks throughout the UK. There were 561 incidents reported including 12 cases of ABO-incompatible red cell transfusion (nine arising from clinical errors and three from laboratory errors), none of which were fatal (📖 see Table 6.1). However, many incidents result in significant morbidity and the most frequently occurring events continue to be due to avoidable errors, often due to failure of correct patient identification resulting in an incorrect blood component being transfused.

Table 6.1 Summary of reported reactions and/or errors

Type of reaction/error	Number of cases	Cases as a percentage of total reactions reported
Incorrect blood component transfused	332	59.1%
Acute transfusion reaction	114	20.5%
Adverse events relating to anti-D immunoglobulin	63	11.2%
Haemolytic transfusion reaction	23	4.1%
Transfusion-related acute lung injury	24	4.3%
Transfusion-transmitted infection	3	0.5%
Post-transfusion purpura	2	0.4%
Transfusion-associated graft versus host disease	0	–
Transfusion-associated circulatory overload	0	–

Incorrect blood component transfused

Blood transfusions involve a complex sequence of activities. To ensure the right patient receives the right blood there must be strict checking procedures at each stage. Administering the wrong blood type is the most serious outcome of error in transfusions. SHOT data have shown that between 1996 and 2004, five patients died as a result of being given ABO incompatible blood. The National Patient Safety Agency (NPSA), the Chief Medical Officer's National Blood Transfusion Committee (NBTC), and Serious Hazards of Transfusion (SHOT) have launched an initiative that offers a range of strategies to ensure blood transfusions are carried out safely.

The initiative aims to implement an action plan involving:
- Competency-based training and assessment for all staff involved in blood transfusions.
- Use of patient wristbands, identity bands, or photo identification cards instead of compatibility form or patient notes as part of the final check.
- Systematical evaluation of local blood transfusion procedures, and appraisal of the feasibility of using:
  - barcodes or other electronic identification and tracking systems for patients, samples, and blood products
  - photo identification cards for patients who undergo regular blood transfusions
  - a labelling system of matching samples and blood for transfusion.

Acute (immediate) transfusion reactions

These occur during or within 1–2 hours of completing the transfusion.

- **Febrile, non-haemolytic reactions** are thought to be caused by antibodies to donor leucocytes. Although definitive evidence is not available, there is sufficient data to suggest that adverse transfusion-associated immunomodulation (TRIM) effects probably exist. In those countries where universal leucodepletion has been implemented for other reasons, anecdotally there seems to be a reduction in these reactions.

- **Hypersensitivity to donor plasma proteins** usually presents as urticaria and is quite common, occurring in up to 1% of transfusions. It may require antihistamines (e.g. chlorpheniramine 10mg IV). A record must be made in the notes, as prophylactic antihistamine may be needed with or without hydrocortisone (100mg IV) before subsequent transfusions. Anaphylaxis from anti-IgA antibody in IgA-deficient subjects is rare, although IgA deficiency occurs in about one in 500 people. Adrenaline (epinephrine) (0.4ml 1:1000 SC or IM), hydrocortisone (100mg IV), fluid volume, and oxygen support may be required. Despite a lack of evidence that intravenous corticosteroids are beneficial for the management of acute anaphylactic transfusion reactions, most clinicians include an infusion of hydrocortisone.

Acute haemolytic immune reaction

Acute immune haemolysis is a life-threatening condition usually caused by ABO incompatibility. Less commonly, there may be other red cell antibodies if the patient has previously been transfused or is a multiparous female. Clinically there is fever and hypotension, and there may be loin pain or pain at the infusion site. In an anaesthetized patient, hypotension and bleeding due to disseminated intravascular coagulopathy (DIC) may be the only findings. Immediate action is to stop the transfusion, but maintain venous access and institute treatment for shock. There may be a need to treat DIC with transfusions of fresh frozen plasma (FFP), pooled cryoprecipitate for fibrinogen, and/or platelet concentrates. A full blood count (FBC), repeat Group & Save, direct Coombs test, coagulation screen, blood cultures, and tests of renal and liver function must be taken. The urine must be tested for haemoglobulinuria and the transfusion pack returned to the laboratory for repeat serological testing.

Acute non-immune haemolytic reactions can also be caused by transfusion of serologically compatible RBCs that have become more fragile as a result of storage. This condition usually does not require rigorous treatment and can be managed with an induced diuresis using Hartmann's solution or 0.9% sodium chloride as tolerated by the patient, until the intense red colour of haemoglobinuria ceases.

Transfusion-related acute lung injury (TRALI)

TRALI is increasingly recognized as a severe acute complication. It is caused by donor leucoagglutinins. Clinically fever, hypotension, non-productive cough, dyspnoea, and hypoxia are seen, typically within 4 hours of the transfusion. Symptoms respond to high flow oxygen administration, in which case the complication is self-limiting. However, if shortness of breath persists after oxygen administration, early respiratory support with intubation, oxygen, and ventilation are required.

Infectious agents transmitted by blood-product transfusion

The actual risk is not high in comparison with the identification/ documentation errors described earlier, but it assumes a high public profile. Careful donor selection and improved testing procedures have further reduced transmission rates. The most serious cause is bacterial contamination of blood causing marked fever and shock. Platelet concentrates are more likely to be infected as they are stored at room temperature and provide an ideal culture medium for any contaminating organism. The contents of the pack may be discoloured. Action should be taken as in acute immune haemolysis but Gram stains of blood and blood cultures are also necessary on both patient and donor blood or platelets. Broad-spectrum antibiotics must be instituted. Infection with viruses, protozoa, prions, and possibly fungi should also be considered. The transfusion-transmitted risks of viral (and parasitic) infections are dramatically increased in countries with a low Human Development Index (HDI) due to a high seroprevalence and underdeveloped pathogen testing and transfusion standards. Reported incidence from SHOT in the UK for 2007 was 0.0001%. All of these transmitted infections were bacterial with one additional case still awaiting completion of investigations.

Post-transfusion purpura (PTP)

PTP is an important, but very rare, delayed immune reaction mediated by anti-platelet antibodies in the recipient, usually a multiparous female. A profound thrombocytopenia develops 5–9 days post-transfusion. Administration of high-dose intravenous immunoglobulin and transfusion of platelets may be necessary with specialist haematology advice.

Graft versus host disease (GvHD)

The potential for transfusion associated GvHD is increasingly recognized as a serious delayed complication in susceptible subjects. These include patients with Hodgkin's disease and those receiving chemotherapy directed particularly against the lymphoid system along with other immunocompromised groups. Mediation is through viable, transfused donor T lymphocytes, which are able to engraft in the host due to the inability of host T cells to recognize donor T cells as foreign and eradicate them. GvHD presents with fever, skin rash, diarrhoea, and abnormal liver function tests, usually within 4 weeks of blood transfusion. This group of patients should receive only irradiated blood, which kills any T cells present in the donor unit.

Transfusion-associated circulatory overload (TACO)

Symptoms include acute respiratory distress, tachycardia, increased blood pressure, and acute or worsening pulmonary oedema. Initial management includes sitting the patient up and administering oxygen. Discontinue the transfusion and consider removing excessive fluid by administration of diuretics. In the management of anaemic patients, post-cardiac surgery transfusion should be used extremely judiciously. The available data indicate that overall, transfusion in this population is associated with significantly worse outcomes as measured by a number of variables: mortality, infection, post-operative duration of mechanical ventilation, and post-operative atrial fibrillation, among others. Although predominantly retrospective in nature, the consistency of these findings supports this position.

Massive transfusion complications

Massive transfusions, of greater than the patient's blood volume administered within 24h, carry additional complications. Dilution coagulopathy as a consequence of early volume replacement with crystalloids and colloids is followed by consumption of coagulation factors, platelets, and fibrinogen due to ongoing bleeding. Baseline FBC and coagulation screens are essential with further monitoring as appropriate to assess response of therapeutic intervention with component therapy. Microvascular bleeding is a good clinical indicator of coagulopathy and should be recognized in order to try and anticipate replacement requirements prior to test results being available from the laboratory. Increasingly, near-patient testing of whole blood coagulation capability plays an important role in the management of massive haemorrhage and transfusion. Hypothermia should be avoided and warmed solutions and blood may be used. Biochemical and ECG monitoring is required for the early recognition of hyperkalaemia, hypocalcaemia, and renal dysfunction.

Complications of coagulation

Surgery with anticoagulation

Increasing numbers of patients present for surgery, emergency and elective, who are on anticoagulant and/or anti-platelet therapy. Antithrombotic therapy is indicated for venous thromboembolic disease (deep venous thrombosis; pulmonary embolism; prophylaxis of DVT or PE; antithrombin III, protein C, and protein S deficiency), arterial thromboembolic disease (prosthetic heart valves, atrial fibrillation, congestive cardiomyopathies, mural cardiac thrombus, acute myocardial infarction, and mitral valve disease), and maintaining patency of vascular grafts, shunts, and bypasses.

Patients with the highest risk of arterial or venous thromboembolism should be off anticoagulation therapy for the minimum period necessary to allow major surgery to proceed with acceptable bleeding risk. Interruption of oral anticoagulants for surgery requires therapeutic-dose heparin with unfractionated (UFH) or low molecular weight heparin (LMWH) during the interval when the international normalized ratio (INR) is subtherapeutic.

High risk patients in whom bridging with therapeutic UFH or LMWH is advised are (Cleveland Clinic Journal of Medicine):
- Known hypercoagulable state as documented by a thromboembolic event and one of the following:
  - protein C deficiency
  - protein S deficiency
  - antithrombin III deficiency
  - homozygous Factor V Leiden.
- Hypercoagulable state suggested by recurrent thromboembolic events (>2).
- Venous or thromboembolic events in the last 1–3 months.
- Rheumatic atrial fibrillation.
- Acute intracardiac thrombus visualized with echocardiogram.
- Atrial fibrillation plus mechanical heart valve in any position.
- Older mechanical valve models (single-disk or ball-in-cage) in mitral position.
- Mechanical valve placed less than 3 months ago.
- Atrial fibrillation with history of cardioembolism.

Minor surgery

Warfarin does not need to be reversed. If the INR is less than 2.5, evidence shows that the risk of bleeding is low and surgery can proceed. If the INR is greater than 2.5 the need for immediate surgery should be balanced against the potential for excessive bleeding. If the surgeon feels the greater risk is from bleeding then the surgery should not proceed until the INR is below 2.5. Options are to withold warfarin and wait for INR to fall, or consider temporary reversal.

Major surgery

Standard practice

Usually warfarin is stopped 4 days before surgery. Standard peri-operative heparin prophylaxis, if indicated, should be commenced when INR is less than 2.0. INR should be checked close to the day of surgery to ensure it has adequately fallen to < 1.5. If INR is > 1.5, then this should be discussed with the surgeon and action should be taken accordingly. Warfarin can be restarted as soon as the patient has an oral intake and post-operative haemostasis is stable.

High-risk patients

For patients at high risk of thromboembolism (TE), management should involve the giving of unfractionated heparin (UFH) by continuous infusion when the INR is less than 2.0, aiming for an APTT ratio of 1.5 and discontinued 2 hours before surgery. Switch to LMWH post-operatively when the patient is haemodynamically stable, and restart warfarin when oral intake is resumed. Heparin can be stopped when the INR is within the therapeutic range. If heparin is continued, the platelet count should be checked at 5 and 10 days.

Assessment for thromboembolism

Risk assessment for TE

This depends on patient factors, the disease, and the surgical procedure. Patient factors that increase the risk of TE include: age, obesity, varicose veins, immobility, pregnancy and the puerperium, previous TE, and thrombophilia. Disease factors include: malignancy, heart failure, trauma, polycythaemia, inflammatory bowel disease, lower limb paralysis, recent myocardial infarction, and nephrotic syndrome. Anticardiolipin syndrome is a less commonly acquired thrombophilic state, which should be suspected if there is recurrent fetal loss, unexplained prolonged APTT, thrombocytopenia, or arterial/venous thrombosis at an early age.

Surgical procedures such as major trauma and orthopaedic surgery, gynaecological and pelvic operations, and any major surgery with a long duration can increase the risk of TE.

Consideration of these factors gives low, moderate, and high-risk groups:

(1) Low risk (<10%):
- minor surgery (<30min), no risk factor other than age
- major surgery (>30min), age <40 years, no other risk factor.

(2) Moderate risk (10–40%):
- major surgery, age >40 years, no other risk factor
- major medical illness, trauma, or burns
- minor surgery, previous TE or thrombophilia with no previous thrombosis.

(3) High risk (40–80%):
- major orthopaedic surgery, fracture, hip, pelvis, lower limb
- major pelvic/abdominal surgery for malignancy
- major surgery, previous TE.

Inherited thrombophilia

This is much less common than the above acquired risk factors, but has assumed a high profile recently, mainly in relation to thrombosis associated with oral contraceptive usage. Thrombosis at an early age (arterial <35 years, venous <40 years), in unusual sites (e.g. mesenteric, retinal), and a strong family history (two or more first-degree relatives) all warrant further testing. Test for antithrombin III (ATIII), protein S, and protein C deficiency, and activated protein C resistance, which is usually associated with the factor V Leiden defect.

Prophylaxis for thromboembolism

Mechanical

Early ambulation is recommended in all patients and may be all that is required for those considered to be at low risk. Elastic stockings and intermittent pneumatic compression can be used in higher-risk patients. Mechanical methods can be combined with anticoagulant therapy to increase the level of prophylaxis.

Anticoagulant

Low dose heparin, both UFH and LMWH, is widely used and effective. LMWH is more convenient (once-daily administration) and has better bioavailability.

Prophylaxis should begin pre-operatively and continue until the patient is reasonably mobile. If the patient requires an epidural, this should be discussed with the anaesthetists as the dose and timing of heparin may increase the risk of critical bleeding due to the epidural and mean that this form of anaesthesia is contraindicated.

Anti-platelet agents

Many patients may already be on anti-platelet therapy with aspirin for vascular disease (IHD, CVA, PVD, HT). Increasingly patients may be on combinations of anti-platelet agents following coronary stent procedures. The maintenance of stent patency may be critically dependent on continuation of this therapy, and changes to treatment should not be undertaken without first discussing with the appropriate cardiologist. If surgery is essential despite the presence of anti-platelet agents then the increased potential for bleeding should be recognized and fully discussed with the patient prior to surgery.

Pre-operative assessment of bleeding problems

The patient history is most important. Details of previous bleeding or bruising episodes should be explored. Sites of bleeding, duration of bleeding, whether the episodes are life-long or recent, family history, response to previous surgery, and requirement for transfusion all need to be recorded together with drug and alcohol history. A suspicion of an abnormal bleeding tendency may be indicated by a history of prolonged bleeding after dental extraction requiring additional intervention or admission, blood transfusion following minor surgery such as tonsillectomy, or excessive menstrual loss.

Examination for petechiae, bruising, stigmata of chronic liver disease, and haemorrhage into joints or muscle compartments is important.

A significant bleeding history should prompt investigation with FBC, prothrombin time (PT), and activated partial thromboplastin time (APTT), and discussion of the case with a haematologist for full clinical assessment of potential bleeding risk and need for further specialist investigations.

Chapter 7

Pressure sores

Aetiology and prevention

The care of patients with pressure ulceration is estimated to cost the NHS £2 billion every year. Treatment is often confined to the wound itself, and the equally important, precise patient risk factors may not be identified and corrected. Patients with advanced pressure ulceration are often referred late to plastic surgeons for myocutaneous flap closure, with significant resource implications. Early referral to multi-disciplinary teams makes services much more efficient, cost effective, and beneficial to patients.

Demographics of those presenting for plastic surgical repair

- Incidence:
  - elderly immobile patients (>25%), with half occurring after the first two weeks of hospital admission
  - quadriplegics (60%)
  - increased in neurologically impaired young and chronically hospitalized.
- Mortality is high due to the overall disease burden.

Risk assessment

- Early risk assessment (ideally within 6 hours of hospital admission) and examination of skin in the 'at risk' areas is important. For risk factors, (📖 see Box 7.1).
- Risk assessments most commonly used are the Waterlow Score (UK) and Braden Scale (USA), but both have limitations (📖 see Box 7.2).

Classification system

The term 'stage' is used in the National Pressure Ulcer Advisory Panel (NPUAP) classification system from the United States, while 'grade' is used in the European Pressure Ulcer Advisory Panel (EPUAP) classification system.

- **Stage/Grade 1: Erythema** – non-blanchable erythema of intact skin. Seen within 30 minutes.
- **Stage/Grade 2: Blistering** – partial thickness skin loss. Seen after 2–6 hours of pressure.
- **Stage/Grade 3: Full thickness loss** – down to fascia. Later presentation.
- **Stage/Grade 4: Muscle/bone involved** – involves muscle, tendon, bone, or joint capsule.

Box 7.1 Risk factors

Extrinsic factors
- **Shear** – mechanical stress parallel to the skin; this causes superficial skin insult and necrosis by compressing the perforating vessels to the skin.
- **Pressure** – a high perpendicular force per unit area causing deep necrosis and vessel blockage.
- **Friction** – when there is resistance to movement between the skin surface and the bed or chair, the outermost layer is lost resulting in desiccation of tissues.
- **Moisture** – this is often overlooked and leads to skin maceration and breakdown. Treat incontinence early, and change sheets often.

Intrinsic factors
- **Ischaemia/sepsis** – these states cause reduced tissue perfusion and increase necrosis.
- **Increased age** – advancing age leads to decreased skin moisture, decreased tensile strength, and increased fragility.
- **Sensory loss** – tissue ischaemia results due to the inability to feel discomfort from prolonged immobility. E.g. spinal cord injury, stroke, epidural anaesthesia, diabetes mellitus.
- **Small vessel microangiopathy** – diabetes, peripheral vascular diseases, and smoking all decrease tissue perfusion leading to necrosis.
- **Anaemia** – decreased wound healing ability, lethargy, and increased immobility.
- **Malnutrition** – lack of trace elements, vitamins, and minerals leads to disordered wound healing.
- **Obesity**

Box 7.2 Risk assessments

Waterlow Score

A daily assessment in every patient including:
- body mass index
- age and sex
- continence
- mobility
- nutrition
- skin changes
- adverse wound healing factors
- neurological deficit
- surgical intervention
- current medications.

Braden Scale

Minimum value of 6, maximum value of 23. Lower scores indicate increased risk of pressure sore development:
- sensory perception
- skin moisture
- activity
- mobility
- friction and shear
- nutritional status.

Management and prevention strategies

- **General measures** – skin care to minimize moisture, care during transfers. Optimize nutrition, address spasticity, attention to incontinence, minimize head of bed elevation to reduce shearing. Optimize blood sugar levels and cessation of smoking. Active treatment of colonization and infection.
- **Pressure relief** – 📖 see Box 7.3.

Box 7.3 Pressure relief

- Static pads on pressure areas – several inches of foam is needed.
- Regular positional changes.
- Customized cushions or wheelchairs.
- Customized air mattresses – exerting less pressure on the patient and facilitating drying of the skin.

Generally Grade I and II pressure sores are treated non-operatively. Grade III and IV pressure ulcers generally require operative intervention but are rarely referred.

Non-operative management

- Debridement at the bedside and appropriate antimicrobial dressings (📖 see Box 7.4).
- Antibiotics where needed.
- Consider investigations:
  - routine blood tests: albumin/pre-albumin for nutrition, inflammatory markers (FBE, CRP, ESR)
  - swabs for microscopy and culture
  - imaging: plain radiography, bone scan, MRI
  - soft-tissue biopsy to rule out malignancy – i.e. Marjolins ulcer in chronic pressure sore, although very rare
  - bone biopsy if deep involvement to rule out osteomyelitis (will then need prolonged antibiotics).
- Strict pressure care, frequent patient turning and body-weight shifting, and use of pressure-reducing mattresses.

Box 7.4 Dressings

Always consider antiseptic/antibiotic dressings in extensive colonization and in addition to antibiotics when there is infection.
- Eschar – Hydrogel
- Erythematous granulation tissue – Hydrocolloid/Hydrogel
- Yellow slough (dry) – Hydrocolloid/Hydrogel
- Yellow slough (moist) – Hydrogel and Absorbent Foam
- Yellow slough (wet) – Alginate-based dressing + Absorbent Foam
- Granulating cavity – consider negative pressure therapy/discuss with tissue viability nurse.

Operative management

- Site-dependent operations can be carried out by plastic surgeons following complete debridement of all devitalized tissues. Grade III and IV pressure ulcers generally undergo flap reconstruction.
- Meticulous haemostasis and obliteration of dead space post-operatively is mandatory. Tension-free closure and pressure offloading from reconstructed area is vital.
- Sacral ulcers: commonly occur after prolonged immobility. Options include local advancement or rotation flaps, pedicled musculocutaneous flaps based on the inferior or superior gluteal muscles, or fasciocutaneous flaps based on the lumbar or gluteal regions.
- Ischial ulcers: commonly occur after prolonged sitting, such as in paraplegics. Local flaps and gluteal flaps are commonly used. The gluteal-thigh flap, hamstring myocutaneous flap, tensor fascia lata flap, anterolateral thigh flap, and gracilis myocutaneous flap are other described options.

Post-operative management

- Pressure relief for 4–6 weeks, antibiotics with microbiology advice, nutritional optimization, seat mapping, and patient and staff education.
- **Complications** – haematoma, infection, wound dehiscence, recurrence.

Chapter 8

Complications related to use of medicines in surgery

General advice on the use of medicines

Medicines bring undoubted benefits to healthcare, but there is always the potential for risk. Strategies to avoid this risk include being aware of the possible risks and reducing the unnecessary exposure of patients to medicines. The maxim that 'more is rarely better – it is usually less safe and always more expensive' is invariably true.

The *British National Formulary* (BNF) is an excellent, comprehensive, and very readable pocket-sized textbook on most aspects of medicine use. It is also provided free of charge to all hospital doctors and pharmacists and is regularly updated. Recently it has also been made available online, and thus accessible wherever there is an internet connection. It is important that all practising prescribers are familiar with it.

Prescriptions should be clear, legible, and indicate precisely what is to be given. For each medicine, the dose, frequency, route, and duration should be specified and with antibiotics it is good practice to specify a review date and continued indication. Always state units clearly, avoiding abbreviations, and writing micrograms, nanograms, and units in full to avoid confusion.

Doses should always be checked, especially for new or unfamiliar medicines, and for patient groups with whom you are not familiar, e.g. paediatrics. Be aware of interactions and the common adverse side effects.

Advice is always available from pharmacists and experienced colleagues. Most hospitals have a medicines information centre in the pharmacy. This is staffed by pharmacists, with access to a range of specialist drug and therapeutics databases, textbooks, and journals. This is a free service, and well worth getting to know, as is your local medical library service.

Use a framework for dealing with prescribing, such as the mnemonic NESCAFE, i.e.:

Is the medicine **N**ecessary?
Is it **E**ffective?
Is it **S**afe?
Is it **C**ost effective?
Is it **A**ppropriate?
Are there **F**ollow-up implications?
Have you **E**valuated the overall benefit of the medicine?

Be aware that medicines prescribed for a patient for a particular purpose will only be required as long as that purpose still exists. Discontinue all medicines that are no longer required. Ensure that *pro re nata* (PRN; when required) medicines, which were used in hospital, are not automatically prescribed on discharge. This is how patients could start using benzodiazepines for night-time sedation at home.

Medicines used in theatres

Theatres are areas that are not subject to usual prescription surveillance, when large amounts of medication are used sometimes rapidly, and as such are also an environment where errors can occur. Injectable medicines account for the majority of medicines used in theatres, incidents involving injectable medicines account for 25% of all medication incidents, and 58% of the most serious incidents according to reports received by the National Patient Safety Agency (NPSA).

The following points should be noted:

- When a particular medicine is routinely used, it is tempting for practitioners to rely on what an ampoule or box looks like (e.g. colour, style, manufacturer's livery) to identify it. This is no substitute for reading the label, noting the drug concentration and its expiry date. Manufacturers often specialize in drugs for a therapeutic area and market drugs with opposing effects in similar packages. Research has shown that one-third of reported medication incidents may be caused by confusion over packaging and labeling.
- Colour coding is often suggested as a way to differentiate between different types of medicines. This approach has difficulties due to the large number of products used, and the number of manufacturers used to source them. Packaging and manufacturers both change very regularly. Colour blindness amongst staff could also be a problem. There is no substitute for reading the label.
- Get all calculations independently checked by another healthcare professional familiar with the calculation. The second check should be done independently without reference to the work of the preparing practitioner, and then confirmed.
- All parenteral solutions should be made up freshly when required. Microbiological considerations generally mean that once made up, solutions should have a maximum shelf-life of less than 24 hours. Often chemical instability will dictate a shorter shelf-life. Wherever possible standardize on ready-made injectable medicines either bought in or made by the Pharmacy Aseptic Unit.
- Unlabelled syringes are obviously dangerous and subject to potential confusion. The NPSA has reccommended that all syringes and infusions containing injectable medicines are labelled if they leave the operator's hand.
- Obtain and use blank labels specifically designed for parenteral drugs.
- All administration of medicines legally requires that a prescription be written. You should ensure that all such details of prescribing and administration are recorded on either the patient's main drug chart or the theatre drug chart.

Adverse drug reactions (ADRs)

ADRs can be divided into two types:
- Predicted:
  - dose-related
  - logical, from a knowledge of their pharmacology.
- Idiosyncratic:
  - allergic reactions
  - autoimmune
  - illogical.

ADRs account for significant morbidity and mortality. They are responsible for 5% of hospital admissions. In hospital, 7% of patients suffer a serious ADR, of which 0.1–0.3% are fatal. The Medicines and Healthcare products Regulatory Agency (MHRA) run the national 'yellow card' scheme whereby healthcare professionals or patients can report ADRs. Reports can be made online or via yellow cards available in any BNF.

Be aware that no matter how good a prescriber you are, your patients will suffer from ADRs. However, a good medication history and knowledge of therapeutics will minimize this risk. Certain patient populations and disease states will pose additional problems for prescribing and such patients are at an increased risk of suffering from ADRs, for example:
- paediatrics
- elderly
- those with renal and hepatic impairment
- multi-organ failure
- multiple drug therapy.

Always consider medicines as a cause of toxicity, and beware of treating one medicine's toxic side effects with another medicine, e.g. the short-term use of opiates causing constipation leading to long-term laxative use, or antinauseants causing Parkinsonism, with the result that the patient is given a diagnosis of Parkinson's disease and treated for this.

Drug interactions

Detailed information on drug interactions is beyond the scope of this text. First refer to the BNF, and then to specialist texts or a medicines information centre.

Drug interactions occur because one medicine interferes with the pharmacokinetics (the effect of the body on the drug, i.e. absorption, distribution, metabolism, and excretion) or pharmacodynamics (the effects of the drug on the body) of another medicine.

Medicines that interfere with (inhibit or induce) the enzymatic (usually hepatic via cytochrome P450) degradation pathways for chemicals cause changes in the pharmacokinetics of other medicines:
- Enzyme inducers include rifampicin, most antiepileptics, and cigarette smoke.
- Enzyme inhibitors include quinolones, chloramphenicol, omeprazole, and cimetidine.

The result of the interaction is that the effects of one medicine are enhanced or reduced.

For those drugs that are toxic at low doses, a drug interaction that further enhances their effect could be very dangerous. (These drugs, with a low ratio of therapeutic dose to toxic dose, are known as drugs with a low therapeutic ratio.)

Medicines with a low therapeutic ratio include:

- warfarin and other anticoagulants
- digoxin
- anti-arrhythmics, e.g. lidocaine (lignocaine) and disopyramide
- methylxanthines, e.g. theophylline and aminophylline
- some antibiotics, e.g. gentamicin and vancomycin
- antiepileptics, e.g. phenytoin and carbamazepine.

Medicines in surgery

Peri-operative maintenance medication for chronic conditions

Medicines taken regularly for chronic conditions may have the ability to cause potential interactions with medicines used peri-operatively; however, few conditions restrict concurrent administration. The peri-operative period can be defined as extending from the pre-operative day, during the procedure, and continuing into the post-operative recovery phase. Thus comprehensive medication management aims to minimize and prevent potential complications, to decrease post-operative pain, and to promote and accelerate recovery. Comprehension and application of general principles of peri-operative medication management can significantly improve the outcomes of the patient undergoing surgery. Therefore it is vital that a pre-operative medicines assessment is carried out to record the patient's medication history. This should include the recent history of:

- medication obtained via the patient's doctor, whether this is regularly or on a 'when required' basis
- inhalers, eye drops, and oral contraceptive pill – patients often don't consider these items to be medicines
- medication purchased over the counter – 'self-medication'
- medication borrowed from relatives or friends
- possible illicit substance use
- herbal or 'natural' remedies
- compliance
- allergic reactions/ADRs
- medication stopped within the last 3 months, e.g. corticosteroids.

The anaesthetist needs to be aware of any medicines being taken by patients prior to surgery. One of the aims of a pre-operative medicines assessment is to ensure that during surgery anaesthetists are aware of potential problems. They can then ensure that patients have a stable and controlled regulation of vital body systems. This is especially so with regard to the cardiovascular, respiratory, metabolic, endocrine, central nervous, and coagulation systems.

Abrupt, temporary discontinuation of medicines due to overzealous 'nil by mouth' (NBM) policies can lead to:

- withdrawal reactions (e.g. benzodiazepines and fitting, and withdrawal symptoms if opiate-dependent)
- rebound effects (hypertensive crisis with withdrawal of antihypertensives)
- impaired reactions to surgery (impaired stress reaction with corticosteroids)
- unmasking of clinical disease (e.g. antiepileptics).

All of these might contribute to a difficult and hazardous post-operative phase. It is essential to optimize the treatment of patients with chronic diseases so that the patients are in the best possible state to cope with the stress of and recovery from surgery.

NBM policies must enable the continuation of vital medicines wherever possible. If the oral route is definitely compromised, then alternative formulations of medicines for other routes of administration are usually available. However, care should be taken to ensure the appropriate dose and frequency is prescribed, as these may not be the same as for the oral route. If alternative routes are not available, then other suitable therapeutic options could be used by the anaesthetist (☐ refer to Table 8.1).

To avoid interrupting long-term oral therapies, oral medication may usually be administered in the NBM period with small amounts (sips) of clear oral fluids.

Hypertension

Antihypertensives (some, not all) can cause a rebound hypertension if abruptly discontinued. These include α-blockers such as prazosin and doxazosin and β-blockers such as propranolol and atenolol. Therefore antihypertensives should be continued throughout the peri-operative period, with a change of formulation or substitution if needed.

Anti-arrhythmics

Most anti-arrhythmics medications are continued throughout the peri-operative period. However, if parenteral formulations are required they may need to be substituted with an anti-arrhythmic from a different class.

Diabetes

It is important to keep tight glucose control prior to elective surgery. Altered insulin and carbohydrate requirements due to fasting and surgery mean that patients need individual assessment. Oral hypoglycaemics (e.g. gliclazide, chlorpropamide, glibenclamide) should be stopped once the patient is NBM (or the day before if they are long-acting drugs) and a sliding-scale insulin regimen used. A sliding scale should also be used for insulin-dependent diabetics.

Corticosteroids

Patients who have been taking systemic glucocorticosteroids (prednisolone, dexamethasone, and hydrocortisone) for at least 3 months (or have completed a long course in the last 3 months) are at risk of an impaired reaction to stress, cardiovascular instability, delayed wound healing, and depressed immune function. An increased dose will be necessary to cover surgery to prevent an Addisonian-like collapse. Routinely it is common practice that replacement therapy is only necessary in those patients on 10mg of prednisolone daily or more.

Oral contraceptives and hormone replacement therapy (HRT)

Oral contraceptives increase the risk of post-operative venous thromboembolism. The action to be taken depends on the type of oral contraceptive being used, and the type of surgery. For minor surgery (e.g. laparoscopic sterilization or tooth extraction), or for contraceptives that do not contain oestrogen, then no action is required. Oral contraceptives containing oestrogen should be discontinued 4 weeks before major elective surgery, or surgery to the legs. Alternative contraceptive methods should also be used. For emergency surgery when this is not possible, prophylactic low-dose heparin should be considered. Current evidence suggests that progesterone-only pills need not be discontinued in the perioperative period.

HRT increases the risk of thromboembolism. However, there is little clear evidence of these risks. Patients on HRT may have additional risk factors because of their age. Therefore, thromboprophylaxis with compression hosiery is recommended for women undergoing elective surgery. In women with other risk factors for thromboembolism it may be worth temporarily stopping HRT.

Anticoagulants

Anticoagulants constitute one of the highest risk areas for medication safety. Appropriate dosing is a key issue for the use of these agents and should be used according to BNF recommendation and national guidance. There is an obvious risk of haemorrhage in patients taking warfarin. Options available include switching to heparin therapy, or for minor operations reducing the INR to 2.0 for the day of the operation. For major operations the INR may need to be less than 2.0, with continuous heparin therapy required. Specialist haematological advice is usually necessary. Aspirin and clopidogrel are usually stopped 7 days prior to surgery.

Antidepressants

Monoamine oxidase inhibitors (MAOIs) (e.g. tranylcypromine, phenelzine) should be stopped 2 weeks before surgery due to the potential for serious interactions with sympathomimetic drugs (e.g. adrenaline (epinephrine) and pethidine). The newer reversible inhibitors of monoamine type A (RIMA), such as moclobemide, are reversible after 24–48 hours.

Tricyclic antidepressants (e.g. amitriptyline, lofepramine) can be continued, but patients are at an increased risk of arrhythmias and hypotension. The effects of exogenous catecholamines (e.g. adrenaline) can be potentiated. Any withdrawal should be planned and gradual in order to prevent a relapse.

Lithium therapy can be continued for minor surgery and stopped 2 days before major surgery. Fluid and electrolytes should be monitored.

Anticonvulsants

These should be continued to enable seizure control. However, usually these drugs have induced hepatic enzyme function so that increased doses of induction agents and opiates may be needed. Some anaesthetic drugs may depress hepatic drug excretion. Close monitoring of anticonvulsants that have a low ratio of therapeutic to toxic effects is needed, e.g. phenytoin.

Anxiolytics

There is a definite risk, especially for short-acting benzodiazepines like lorazepam, of a withdrawal reaction. In addition, there may be a possible additive effect with other sedative agents used in anaesthesia, or conversely tolerance may be a problem.

Respiratory therapy

Patients with asthma or chronic obstructive pulmonary disease (COPD) require bronchodilators or corticosteroids to maintain good pulmonary function. This therapy should be continued peri-operatively.

Glaucoma therapy

Ocular therapy for glaucoma can be continued without compromising a NBM policy. You should be aware that systemic absorption of some eye drops can occur, especially with β-blockers, e.g. timolol.

Medicines affecting thyroid function

Thyroxine or antithyroid drugs should be continued if possible to avoid metabolic changes. However, thyroxine has a long half life (7 days) and may be omitted for a single day or two.

Immunosuppressants

Immunosuppressants, e.g. methotrexate and azathioprine, impair tissue healing. There is obviously a balance between risk and benefit about temporarily discontinuing these medicines peri-operatively.

Table 8.1 Oral drug therapy guidelines for surgical patients

BNF class	Drug group (examples)	Risk	Use pre-operatively when nil by mouth	Alternative post-op. if unable to take oral medication	Management
Gastrointestinal	Antispasmodics, motility stimulants (mebeverine)	Increased risk of ileus	Omit pre-operative dose		Monitor U+E
	H₂-receptor antagonists (ranitidine)	Reduce risk of acid aspiration	Give 2h pre-operatively	IV ranitidine	
	Proton-pump inhibitors (omeprazole)	Reduce risk of acid aspiration	Give 2h pre-operatively	IV ranitidine	
Cardiovascular	ACE inhibitors (ACEI) (lisinopril, enalapril)	Hypotension Renal failure Reduced cerebral blood flow	Minimum withholding time depends on ACEI (>12h captopril, >24h lisinopril). Can be continued with caution. Discuss with anaesthetist	Alt. IV antihypertensive agent/IV diuretic. Some ACE inhibitors absorbed sublingually, e.g. captopril	Monitor BP and U+E. Avoid NSAIDs
	Angiotensin II antagonists (losartan)	Hypotension Renal failure	Can be continued with caution. Discuss with anaesthetist	Alt. IV antihypertensive agent/IV diuretic	Monitor BP and U+E. Avoid NSAIDs
	Alpha-blockers (doxazosin)	Hypotension	Continue—improves C/V stability	Alt. IV antihypertensive	Monitor BP

Anti-arrhythmics	Prolong n/m block Bradycardia Reduce cardiac output	Continue	Use IV alternative within same class	ECG monitoring Monitor U+E
Anticoagulants (warfarin)	Haemorrhagic risk	*Minor:* INR 2.0 on day of op. *Major:* stop 3 days before. Aim or INR <2. High-risk patients start on continuous heparin infusion or treatment dose of LMWH. (See local haematology guidelines)	Heparin (UFH or LMWH) prophylaxis until oral intake resumed and INR within therapeutic range for 2 consecutive days	INR, APTT (if on UFH), platelet counts (>5 days UFH). Check BNF for interacting drugs
Anti-platelets (aspirin, clopidogrel, dipyridamole)	Haemorrhagic risk	Usually stop 7 days prior to surgery. Seek advice in patients with severe IHD or history CVA/TIA and coronary stents.		
Beta-blockers (atenolol, propranolol)	Hypotension Bradycardia Bronchospasm	Continue—improves C/V stability. Rebound if withdrawn	Give alt. IV β-blocker or GTN patch if patient symptomatic	Monitor BP and pulse

(continued)

Table 8.1 Oral drug therapy guidelines for surgical patients (*continued*)

BNF class	Drug group (examples)	Risk	Use pre-operatively when nil by mouth	Alternative post-op. if unable to take oral medication	Management
	Calcium-channel blockers	Hypotension Bradycardia (verapamil)	Continue	IV antihypertensive	Monitor BP and pulse
	– diltiazem, verapamil	Additive effect with enflurane, halothane			
	– dihydropyridines	Additive effect with isoflurane			
	Central-acting hypertensives (clonidine, methyldopa)	Hypotension	Rebound if withdrawn—hypertensive crisis with one missed dose. Continue		Monitor BP
	Digoxin	Increased toxicity with suxamethonium Arrhythmias	Continue	IV digoxin. Note: different routes have different bioavailabilities therefore doses may need to be adjusted	Monitor digoxin level and K+
	Diuretics— thiazide and loop (bendroflumethiazide, furosemide)	Arrhythmias Prolonged n/m block	Continue	IV diuretics	Monitor BP, fluids, U+E
	Diuretics—potassium-sparing (amiloride, spironolactone)	Tissue damage Reduced kidney perfusion Hyperkalaemia	Omit on morning of surgery	Add potassium to fluids where needed	Monitor U+E

Nitrates	Hypotension	Continue	Topical, buccal, sublingual, and IV forms available	Monitor BP
K+channel activators (nicorandil)	Hypotension	Continue	Alternative anti-anginals (see nitrates)	Monitor BP
Vasodilators (hydralazine)	Reflex tachycardia Hypotension	Continue	IV alternatives available	Monitor BP and pulse
CNS Anticonvulsants	Induce hepatic enzymes (phenytoin, barbiturates, carbamazepine) Anaesthetics may depress hepatic drug elimination Resistance to non-depolarizing muscle relaxants	Continue	Phenytoin—different routes have different bioavailabilities therefore doses may need to be adjusted	May need increased doses of induction agents and opiates. Phenytoin levels pre- and post-op.
Antipsychotics (haloperidol, thioridazine)	Sedation Arrhythmias	Continue (anti-emetic effect useful)	IV alternatives available	
Benzodiazepines (diazepam, temazepam)	Tolerance Additive effects Withdrawal syndrome	Continue	IV and rectal forms if necessary	May need lower/higher doses for sedation

(continued)

Table 8.1 Oral drug therapy guidelines for surgical patients (continued)

BNF class	Drug group (examples)	Risk	Use pre-operatively when nil by mouth	Alternative post-op. if unable to take oral medication	Management
	Lithium	Prolongs n/m blockade Toxicity	Discontinue 24–48h before major operations. Restart post-op.	Haloperidol±lorazepam in some cases	Check levels, monitor fluids and U+E. Avoid NSAIDs
	Monoamine oxidase inhibitors (MAOIs)	Hypertension, hyperthermia, convulsions, coma with opioids, esp. pethidine and sympathomimetics. Can be fatal	Stop 2 weeks before surgery. Newer reversible MAOIs are reversible after 24–48h. Psychiatric advice needed. Alternatively, use 'safe' anaesthesia. Discuss with anaesthetist	Withhold whilst on opioids	
	Tricyclic anti-depressants (TCAs)	Increase effect of exogenous catecholamines, e.g. adrenaline resulting in arrhythmias	Ideally withdraw but this may not be possible or clinically appropriate. Avoid proarrhythmic anaesthetic agents. Use reduced doses of sympathomimetic agents	Extended half-lives so can be omitted for few days	
	Selective serotonin-reuptake inhibitors (SSRIs)	Serotonin syndrome, e.g. pethidine, pentazocine	Continue until day of surgery. Omit preoperative dose. Avoid interacting agents	Extended half-lives so can be omitted for few days	

	Anti-Parkinsonian drugs	Arrhythmias Hypertension (L-dopa) Symptoms exacerbated by some anti-emetics	Continue	No IV but ng L-dopa possible. SC apomorphine may be available, but seek consultant neurologist advice	Avoid metoclopramide and prochlorperazine
Endocrine	Insulin	Increased risk of post-op. infection Altered requirements	Glucose, potassium, insulin (GKI)	GKI (see local protocol)	Monitor blood glucose and K+
	Oral hypoglycaemics (tolbutamide, gliclazide)	Peri-operative hypoglycaemia Lactic acidosis (metformin)	Minor surgery—omit on day of op. Major surgery—stop once patient NBM either on day of op. or day before if long-acting agent or metformin used	GKI for major surgery (see local protocol)	Monitor blood glucose and K+
	Corticosteroids (long-term/last 3 months)	Hypotension. Impaired stress reaction. Delayed wound healing. Altered immune function. Risk of bleeding with NSAIDs	Continue at increased dose	Increase dose to cover surgery. Dose depends on usual steroid dose, duration, indication, e.g. 25–50mg IV hydrocortisone every 6–8 hours, dependent on type of surgery	Monitor blood glucose and K+

(continued)

Table 8.1 Oral drug therapy guidelines for surgical patients (continued)

BNF class	Drug group (examples)	Risk	Use pre-operatively when nil by mouth	Alternative post-op. if unable to take oral medication	Management
	Combined oral contraceptive (COC) (oestrogen-containing)	Increased risk of DVT/PE in major surgery	Discontinue 4 weeks prior to major surgery. Progestogen-only pill is suitable alternative	Restart with first menses that occur at least 2 weeks after discharge	Thromboprophylaxis
	Progestogen-only contraceptives (includes injectables)	No added risk of thrombo-embolic risk	Continue		
	Hormone replacement therapy	Slight increased risk of DVT/PE	May be continued. If patient has other risk factors and therefore wishes to discontinue then need to stop 4 weeks prior to surgery	Restart after discharge as for COC	Thromboprophylaxis
	Thyroxine and anti-thyroid drugs (carbimazole)	Impaired stress reaction if hypothyroid	Continue	May discontinue therapy for several days due to long half-life	TFTs to ensure dose adequate
Musculoskeletal/ joint disease	NSAIDs (diclofenac, piroxicam)	GI haemorrhage Impaired wound healing Renal impairment	Stop to allow platelet recovery, 1 day prior to surgery for short-acting drugs, 3 days for long-acting	PR preps available	U+E

	Impaired wound healing Renal impairment	Stop prior to surgery	Restart once wound healed	U+E. Caution with NSAIDs
Methotrexate			Restart once wound healed	
Azathioprine	Major wound complications	Stop 3 weeks before surgery		
Topical eye preps	Bradycardia due to systemic absorption (β-blockers)	Continue		
Steroids pilocarpine, β-blockers (timolol)				

The above table is not exhaustive, although most drug groups not included in the above table can be omitted pre/peri-operatively. In all cases the anaesthetist responsible for the patient should be consulted regarding medication to be stopped prior to surgery.

Abbrev.: NBM, nil by mouth; pre-op, pre-operatively; post-op, post-operatively; U+E, urea and electrolytes; IV, intravenous; PO, orally; PR, rectally; ACE, angiotensin-converting enzyme; BP, blood pressure; NSAIDs, non-steroidal anti-inflammatory drugs; CV, cardiovascular; n/m, neuromuscular; ECG, electrocardiogram; INR, International normalized ratio; LMWH, low molecular-weight heparin; UFH, unfractionated heparin; APTT, activated partial thromboplastin time; BNF, British National Formulary; IHD, ischaemic heart disease; CVA, cerebrovascular accident; TIA, transient ischaemic attack; GTN, glyceryl trinitrate; DVT, deep vein thrombosis; PE, pulmonary embolus; TFTs, thyroid function tests; GI, gastrointestinal.

Commonly used peri-operative drugs

Opiates

Most patients who have not had opiates before suffer from nausea and vomiting, especially when ambulatory. An anti-emetic like cyclizine or prochlorperazine should be prescribed at the same time as any opiate.

- All opiates can cause respiratory depression; this is dependent on their potency and the dose used. Care should be taken in those patients with a decreased respiratory reserve.
- All opiates can also cause constipation, including codeine, so it is advisable to prescribe laxatives at the same time as opioids. A stimulant laxative such as senna and a stool softener such as sodium docusate should be used. Beware of patients with an acute abdomen as the purgative effect may result in perforation.
- All opiates can cause behavioural toxicity, particularly dysphorias. This may be a problem especially in older patients.
- Doses of opiates should be appropriate to the patient, their body weight, and any concomitant disease. All patients should be monitored for efficacy and side effects:
  - start with low doses in the elderly and debilitated patient
  - use low doses or avoid opiates in patients with renal or hepatic impairment
  - avoid the use of opiates in patients with a head injury or raised intracranial pressure (can interfere with pupilliary responses).

Anti-emetics

There are four main classes of agents used as anti-emetics: anticholinergics, antihistamines, dopamine antagonists, and 5HT3 antagonists. However, because of the many ways in which the vomiting centre can be triggered, no single medicine or class of medicine is completely effective in controlling post-operative nausea and vomiting.

Anticholinergic drugs inhibit stimulation of the vomiting centre by blocking the action of acetylcholine at the muscarinic receptors in the vestibular system. They also reduce gastric motility and afferent stimulation of the vomiting centre.

Antihistamines such as cyclizine are suitable alternatives to prochlorperazine and metoclopramide, although not as efficacious. They can cause drowsiness and often show anticholinergic side effects such as dry mouth and blurred vision.

Anti-emetics, which block central dopamine receptors (e.g. metoclopramide and prochlorperazine), can cause significant behavioural toxicity, sedation, and acute dystonic reactions. These facial and skeletal muscle spasms are more common in the young, in females, and in elderly and debilitated patients. They tend to occur soon after therapy has started. The dystonias, such as oculogyric crisis or torticollis, can be treated if severe by parenteral antimuscarinics, e.g. procyclidine or benzatropine. Other extrapyramidal side effects can occur on prolonged therapy, e.g. Parkinsonian symptoms with tremor and akathesia. 5HT3 antagonists, such as ondansetron, are useful as second- or third-line therapy in patients who cannot tolerate standard antinauseants, and they also have a specific use in cytotoxic chemotherapy. They should be considered as prophylaxis in patients known to be at risk of a decreased level of consciousness (oral surgery), or who have a history of uncontrolled post-operative nausea and vomiting.

Non-steroidal anti-inflammatory drugs (NSAIDs)

Although these medicines are devoid of the respiratory depression and drowsiness caused by opiates, and are very effective analgesics, there are specific safety concerns, especially with their long-term use.

NSAIDs cause gastric irritation and should be avoided in patients with active peptic ulceration who are at an increased risk of haemorrhage or perforation. NSAIDs are contraindicated in patients with a history of hypersensitivity (asthma, urticaria, angioedema, and rhinitis) to aspirin or other NSAIDs and in patients with inflammatory bowel disease.

Caution is required with the use of NSAIDs in patients with renal, hepatic, or cardiac impairment, as NSAIDs may cause a decrease in renal function. Patients also taking angiotensin-converting enzyme (ACE) inhibitors (e.g. captopril, enalapril, lisinopril) may be at a higher risk of renal impairment due to a drug interaction.

When used intravenously, additional contraindications include bleeding diathesis, operations with a high risk of haemorrhage, history of confirmed or suspected cerebrovascular bleeding, history of asthma, hypovolaemia, and dehydration.

NSAIDs are more effective when used regularly rather than on a PRN basis. They have a useful opiate-sparing effect and have additive effects in combination with simple analgesics such as paracetamol.

Paracetamol/opiate combinations

In order to gain maximum benefit from paracetamol it is better to use it on a regular basis rather than a 'when required' regimen. If the patient is in constant pain, paracetamol is very effective when used either as a stand-alone medicine or when used in combination with other simple analgesics or opioids.

Combinations of paracetamol with a low-dose opiate, such as dihydrocodeine and codeine, are popular as minor to moderate analgesics. However, the evidence for the efficacy of adding low-dose opiates to paracetamol is limited and controversial. Increasing the dose of opiates will of course improve efficacy and allows easy dose titration of doses but the unwanted side effects of opiates may still occur as discussed earlier.

Thromboprophylaxis

Consider appropriate therapeutic and mechanical measures to prevent deep vein thromboses (DVTs) and pulmonary embolism (PE). The use of either unfractionated heparin or low molecular weight heparin (LMWH) should be encouraged. Costs of both are approximately equal; LMWH may be slightly more effective, especially in orthopaedic surgery, and is easier to administer once a day. Thromoprophylaxis measures should be adopted in line with national guidelines, which are available from NICE and the Department of Health.

IV therapy

Correct fluid replacement is vital if a patient is NBM. However, the volume and type of fluid should be appropriate. Total volume, tonicity, and electrolyte content are important.

Requirements

For an 80kg adult this equates to 2–3 litres a day, incorporating 150mmol of sodium and 40–60mmol of potassium. This maintenance therapy can be achieved by prescribing 1 litre of sodium chloride 0.9% infused over 8 hours followed by 1–2 litres of dextrose 5% each infused over 8 hours. Both dextrose 5% and sodium chloride 0.9% are available with 20mmol/l or 40mmol/l of potassium chloride.

Prescribing

It is good practice to prescribe each individual bag of IV fluid separately on the fluid prescription chart. This forces a daily review of IV fluid therapy. IV fluids should be prescribed on the current day's chart: 'flicking' back over previous charts to find the next solution can result in adverse events. Systems that allow a prescription to cover an unlimited period of administration are inherently dangerous, and can lead to unintentional fluid overload. Fluid overload in the elderly with concomitant congestive heart failure can be fatal. Note that a number of medicines (IV and oral) contain quite large amounts of sodium, which need to be considered when calculating electrolyte requirements.

Intravenous additives

IV therapy, which involves a sealed sterilized system (i.e. a bag of infusion fluid) is generally safe and free from contamination. However, all bags should be inspected for the presence of particles or other contamination, including if the bag has crystallized or if it is a different colour from normal.

Once sealed systems are breached, e.g. by adding medicines to a bag of fluid for infusion, then microbial contamination becomes a potential problem. The physical and chemical stability of adding medicines and nutrients to infusion fluid is of key importance, and if in doubt you should always refer for confirmation of additions to pharmacy.

The guidelines are:
• Only add a medicine to an infusion if it is really necessary (i.e. constant plasma concentration required; avoidance of a high, potentially toxic plasma concentration; dilute concentration required to avoid local tissue damage).
• Always use a commercially available preparation if suitable (e.g. dopamine and potassium infusions are available premixed and sterilized).
• Use a strict aseptic technique, wash your hands, and use gloves.
• All preparations should be freshly made and used immediately.
• After adding additives, shake the infusion well. Some additives are denser than the infusion fluid and can settle unseen at the bottom of an infusion bag. This readily happens with potassium chloride solutions,

and can result in a bolus of all of the additive being infused – with potentially lethal consequences.

- After adding additives check for signs of incompatibility immediately and then periodically afterwards. Look for precipitates, colour changes, and hazy or cloudy solutions. Look in the bag and the intravenous line. Some incompatibilities are often only seen after the fluid has mixed with other fluids being infused at the same time through Y sites, for example.
- Clearly label the infusion solution with the name of the medicine, the amount added, the date and time of addition, the patient's name, and the date and time of expiry. Labels designed for this are usually available from the pharmacy.
- Always seek expert advice from the pharmacy as some medicines are inherently unstable.
- Wherever possible use a centralized intravenous additive service. Contamination of parenteral fluids is a problem from which patients still suffer morbidity and mortality.
- Total parenteral nutrition (TPN) is expensive, complicated to make, and is an ideal medium for the growth of microorganisms if contaminated. The compounding of TPN should be carried out within the pharmacy under strict aseptic conditions.
- Never add medicines to blood, albumin, colloids, mannitol solutions, sodium bicarbonate, or lipid solutions due to the risk of instability or haptan formation.
- Some IV medicines are chemically incompatible when when given together, e.g. infused through a 'Y' connector. Check with the pharmacy before running IV medicines together.

The BNF contains much useful information on this topic.

Using the oral route of administration

The IV route of administration is obviously mainly used peri-operatively. However, consider switching to oral as soon as possible. The oral route reduces the risk of adverse events, decreases the administration work-load, and reduces the cost, but is only to be used when the gut is effective. Oral and IV doses are not always interchangeable. Check with the BNF/pharmacy if unsure.

Antibiotics

Antibiotic guidelines for treatment and prophylaxis should be agreed, implemented, and subjected to regular updates and audits.

Principles of antibiotic prophylaxis

The decision regarding the benefits and risks of prophylaxis for an individual patient will depend on:
- the patient's risk of surgical site infection
- the potential severity of the consequences of surgical site infection
- the effectiveness of prophylaxis in that operation
- the consequences of prophylaxis for that patient (e.g. increased risk of *Clostridium difficile* infection).

Selection of agent should reflect professional body recommendations, local antibiotic sensitivities, drug costs, and consultant experience.
- The selected antibiotic for prophylaxis must cover common pathogens.
- Patients with a history of anaphylaxis, urticaria, or rash occurring immediately after penicillin or cephalosprin therapy are at an increased risk of immediate hypersensitivity and should not receive prophylaxis with a beta-lactam antibiotic.

In order to keep the risk of surgical site infection to a minimum antibiotic prophylaxis should be administered to ensure maximum blood and tissue levels coincide with the time of surgical incision. The timing of the first dose is crucial and should be up to 60 minutes prior to incision. An ideal time would be to give the antibiotic at the same time as the induction of anaesthesia.
- In most cases prophylactic antibiotics should be administered intravenously.
- An additional dose of antibiotic may be indicated if surgery is prolonged or there is blood loss during surgery of 1500ml or haemodilution of up to 15ml/kg.
- For most procedures requiring antibiotic prophylaxis, a single dose is satisfactory.
- Prophylaxis should not normally extend beyond 24 hours after the procedure.
- Fluid replacement bags should not be primed with prophylactic antibiotics because of the potential risk of contamination and calculation errors.

Treatment of infections
Antibiotic regimens for treatment should be:
- Targeted at the pathogens likely to cause surgical site infections.
- Chosen according to culture and sensitivity results and local sensitivity patterns for likely organisms.
- Of short duration to minimize adverse drug reactions and reduce antibiotic resistance, *Clostridium difficile* infection, and environmental exposure.
- Reviewed daily and switched to an oral equivalent at the earliest opportunity. Patients who are colonized should not be treated unless they have signs of an active infection.

Surgery altering the pharmacokinetics of medicines

Pharmacokinetics relate to the effect of the body on the drug (absorption, distribution, metabolism, and excretion). Absorption of drugs from IM injections and the gastrointestinal tract are affected by fluid balance changes, changes in gastrointestinal motility, and shifts in vascular perfusion. Fluid balance changes and shifts in vascular perfusion affect the distribution of drugs. Metabolism and excretion of medicines are affected by changes in hepatic and renal function.

Complications after specific types of surgery

Complications of gastrointestinal surgery

General principles

Gastrointestinal surgery is performed for a range of benign and malignant pathologies, in both elective and emergency settings. It is essential to appreciate the normal post-operative course for these patients and be able to detect those who are not progressing as well as they should. Whilst deterioration can be rapid and obvious, gastrointestinal-specific complications can be delayed or covert in presentation; for example anastomotic leak commonly presents between 7–10 days. A high index of suspicion is required to detect the development of complications at an early stage, and to act in a timely fashion in order to prevent the potentially disastrous sequelae of gastrointestinal complications.

Assessment of the post-operative abdomen

The commonest gastrointestinal complications are bleeding, inflammation or infection, anastomotic leak, infarction, obstruction, and perforation. The patient who is unwell after gastrointestinal surgery can seem complex to assess, and the presence of various abdominal drains, feeding tubes, and intestinal stomas can be distracting. A systematic approach is recommended:

Clinical assessment

- Airway, Breathing, Circulation. Always consider the need for simultaneous resuscitation and assessment.
- Nature of deterioration – a full history and thorough examination should enquire about any abdominal pain, the presence of vomiting or diarrhoea, and whether there is any abdominal distension. Establish if there is pyrexia and whether it has a pattern. Relate any confusion to early sepsis or cardiorespiratory compromise, and establish whether there is hypotension, tachycardia, or hypoxia.
- Duration of deterioration – this needs to be related to the nature and date of surgery and whether there is an anastomosis. At the same time, consider any relevant cardiac, respiratory, or hepatic disease. Review the case notes, the nursing record, and operation note as soon as the patient's condition is stable and permits, including post-operative instructions and observations and recent progress. Review any medication; specifically, has the patient continued to receive their usual medication, e.g. cardiac drugs if 'nil by mouth', antibiotics, anti-thrombotic measures, or steroids (which can further mask abdominal signs)?
- Observation charts – systematically look for:
  - temperature – persistently raised, spiking, hypothermia
  - tachycardia
  - tachypnoea
  - hypotension
  - oliguria
  - the fluid balance chart, including drain output and naso-gastric losses.
- Ask yourself does the patient have systemic inflammatory response syndrome (SIRS), which is comprised of two of the following:
  - temperature >38°C or <36°C
  - heart rate >90 beats/min
  - respiratory rate >20 breaths/min
  - white blood cell count >12 $\times$ 10^9/l or <4 $\times$ 10^9/l or >10% immature neutrophils.

- From the initial assessment, assess if the patient is pale (blood loss), diaphoretic (pyrexia, shock), dehydrated, oedematous (sepsis, malnourished), or in pain. General examination of the whole patient must also be undertaken to assess co-morbidity or the early signs of organ dysfunction. This should include the cardiovascular and respiratory systems, and the abdomen.
- If there is a naso-gastric tube, ask yourself if it is necessary at all if drainage or aspirate is minimal. If aspirates are persistent, measure their volumes and assess if they are bloodstained, bilious, or faeculent.
- If there are abdominal drains determine where they are placed and what they are intended to drain. Refer to the operation note. Assess the volume of fluid in the drain and the rate of loss of fluid (especially blood). Assess the nature of drain fluid – blood, bile, faeces (anastomotic leak).
- Review any stomas – are they well perfused or ischaemic; has the stoma functioned yet?
- Examine any wounds for cellulitis and whether they are healing satisfactorily. If a wound is discharging haemoserous fluid, consider the 'pink sign' of impending wound dehiscence. If dark red 'blood' is discharging consider a liquefying haematoma. Pus signifies an infected wound where infection is being localized. Bowel contents leaking from a wound or drain may indicate a fistula.
- Abdominal tenderness in the post-operative period is difficult to interpret, except in the case of generalized peritonitis. Pain and tenderness near recent incisions are a distracting factor. Do not routinely withhold analgesia before examining the abdomen. However, an epidural can mask peritoneal irritation – if in doubt, turn it off. In the paralysed, ventilated patient on ITU, abdominal tenderness is clearly absent and other signs have to be relied on (pulse, bowel sounds, etc.).
- Listen for bowel sounds; their absence suggests paralytic ileus or peritonitis. They may be normal but if hyperdynamic there may be obstruction. A succussion splash may indicate there is gastric dilatation, which needs urgent decompression to prevent the risk of aspiration.
- Undertake a rectal examination with extreme caution if there is a recent colorectal anastomosis. Is the rectum empty or impacted? Is there melaena, pelvic tenderness (pelvic abscess), or disruption of a low anastomosis?
- Consider the need for a higher level of care (HDU/ITU) if there is impending or actual organ failure. Reassess the patient frequently for evolution of new signs and response to treatment.
- Make a definitive plan of action.
- Consider the need for an early return to theatre or further appropriate investigations.
- Communication is vital – involve senior staff, nurses, and the patient's relatives early.

Investigations

Biochemical
- plasma urea and creatinine (raised in dehydration or renal failure)
- plasma sodium/potassium/chloride (low if excessive GI losses through diarrhoea, vomiting, or NG tube losses)
- arterial blood gas analysis (metabolic impact of fluid loss or sepsis)
  - metabolic acidosis (poor perfusion/tissue ischaemia) – in proportion to base deficit
  - metabolic alkalosis (vomiting – acid losses)
- high lactate (poor perfusion or tissue ischaemia) – needs aggressive resuscitation if >4mmol/l
- drain fluid analysis
  - amylase (in pancreatic fistula the amylase level is greater than three times the serum amylase activity)
  - electrolytes (in a urinary fistula there is low sodium, <20mmol/l, and a raised urea and creatinine).

Haematological
- haemoglobin level (may be preserved in acute haemorrhage)
- white cell count (total and differential)
  - normal transient rise after surgery (<13 × 10^9/l)
  - WCC above 20 × 10^9/l (consider gut infarction)
- coagulation
  - disseminated intravascular coagulopathy (DIC) in sepsis (low platelets/low fibrinogen/high thrombin time/high prothrombin time/ high APTT/raised fibrinogen degradation products or D-dimers). This needs correction before reoperation or therapeutic radiology
- C-reactive protein – normal transient rise post-surgery (inflammation). Trends are more use than absolute value but a sustained level >150mg/ ml implies significant complications.

Microbiological
- cultures of sputum, urine, blood, faeces, and wound or drain fluid may be relevant in sepsis or if there is a persistent pyrexia
- have cultures taken at time of surgery or earlier been appropriately reviewed and considered in treatment?

Radiological
- chest X-ray (a pneumoperitoneum may be normal up to 5 days after laparotomy) but high index of suspicion should be maintained
- abdominal X-rays are of little value in the post-operative period
- ultrasound:
  - user dependent, dynamic modality
  - areas of interest may be obscured by dressings/bowel gas
  - there is 43% sensitivity and 100% specificity in post-operative abdominal abscess.

- CT scan:
  - 93% sensitive and 100% specific for intra-abdominal collections
  - oral contrast of value in distinguishing ileus/obstruction (a cut-off point may be seen with the latter)
  - rectal contrast can be used in diagnosis or determining extent of colorectal anastomotic leaks.
- a radiolabelled white cell scan is occasionally helpful in localizing occult infection that cross-sectional imaging has failed to locate (100% sensitive and 73% specific)
- contrast studies – gastrograffin swallow or enema to confirm anastomotic integrity
- fistulography can delineate the anatomy of proximal and distal bowel before reconstruction of an entero-cutaneous fistula.

Post-operative pyrexia – investigation and management

(📖 See Chapter 2 Infection, p.29.)

Pyrexia demands careful evaluation as it can accompany potentially serious complications. Careful physical examination invariably reveals the cause of fever supported by judicious microbiological and radiological investigation.

There is little role for blind antibiotic treatment in the absence of a diagnosis unless the patient remains unwell and cultures have been obtained. Treat the patient not the fever.

Early causes (<48 hours)

Pyrexia in the first 12–24 hours can be a physiological response to tissue trauma. This is particularly the case if localized infection has been disturbed or an inflammatory mass resected.

- Basal atelectasis of the chest is the commonest cause in the early post-operative period and is prevented by early mobilization and chest physiotherapy.
- Malignant hyperpyrexia is a rare but important cause of immediate pyrexia and is caused by volatile anaesthetic agents in susceptible patients.
- A transfusion reaction should also be considered where blood has been administered.

Late causes (>48 hours)

- Pulmonary consolidation (consider atypical infections if immunocompromised).
- Breach in skin defences (IV cannulas, epidural site, central line/Hickman line).
- Urinary infection after prolonged bladder catheterization.
- Abdominal wound cellulitis or abscess. Don't forget concealed wounds such as perineal and thoracic wounds.
- Intra-abdominal collections must be considered (pelvic abscess, subphrenic abscess, liver abscess, infected haematoma at the operative site, foreign body, or retained swab).
- Anastomotic leak (exclude by water soluble contrast study or CT).
- Biliary cholangitis or acalculous cholecystitis.
- Enteric infection (*C. difficile* or vancomycin-resistant *Enterococci*).
- Thrombophlebitis, deep vein thrombosis, or pulmonary embolism.
- Infective endocarditis (particularly after prolonged central venous cannulation).
- Sinusitis – (after prolonged NG placement).
- Certain malignancies can give rise to pyrexia.

Investigation of post-operative fever

- Microbiological – culture all potential sources of infection:
  - urine
  - sputum
  - wound
  - drain fluid
  - stool
  - blood – peripheral and central catheter sampling.
- Radiological – consider:
  - CXR
  - abdominal CT
  - radiolabelled white cell scan
  - echocardiography
  - deep venous ultrasonography.
- Re-look laparotomy (without undue delay) may ultimately be required if there is ongoing concern.

Management of bleeding

Intra-operative bleeding during the course of gastrointestinal resection varies from troublesome oozing to life-threatening haemorrhage. The mesentery may be thickened as a result of the disease process, for example in Crohn's disease, increasing the risk of bleeding. Knowledge of arterial and venous anatomical variation with an awareness of the 'danger areas' encountered during dissection limit unexpected blood loss.

Intra-operative bleeding

Pelvic bleeding

Sites
- lateral pelvic sidewall or internal iliac branches
- prostatic
- presacral venous plexus.

Control
- suture (for example iliac vessel repair or internal iliac ligation)
- diathermy (use caution near pelvic nerves or ureter)
- argon plasma coagulation (APC) for pelvic sidewall or prostatic bleeding
- Presacral bleeding is particularly difficult to control and can result in several litres of blood loss. Suture and diathermy are rarely effective. Options in this situation are the use of sterile pins or tacks pushed into the sacrum to tamponade the space, or to pack the pelvis with wide ribbon gauze for 48 hours.

Splenic bleeding

Causes
- mobilization of the splenic flexure of the colon
- subtotal gastrectomy
- distal pancreatectomy.

The greater omentum is adherent to the lower pole of the spleen and traction on this can lead to capsular bleeding.

Control
- direct pressure
- haemostatic gauze
- fibrin glue
- diathermy
- splenectomy should be a last resort because of the risk of overwhelming post-splenectomy infection (OPSI).

Post-operative bleeding

Intraluminal

Anastomotic bleeding may be managed expectantly but is more likely to need direct suture if accessible (and recognized before closure).

Gastroduodenal ulceration

Stress response or the use of NSAIDs are the commonest causes and early gastroscopy and endotherapy is essential for bleeding control:
- injection of adrenaline and saline
- heater probe
- endoclipping.

Surgery for failure of endoscopic therapy or re-bleeding can be a challenging operation:
- underunning of the bleeding vessel
- partial gastrectomy.

Intra-abdominal

Occult blood loss such as intra-abdominal bleeding from the operative field can present with unexplained tachycardia and oliguria. Late signs are hypotension and abdominal distension. This will invariably require an expeditious re-exploration to control the bleeding.

Pelvic bleeding can lead to the formation of a haematoma. This can present later as a pelvic abscess if infection ensues, and is thought to be a leading cause of colorectal anastomotic leak following erosion through the suture line.

Paralytic ileus

After surgery there is a delay in return to normal bowel function. Generally there is gastric stasis for <24 hours, small bowel ileus for 2–3 days, and a colonic ileus for 4–5 days. Traditionally patients had oral intake withheld until passage of flatus, heralding resolution of ileus. There is little evidence to support this practice and patients are increasingly encouraged to take oral fluids and diet. Enhanced recovery programmes that include epidural anaesthesia, early mobilization, and avoidance of opiates have done much to ameliorate the problem of paralytic ileus. A small proportion of patients do not tolerate early feeding and develop paralytic ileus, which can be prolonged. It is usually diagnosed more than 48 hours after laparotomy.

Clinical features

- Absence of abdominal pain.
- No passage of flatus.
- Abdominal distension.
- Vomiting – often effortless with high output naso-gastric aspirates if an NG tube is in place. Early placement of a naso-gastric tube helps to reduce the risk of aspiration.
- Respiratory compromise if abdomen is tympanic.
- Bowel sounds are usually absent.

Risk factors for post-operative paralytic ileus

- duration of surgery
- peritonitis
- open versus laparoscopic approach
- excessive saline infusion, third space sequestration, and mesenteric oedema
- opiate analgesia
- post-operative immobility
- electrolyte disturbances (hypokalaemia, hyponatraemia, hypomagnesaemia)
- uraemia
- hypoproteinaemia

The predominant cause of prolonged ileus is persistent peritoneal sepsis or an anastomotic microleak, which is probably under-diagnosed.

Management

Treatment of the precipitating cause usually leads to spontaneous resolution. This involves intravenous fluid resuscitation with electrolyte correction and prompt naso-gastric decompression, particularly if gastric dilatation is suspected. Plain radiographs of the abdomen are of little value but may exclude acute gastric dilatation.

If there is concern that the patient may have mechanical obstruction (colicky pain and hyperdynamic bowel sounds) or an anastomotic leak, then a CT scan with positive oral gastrograffin aqueous contrast is of value. The oral contrast may have a stimulating effect and resolve the ileus.

Consideration of nutritional support should be made if ileus is prolonged for 5 days, or earlier if the patient is malnourished and there are other complications that may delay recovery.

Nutritional support

(📖 See Chapter 5, Complications of nutrition, p.99.)

The enteral route of feeding is always preferable if the gut is accessible and functioning. Enteral nutrition modifies antibacterial host defences, blunts the metabolic response to trauma, and maintains gut mucosal mass, gut barrier function, and normal enteric flora. Enterocytes derive their nutrients directly from the lumen, particularly in the case of glutamine. Signs of inadequate function includes abdominal distension, vomiting, and large naso-gastric aspirates. There may be some benefit in even low volume feed rate (30ml/hr for example) in these circumstances. Use of prokinetics and agents such as metoclopramide to promote gastric emptying may assist this aim. Patients must be carefully monitored and fed upright because of the risks of feed aspiration. This risk can be reduced by post-pyloric, nasojejunal feeding via a specific tube placed at laparotomy. Similarly (routine after oesophagectomy), a feeding jejunostomy can be placed so that enteric feeding can commence immediately after surgery. Complications of this technique include tube displacement with leakage of feed into the peritoneal cavity and failure of the tract to close upon removal.

It is now accepted practice that it is safe to feed patients in the presence of a newly created anastomosis without an increase in complication rates or anastomotic dehiscence. An exception would be upper GI anastomoses (for example oesophago-gastric) where more caution is currently exercised.

As a general rule, patients not established on enteral feeding 5 days after gastrointestinal surgery must be considered for parenteral support. If TPN is anticipated to be used for less than 2 weeks then peripheral parenteral nutrition is more appropriate than obtaining central venous access with its attendant complications. Fewer calories and nitrogen can be supplied by the peripheral route. Neither technique is as successful as enteric feeding, which should be instituted as soon as possible.

Anastomotic leak

Presentation may be subtle with extra-intestinal signs but a high index of suspicion is required to avoid delay in diagnosis.

Clinical features

- 'failure to progress', lethargy, anorexia
- cardiac dysfunction – atrial fibrillation, dysrhythmia, hypotension, or circulatory collapse
- respiratory signs – dyspnoea or tachypnoea
- fever
- prolonged ileus, abdominal distension, or hiccups
- high WCC and CRP
- low albumin
- metabolic acidosis.

Risk factors

- poor blood supply to the anastomosis
- tension at the anastomosis
- distal obstruction
- imprecise surgical technique
- poor nutrition
- steroids
- local infection or haematoma.

Oesophageal leak

Presentation

Respiratory decline, pleural effusion or atrial fibrillation, and SIRS.

Diagnosis

Can be made on CXR, water-soluble contrast swallow, or endoscopy showing necrosis of the conduit.

Types

Subclinical and locally contained; or uncontained with conduit necrosis. A stable patient needs a chest drain, nil by mouth, retention of the naso-gastric tube (do not replace it if it has been removed as the anastomosis may be further disrupted), broad-spectrum antibiotics and antifungals, and a feeding jejunostomy.

An unstable patient needs surgery:

- diversion-cervical oesophagostomy, closure of gastric remnant, and drainage of the mediastinum and pleura
- consider placing a percutaneous T-tube into the anastomotic defect to create a controlled fistula. Ensure enteral nutrition is addressed through a feeding jejunostomy.

Pancreatic leak or fistula

This is defined as a drain output of any measurable volume of fluid on or after post-operative day 3 with an amylase content greater than three times the serum amylase activity. Also, a collection may be seen on CT scan and there may be SIRS.

Most settle with conservative management (nutrition via feeding jejunostomy, CT-guided drainage, pancreatic suppression). The need for reoperation is rare. Prophylactic use of somatostatin analogues does not prevent a pancreatic fistula, although it may have benefit in an established fistula. Routine drainage of the pancreatic stump does not prevent post-operative abdominal collections. Pancreatic duct stenting does not prevent fistula formation.

Colorectal leak

There are usually early signs and symptoms of loose bowel action with increased frequency or incontinence with distension but the leak may be covert. Abdominal pain may relate to local or generalized peritonitis, usually with sepsis.

Types

- Subclinical, where there is a radiological detection of leak in the absence of abdominal signs or symptoms. This usually occurs in the presence of a proximal diverting stoma and is discovered on routine contrast enema prior to stomal closure.
- Clinical leak, when there are signs of peritonitis, abscess, sepsis, or faecal discharge from the drain or wound.

There is evidence from large meta-analyses that mechanical bowel preparation may be unnecessary prior to colorectal resection as the incidence of anastomotic leak is the same. Bowel preparation does not prevent anastomotic leak but may mitigate against its consequences. Similarly there is no evidence that early enteral feeding increases the risk of anastomotic disruption.

Management

Intraperitoneal anastomosis (colo-colic/ileo-colic)

When there is an unstable patient with peritonitis, resuscitation is needed with reoperation at which the anastomosis is taken down with proximal stoma formation and peritoneal lavage.

In low grade sepsis and localized peritonitis confirmed on CT scan or contrast enema, percutaneous drainage of a perianastomotic abscess may be possible. If an intraperitoneal free leak is identified then operation is advisable.

Subclinical leaks can be managed conservatively and abscesses <3cm may be treated successfully with broad spectrum antibiotics.

Extraperitoneal leak (colorectal/coloanal pelvic anastomosis)

Patients with generalized peritonitis and septic shock need resuscitation and surgery to take down the anastomosis. Stable patients with minimal sepsis and CT scan and/or water-soluble contrast enema evidence of a leak may be treated conservatively. Patients with a pelvic abscess should have proximal diversion and abscess drainage, but the latter may be possible either radiologically or at examination under anaesthetic (EUA).

Management of the open abdomen

In cases of severe intra-abdominal sepsis it may be preferable to leave the abdominal cavity open, as one would in treatment of other abscesses (laparostomy). Alternatives are abdominal closure with either planned re-look laparotomy at 48 hours to drain further sepsis or confirm bowel viability, or 'on-demand' laparotomy only if clinically indicated. A multi-centre study of these two techniques suggests that on demand laparotomy is preferable in terms of costs with no difference in mortality.

Indications for laparostomy
• Inability to close the abdomen primarily.
• Gross peritoneal contamination.
• Abdominal compartment syndrome.
• Planned second look procedure.

Methods of coverage of intra-abdominal contents
• Saline soaked gauze roll.
• Abdominal wound manager device.
• The Bogota bag is a sterile 3 litre saline bag cut to size to contain mobile viscera and sutured to wound edges.
• Mesh coverage can incorporate an absorbable mesh (Vicryl) or Gore-tex-coated non-absorbable mesh or porcine collagen (Permacol).
• Vacuum-assisted closure (negative pressure therapy (NPT)).

Most surgeons initially use a temporary coverage technique (gauze roll/Bogota bag) and convert to a longer-term coverage method (mesh or NPT) once the bowel is protected by a fibrinous coat or granulation tissue.

There are reports of small bowel fistulation following early application of negative pressure wound devices, although these may be related to the initial injury or procedure. It is recommended to use polyvinylalcohol (PVA) foam or polyethylene sheet to protect the bowel before placement of the standard sponge dressings and use of NPT.

Enterocutaneous fistula

Post-operative intestinal fistulas, defined as drainage of intestinal contents for >48hrs through a wound or drain, are more common than fistulas arising from diseased bowel.

Causes
- unrecognized intestinal injury
- breakdown of enterotomy repair
- breakdown of anastomosis
- breakdown of exposed bowel in a laparostomy wound.

Risk factors
- malnutrition
- immunocompromised state
- peritonitis
- previous surgery.

Management

Resuscitation
Patients are often unwell as a result of sepsis and fluid depletion and may need basic ABC resuscitation, with high inspired oxygen and IV fluid resuscitation (with 0.9% saline with added potassium). Strict fluid balance is needed with accurate fluid balance monitoring, which may need to be on HDU/ITU.

Wound care is needed to protect the skin against excoriation. Microbiological sampling of blood cultures and swabs may help with antibiotic therapy if indicated.

Restitution – remember the acronym 'SNAP'

Sepsis
An intra-abdominal abscess is associated with a high mortality if it is left untreated. All patients should have an abdominal CT scan to exclude an intra-abdominal collection if it is suspected. If present this should be drained, preferably using an interventional radiology technique, or surgically if necessary.

Nutrition
Malnutrition is also associated with high mortality. High fistula output and persistent sepsis exacerbates malnutrition. Vitamin, mineral, and trace element deficiencies commonly coexist, for example magnesium, zinc, cobalt, vitamin C, vitamin B12, folate, and iron.

If the gut is available for normal absorption of enteral feeds, such as in low output distal fistulas, then the enteral route is always preferable. This can be given as normal diet, naso-gastric feeding, elemental diet, or low residue diet. Even in proximal fistulas the gut can be used – fistuloclysis is feeding distal to a fistula through intubation of the distal limb of a fistula if it can be identified. If the patient cannot be fed enterally then total parenteral nutrition is needed. This must supply all energy, protein, lipid, electrolyte, and mineral requirements. If TPN is needed for greater than 2 weeks a dedicated offset Hickman or Broviac line is required to the risk of catheter infection and the risk of bacteraemia. It is vital that intra-abdominal sepsis is controlled as nutrition will not be effective in the face of an ongoing catabolic negative nitrogen state.

*A*natomy

Contrast studies can be performed once the patient is stable to define the anatomy of the fistula and the condition of the proximal and distal gut. The aims are to define an associated abscess cavity and exclude distal obstruction. This can be achieved by direct fistulograms, barium follow through, or barium enema/retrograde enema via a stoma. A distal loop may be identified for fistuloclysis.

*P*lan

It can be predicted whether the fistula will close by conservative or surgical measures. Spontaneous closure of a post-operative fistula is likely if there is:
- no distal obstruction
- no diseased bowel
- no abscess or foreign body
- no muco-cutaneous continuity.

Adverse factors include persistent sepsis, duration of the fistula for >6 weeks despite TPN, diseased bowel at the fistula site (for example Crohn's disease or cancer), an initial fistula output of >1 litre/day, and a complex rather than a simple fistula. There is no good evidence that somatostatin or its analogue octreotide promotes closure of a post-operative fistula.

Reconstruction

Closure of a fistula should be seen as an elective operation; attempts to resect a fistula when the patient is nutritionally replete or septic is associated with high mortality. Entry to the peritoneal cavity before 6 months is extremely difficult because of adhesions. When the fistula prolapses it is a good indication that the peritoneal cavity has been re-established. Resection and end to end anastomosis restores continuity. Abdominal closure is essential but may be difficult if the patient has previously had an open abdomen. Use of mass abdominal wall closure is recommended although mesh closure or laparostomy may occasionally be required.

Rehabilitation

It is essential to maintain the morale of the patient, their family, and the nursing staff during this prolonged treatment.

Short bowel syndrome

Short bowel syndrome is defined as an insufficient length of functioning gut to allow adequate absorption. The severity of malabsorption depends on the length of remaining small bowel and whether the colon is in continuity. Requirements for water, electrolytes, and nutrition vary from oral supplementation to total dependency on a parenteral route of administration.

High output stoma is defined as a loss greater than 1 litre per day. The fluid is electrolyte rich, often containing 100mmol/l sodium along with potassium and magnesium. Patients can rapidly become dehydrated to the point of pre-renal failure. Thirst is stimulated and ingestion of hypotonic water promulgates the stomal output.

Types of short bowel syndrome

- Jejunum-colon type – following jejuno-ileal resection with jejunocolic anastomosis.
- Jejuno-ileal type – following jejunal resection, >10cm terminal ileum remaining, colon remains.
- End jejunostomy – following jejunum/ileum/colon removal.

Patients who have jejunum-colon short bowel syndrome have steatorrhoea and diarrhoea and develop incipient malnutrition, whereas patients with a jejunostomy may have severe water and electrolyte disturbances from the outset.

Causes leading to short bowel syndrome

- ischaemia – extensive after superior mesenteric artery thrombosis resection
- Crohn's disease
- radiation enteritis
- adhesions/volvulus
- adjuvant chemotherapy in the presence of an ileostomy/jejunostomy can induce high output losses.

Clinical features

- weight loss
- dehydration/pre-renal failure/postural hypotension
- malnourishment
- diarrhoea
- steatorrhoea
- lethargy or tinnitus related to hyponatraemia
- 'cramps' or tetany related to hypomagnesaemia.

Management

This requires early parenteral replacement of fluid and electrolyte deficit. Patients can lose 100mmol/l sodium and 15mmol/l potassium in the jejunostomy/ileostomy fluid. Initial resuscitation needs 0.9% saline (as much as 2–4 litres in the first 24 hours may be needed). There should be accurate fluid balance with measurement of weight daily.

Nil by mouth should be instigated for 24–48 hours if there is severe dehydration whilst deficits are corrected parenterally. Thereafter oral intake of hypotonic fluid should be restricted to 0.5l per day as this may increase stomal sodium losses. Oral fluid should be electrolyte rich, such as an oral rehydration solution (ORS) or St Mark's solution.

ORS	St Mark's solution
Sodium 90mmol/l	Sodium chloride 3.5g/l (60mmol/l)
Potassium 20mmol/l	Sodium bicarbonate 2.5g/l (30mmol/l)
Chloride 80mmol/l	Glucose 20g/l (110mmol/l)
Citrate 10mmol/l	
Glucose 111 mmol/l	

Plasma sodium, potassium, and magnesium need regular monitoring with the urinary sodium kept above 20mmol/l. A low residue or low fibre diet can be given to help thicken the effluent.

Other causes of high output, such as intra-abdominal sepsis, partial bowel obstruction, infective enteritis, recurrent disease (particularly Crohn's disease), sudden drug withdrawal (opiates, steroids), and use of prokinetic drugs need to be excluded.

Drug treatment

- Titrate loperamide (2–4mg 1 hour before meals four times a day; higher dosage has been suggested) and codeine phosphate (30–60mg up to four times a day) to reduce output.
- Proton pump inhibitors (for example omeprazole 80mg/day) can reduce gastric secretions.
- Octreotide 50–200µg given subcutaneously three times a day to reduce gastric/biliary/pancreatic secretions.
- Cholestyramine can reduce diarrhoea due to bile salt malabsorption.

Regular electrolyte estimations guide resuscitation. Once the patient is rehydrated and the stoma output normalized, fluid restriction can be relaxed and parenteral fluid discontinued.

- Aim for a stoma output of <2 litres/day, a urine output of >1 litre/day, urinary sodium >20mmol/l, and magnesium 0.7–1mmol/l.
- Treat hypomagnesaemia with oral magnesium oxide, 12–24 mmol/day.
- Trace element replacement needs to be monitored and replaced, particularly selenium.
- Remember to give vitamin B12 injections, also vitamins A, D, E, and K.

Nutritional assessment (⊞ See Chapter 5 Complications of nutrition, p.99.)

A BMI <18.5, weight loss >10%, and mid-arm muscle circumference of <19cm in women and <22cm in men indicates significant malnutrition.

Nutritional support

Jejunal length (cm)	Jejunum-colon	Jejunostomy
0–50	Parenteral nutrition	PN and parenteral saline
51–100	Oral nutrition	PN and parenteral saline
101–150	None	Oral nutrition and oral glucose/saline
151–200	None	Oral glucose/saline solution

Adhesions

Peritoneal adhesions are an inevitable consequence of abdominal surgery. Over 90% of patients develop adhesions following surgery, although not all are symptomatic. Adhesions are responsible for 75% of cases of small bowel obstruction and a 5% five-year readmission rate after surgery. They are also thought to cause chronic abdominal and pelvic pain and be a cause of female infertility. There is no accurate diagnostic test for adhesions besides inference from small bowel obstruction.

Causes
- congenital (band adhesion)
- surgical trauma-denuded peritoneal membrane
- foreign body reaction – starch on gloves, lint from swabs, suture material
- peritoneal blood

Prevention
- good surgical technique to minimize tissue trauma with meticulous haemostasis
- laparoscopic surgery
- there is no good evidence for routine use of anti-adhesion barriers at present, although these are in widespread use.

Treatment
Small bowel obstruction
- Resolution by conservative treatment is usual.
- Resuscitation, intravenous rehydration, electrolyte correction.
- Naso-gastric tube with free drainage and 4-hourly aspiration (to exclude the risk of aspiration).
- Give 200ml dilute water-soluble contrast on admission. This is a good predictive test of likely resolution by conservative treatment if it enters the colon by 24 hours.
- Indications for surgery: tachycardia, raised inflammatory markers, abdominal tenderness, and failure of conservative management (48 hours is the usual allowed time).
- Laparoscopic division of adhesional small bowel obstruction has been reported and shown to be safe.

Chronic abdominal pain or intermittent obstructive symptoms after previous surgery
After radiological imaging has excluded other pathology it may be appropriate to perform a diagnostic laparoscopy with division of adhesions if they are found; however, this approach may be no more beneficial than diagnostic laparoscopy alone.

Enteric infections

Any patient who has post-operative diarrhoea must have an infective cause excluded, particularly *Clostridium difficile*-associated diarrhoea (CDAD).

Symptoms

- watery green, offensive-smelling diarrhoea
- fever, anorexia, malaise
- 'cramping' abdominal pain.

Risk factors

Elderly patients, particularly after a long hospital stay, are most at risk. There is usually a history of multiple antibiotic use and lengthy or multiple courses (any broad spectrum antibiotic can be responsible, particularly cephalosporins, fluroquinolones, and clindamycin). The presence of an NG tube or anti-ulcer medication (non-acidic pH) is also typical.

Complications

- pseudomembranous colitis
- toxic megacolon
- colonic perforation
- death.

Diagnosis

This is made by stool culture – specific for *C. difficile* enterotoxin A/cytotoxin B (enzyme immunoassay). At endoscopy or rigid sigmoidoscopy pseudomembranes may be seen (this risks perforation and is not recommended). An abdominal radiograph may show toxic megacolon in severe cases or free peritoneal gas if there is a perforation.

Treatment

- Stop unnecessary antibiotics.
- Urgent attention to fluid and electrolyte balance, and hydration.
- Early isolation with cohort nursing of infected cases.
- Avoid anti-diarrhoeal agents.
- If symptomatic (severe diarrhoea) treat with oral metronidazole or vancomycin.
- Surgery (subtotal colectomy) is indicated if megacolon or perforation develops.

Prevention

- Good antibiotic prescribing practices with short courses and avoidance of broad spectrum prescribing are crucial. There is some evidence that probiotics prevent infection.
- Avoidance of transmission – source isolation, with appropriate infection control through hand hygiene (washing, not alcohol gel), gloves and aprons, and adequate environmental cleaning need to be instituted.

Surgical site infection (SSI)

This is covered in an earlier chapter (📖 see Chapter 2, Infection, p.29). However, the possibility of synergistic or necrotizing wound infection needs special mention as it is more common after GI surgery. It presents as a rapidly spreading cellulitis, later developing necrotic patches within. It is usually due to the synergistic actions of microaerophilic non-haemolytic *Streptococci* with anaerobes. Infection spreads along fascial planes but not usually through them. Thrombosis within subcutaneous vessels is pathognomic and limits penetration of antibiotics. The patient often has signs of toxaemia out of proportion to simple cellulitis.

Early recognition is essential and may need early admission to ITU for monitoring and organ dysfunction support. The treatment is immediate surgical debridement back to healthy bleeding tissues. An aggressive initial debridement is often life-saving. Broad spectrum antibiotics should be instituted and fresh tissue sent for culture. The wounds should be assessed under anaesthetic on a daily basis and debrided further as required. Skin grafts may be necessary once the infection has resolved. The use of hyperbaric oxygen is controversial.

Intra-abdominal abscess

Radiological drainage of deeper intra-abdominal collections where feasible is preferable to open drainage (CT/USS guided). Anastomotic leak as a cause of intra-abdominal abscess needs early recognition and management with reoperation and drainage if inaccessible by interventional radiology.

Burst abdomen

Burst abdomen should be seen much less commonly in modern surgical practice now that mass closure of laparotomy wounds with synthetic polymer, non-absorbable, monofilament sutures is used (although success with synthetic polymer absorbables has also been shown). It is recommended that a suture length four times the length of the wound is used (Jenkin's rule). Burst abdomen presents on day 6–10 with a serosanguinous discharge from the wound followed by complete all-layer dehiscence with prolapse of bowel through the wound. The serosanguinous discharge is often present as a precursor and its appearance should suggest the removal of 1–2 skin clips or sutures and gentle exploration of the wound with a sterile glove on the ward to ensure underlying abdominal wall is intact. The skin may remain intact without prolapse, but if treated conservatively without resuture a full length incisional hernia is likely to result.

Risk factors

This is viewed by many as a technical failure but certain patients are more at risk, such as those with:
- malnutrition
- malignancy
- abdominal distension
- wound infection
- diabetes
- steroid use.

Management

Cover the bowel with moistened gauze packs and arrange an early return to the operating theatre to close the wound. Localized closure with single sutures almost inevitably fails as the underlying cause affects the full wound length. The most reliable methods for closure include the interrupted near-and-far technique with heavy nylon in addition to conventional mass closure suture (💭 see Figs. 9.1 and 9.2) or if too much tension is present, a mesh may be required as used in abdominal compartment syndrome. Deep tension sutures with plastic tube collars are generally to be avoided if possible due to the damage they cause to the skin.

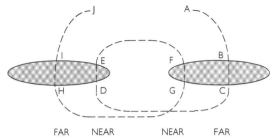

FAR   NEAR   NEAR   FAR

Fig. 9.1 Technique of Cardiff repair (transverse section).

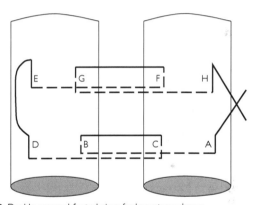

Fig. 9.2 Double near-and-far technique for laparotomy closure.

Abdominal compartment syndrome

This is defined as a sustained increase in intra-abdominal pressure (IAP >20mmHg) associated with new organ dysfunction.

Measurement

Measuring IAP is simple using the transvesical pressure by connecting a urinary catheter to a transducer after instillation of 25ml saline. As with central venous pressure the observation of trends in value is more informative than individual readings.

Diagnosis is based on more than three of:
- IAP >20mmHg
- pCO_2 >45mmHg
- increase in airway pressure with a decrease in tidal volume
- sudden drop in urine output.

Causes

- visceral oedema
- paralytic ileus
- ascites
- retroperitoneal haematoma
- pneumoperitoneum.

Management principles

These involve serial monitoring of IAP with optimization of systemic perfusion and organ function. Appropriate medical procedures to reduce IAP and end-organ consequences of ACS should be instituted with prompt surgical decompression for refractory intra-abdominal hypertension.

Medical treatment

Improve abdominal wall compliance by:
- Sedation/analgesia; neuromuscular blockade; supine body positioning.
- Naso-gastric decompression and decompression of colonic pseudo-obstruction if present.
- Prokinetic agents such as metoclopromide or erythromycin.
- Drainage of any intra-abdominal fluid collection.
- Correct positive fluid balance by fluid restriction, diuretics, colloids, and if necessary haemofiltration.

Surgical treatment

This involves a technique of open abdomen followed by a temporary closure. This is often best achieved by a Bogota bag-type approach as early closure of the abdomen when the problem has eased is the aim. Alternatively a mesh can be sewn into the wound edges to decompress the abdomen followed by surgical repair when the condition has resolved. The use of vacuum assisted closure (negative pressure therapy) of the abdominal wall wound can aid in recovery and make later closure easier.

Complications of laparoscopic surgery

Classification
- Access or trocar-related injuries.
- Pathophysiological due to pneumoperitoneum, CO_2 insufflation, or patient position.
- Energy source or specific procedure-related complications.

Access or trocar-related injuries
The two main forms of abdominal access are Veress needle or open (sometimes called the Hasson) techniques. It is important to realize that both methods can result in a visceral injury. The early recognition of such an injury, particularly to the small or large bowel, allows repair either laparoscopically or by open conversion, and minimizes the consequences of injury. A major vascular injury necessitates immediate conversion leaving the trocar *in situ* and often the help of a vascular surgeon.

Other complications related to access
- Epigastric vessel injury – this can result in significant bleeding at surgery or a significant post-operative haematoma. Bleeding may only become apparent at the end of the procedure on trocar removal, as the port may have been tamponading the vessel. Resolution is achieved by simple suture on a straight needle passed from outside to in and back out again laparoscopically, or by use of a port site closure device.
- Port site hernia – this is a late complication and is avoided by direct fascial closure of all ports greater then 5mm in diameter, regardless of manufacturers' claims!

Pathophysiological effects
Cardiovascular and respiratory effects
The pneumoperitoneum causes pressure effects on the venous return and as a consequence decreases cardiac output and may have an effect on blood pressure. The rapid expansion of the peritoneal cavity can also induce a vagal effect and therefore slow insufflation is recommended in elderly or other vulnerable patients. There is no reason for the intra-abdominal pressure in laparoscopic surgery to exceed 12mmHg in the vast majority of cases.

Splinting of the diaphragm due to the pneumoperitoneum, as well as the extreme Trendelenburg position adopted in some pelvic cases, may lead to an increase in ventilatory pressure.

Gas embolus
This occurs where intraperitoneal carbon dioxide enters an open vein causing gas to pass from the right side of the heart to the pulmonary artery. Massive embolus causes an underperfused lung with a sudden drop in $ETCO_2$. Progressive embolus causes a rise in blood pCO_2 with an abnormal rise in $ETCO_2$ before suddenly falling.

Other signs are of acute right heart failure with hypotension and a fall in cardiac output, hypoxaemia, bradycardia, a millwheel machinery heart murmur, and a widened QRS complex.

Treatment is to release the pneumoperitoneum, give 100% oxygen, apply a steep Trendelenberg position, and position the patient in left lateral to allow the gas bubble to move back to the right ventricle. Aspiration through a central venous catheter may be attempted.

Positional effects

Complex laparoscopic procedures often require the use of extreme positioning on the operating table and due attention must be paid to sites of potential nerve damage or neurapraxia. Particular areas at risk are the brachial plexus and lateral peroneal nerve in steep head down. Venous stasis in the legs is a risk in reverse Trendelenberg position in association with the abdominal effects of the pneumoperitoneum and hence thromboprophylaxis measures are important.

Specific operations – indications, complications, alternatives

Oesophagectomy

Indications
Operable oesophageal or gastro-oesophageal junction adenocarcinoma or high grade dysplasia in Barrett's oesophagus. Either two-stage, Ivor-Lewis approach – abdominal then transthoracic – or transhiatal (cervical approach).

Post-operative complications
General
- Respiratory complications (25–50%) include atelectasis, lobar collapse, and bronchopneumonia. Prevention is through effective analgesia, chest physiotherapy, and early mobilization.
- Thromboembolic complications (10%).
- Cardiovascular or cerebrovascular events.

Specific
- Haemorrhage – secondary haemorrhage associated with mediastinal sepsis.
- Gastric stasis or aspiration pneumonia can be prevented by pyloroplasty and naso-gastric intubation.
- Anastomotic leak (📖 see Anastomotic leak, p.172). The incidence is 12%, with a mortality of 43–86%. No difference in incidence between stapled and hand-sewn anastomosis has been shown.
- Chylothorax – this is a leak of chyle from the patent thoracic duct with an incidence of 0.2–10%. Management – initial conservative management if <400ml/day; stop enteric feed, trial of etilefrine (sympathomimetic drug). If lymphopenia develops (common), commence co-trimoxazole to prevent *Pneumocystis* pneumonia. If the chyle leak is more than 400ml/day or is persistent, consider thoracotomy and ligation of thoracic duct. Give lipid-rich feed peri-operatively to promote the leak and assist in identification of duct.
- Benign anastomotic stricture – there is a reduced incidence following hand-sewn anastomosis. Treatment is by gentle endoscopic dilatation.
- Tracheobronchial injury or fistula.

Alternatives to surgery
- Malignancy – chemoradiotherapy; stenting; laser treatment.
- Barrett's oesophagus – photodynamic therapy.

Fundoplication

Indications

Gastro-oesophageal reflux disease (GORD) with complications (oesophageal ulcer/stricture/recurrent aspiration/Barrett's oesophagus) or failed medical management.

The fundus of the stomach is mobilized (with or without division of the short gastric vessels) and wrapped behind or in front of the gastro-oesophageal junction to limit reflux episodes.

Types

- Nissen fundoplication with a 360 degree wrap. Commonly performed laparoscopically.
- Posterior partial fundoplication (Toupet) – 270 degree partial wrap.
- Anterior partial fundoplication (Belsey mark IV) – 240 degree partial wrap.

Complications

- Oesophageal perforation – posterior dissection or traumatic insertion of calibrating oesophageal bougie.
- Pneumothorax/pneumomediastinum.
- Pulmonary embolus.
- Vascular injury – IVC/aorta/left hepatic vein.
- Dysphagia – related to tightness of the wrap.
- Gas bloat syndrome – inability to belch due to restriction of wrap with an incidence of 60% in 360° Nissen, 25% in 270° Toupet.
- Hiatus hernia –prevented by cruroplasty.
- Failure – early (technical); late – 12% of patients require antisecretory medication at 5 years follow-up.

Gastrectomy

Indications

- gastric malignancy
- gastric ulcer (bleeding or perforation) – elective gastrectomy for peptic ulcer disease now rare.

Types

- distal gastrectomy (Bilroth I/II/Polya)
- subtotal gastrectomy
- total gastrectomy.

Complications

Early
- Haemorrhage.
  - Reactive (early) or secondary haemorrhage – usually due to intra-abdominal sepsis.

- Duodenal stump leak – technical error; distal obstruction; duodenal ischaemia. Early leak (bile in drain) – re-exploration; late leak (bile in drain) – leave drain and allow fistula tract to form.
- Abscess – radiological drainage.
- Sepsis – re-explore, place paraduodenal drain or catheter into defect with HDU or ITU admission.
- Anastomotic leak. Early – re-explore, place a drain, feeding jejunostomy, and consider repair or revision of anastomosis; late – if patient is well, conservative treatment. If patient is unwell, reoperate, place drain and construct feeding jejunostomy.
- Pancreatic fistula.

Late
- Early fullness – loss of gastric reservoir.
- Dumping syndrome – post-prandial pain/fullness/diarrhoea.
- Hypoglycaemia.
- Diarrhoea – truncal vagotomy/dumping syndrome/bacterial overgrowth.
- Bile reflux.
- Stomal ulceration.
- Nutritional deficiencies – vitamins B12, A, D, iron.

Oesophagogastroduodenoscopy (OGD)

Indications
- dyspepsia >45 years old
- dysphagia
- iron deficiency anaemia
- stenting of malignant strictures
- dilatation of benign strictures.

Complications
- Bleeding/pain/aspiration pneumonia.
- Oesophageal perforation – if detected early with no solid food contamination then it may be possible to manage non-operatively. Investigations include CXR, contrast study, and repeat endoscopy. Management – broad spectrum antibiotics, antifungal treatment, an anti-secretory drug such as a proton pump inhibitor, NG tube, drainage of any pleural effusion, PEG tube for drainage, enteral feeding – NJ tube. Serial contrast swallows can be used to monitor healing. There should be a low threshold for intervention.

Indications for surgery include large perforations into pleural or peritoneal cavity or missed perforation with gross contamination. Perforation of malignant stricture can be managed with a covered expandable metal stent if there is disseminated disease, or if the patient is unfit for surgery. If the patient is fit and being considered for curative surgery then consider proceeding to oesophagectomy.

Endoscopic retrograde cholangiopancreatography (ERCP)

Indications
- bile duct calculi
- diagnosis and treatment of benign/malignant bile duct strictures.

Complications
- Bleeding after sphincterotomy – adrenaline injection.
- Perforation, usually retroperitoneal – conservative management.
- Pancreatitis – cause of 1% mortality. Supportive care.

Cholecystectomy (laparoscopic)

Indications
- symptomatic cholelithiasis.

Complications
- bleeding
- gallbladder perforation leading to spilled gallstones
- bile duct injury – 0.2–0.5% incidence (open cholecystectomy: 0.06%).

Types of injury to bile duct
- complete transection
- complete transection with missing segment
- partial transection
- clip occlusion
- diathermy injury
- sectoral or accessory duct leak.

Presentation
Intra-operative recognition (abnormal cholangiogram). There may be bile in the drain or there may be a delayed presentation with abdominal pain, nausea and vomiting, fever, jaundice, and sepsis.
- Investigation – LFTs, WCC, USS of abdomen (when a collection or proximal duct dilatation may be seen).
- Define anatomy – ERCP (+ stent if there is a cystic duct or lateral duct leak) or PTC ± drain.
- Management – broad spectrum antibiotics with percutaneous drainage of a collection or biliary drainage.
- More complex management requires the input of a specialized hepatobiliary unit where reconstruction using Roux-en-Y hepaticojejunostomy may be one of the techniques considered.

Pancreatectomy

Indications
- operable pancreatic or ampullary cancer
- cystic neoplasms
- chronic pancreatitis
- trauma.

Types
- pylorus-preserving pancreaticoduodenectomy (PPPD)
- Whipple's procedure – includes resection of distal stomach
- distal pancreatectomy.

Complications
- Haemorrhage – associated with post-operative infection or pancreatitis.
- Intra-abdominal infection and sepsis.
- Gastric outlet obstruction.
- Leak from pancreatic anastomosis or biliary anastomosis.
- Splenic injury.

Small bowel resection

Indications
- congenital lesions
- perforation
- ischaemia
- Crohn's disease
- tumour.

Complications
- bleeding, including mesenteric haematoma and anastomotic bleeding
- anastomotic leak
- recurrent disease – particularly in Crohn's disease
- internal hernia – mesenteric defects need closing after resection and anastomosis.

Colonoscopy

Indications
- investigation of rectal bleeding/altered bowel habit
- surveillance – colonic polyps, family history of bowel cancer
- colorectal cancer follow-up
- inflammatory bowel disease.

Complications
- Bleeding after biopsy or polypectomy. Treat by adrenaline injection (1 in 10 000) or application of endoscopic clips. Try to avoid using diathermy.
- Perforation – (1:1000 diagnostic; 1:500 therapeutic) there is an increased incidence after right-sided (compared to left-sided) biopsy or polypectomy. Right-sided 'hot' biopsy should be avoided for this reason. Early detection with no systemic signs and after good bowel preparation can be considered for conservative management (small defect, therapeutic colonoscopy). Early surgery and primary repair should be considered if there is a large defect (diagnostic colonoscopy). When diagnosis is delayed then surgery is needed and defunctioning if there is faecal soiling.

Intestinal stomas

Ileostomy
Indications
- panproctocolectomy for inflammatory bowel disease
- defunctioning of distal anastomosis or obstruction.

Complications
- retraction
- prolapse
- parastomal hernia
- fistula.

Colostomy
Indications
- segmental colonic resection without anastomosis
- defunctioning loop colostomy for perianal pathology, e.g. fistula/incontinence.

Complications
- hernia
- prolapse
- stenosis
- necrosis.

Right hemicolectomy/ileocaecal resection

Indications
- colon cancer
- neuroendocrine tumours such as carcinoid
- Crohn's disease
- solitary caecal diverticulum and other rare pathologies such as caecal volvulus.

Complications
- injury to other organs: ureter (rare), gonadal vessels, duodenum
- anastomotic leak
- disease recurrence
- vitamin B12 deficiency.

Left hemicolectomy/sigmoid colectomy

Indications
- colonic cancer or large polyps not resectable at colonoscopy
- diverticular disease
- sigmoid volvulus, particularly with ischaemia.

Complications
- injury to ureter may require repair over double J stent
- injury to spleen usually due to injudicious retraction during splenic flexure mobilization
- anastomotic leak.

Anterior resection

Indications
- rectal cancer
- rarely for endometriosis invading the rectum.

Complications
- injury to ureter/gonadal vessels
- injury to hypogastric nerves – impotence/urinary problems
- pelvic bleeding
- anastomotic leak
- anterior resection syndrome – frequency/urgency/tenesmus – exacerbated by neoadjuvant radiotherapy
- incontinence if poor sphincter pressures
- local recurrence.

Abdomino-perineal resection

Indications
- low rectal cancer
- recurrent anal cancer.

Complications
- injury to ureter/gonadal vessels
- injury to hypogastric nerves – impotence/urinary problems
- pelvic bleeding
- colostomy complications
- perineal wound – poor healing or sinus formation if previous radiotherapy
- female complications, including dyspareunia, vaginal stenosis if concomitant excision of posterior wall of vagina.

Proctectomy

Indications
- proctitis unresponsive to medical management after subtotal colectomy
- severe perianal Crohn's disease.

Complications
- Pelvic nerve damage – incidence might be reduced by a close rectal plane of dissection.
- Perineal wound – infection/poor healing. Exacerbated by steroids.
- Pelvic abscess/haematoma.

Ileo-anal pouch

This is a procedure to restore intestinal continuity following proctocolectomy for chronic ulcerative colitis (UC) or familial adenomatous polyposis (FAP). It involves creation of an ileal reservoir (usually in a J-shaped configuration), which is anastomosed to the upper anal canal. For FAP the epithelium above the dentate line is removed (mucosectomy) to prevent malignant change. The procedure is generally not performed in Crohn's disease because of an unacceptable complication rate.

Complications
- Inflammation and sepsis affects 3–25% of ileo-anal pouches and is a frequent cause of pouch failure. It is classified into acute and chronic types. Chronic sepsis is implicated in a pouch-vaginal fistula. This has an incidence of 2.6–16% and affects ulcerative colitis patients more than FAP.
- Poor function – defined as >10 bowel actions per day and affects 20–40% of patients. This may occur due to anastomotic stenosis, a poor pouch volume, retained rectum, or pouchitis.

- Pouchitis or inflammation of the pouch only affects UC patients (9–50%). Presents with frequency, urgency, bleeding, and pain. Pouchoscopy demonstrates mucosal oedema, erythema, and ulceration. Antibiotic treatment is of use in the short term, either ciprofloxacin or metronidazole. Topical mesalazine or cortisone may also help. There may be a role for probiotics.
- Neoplastic transformation – dysplasia or carcinoma can occur in the retained epithelial cuff in ulcerative colitis and surveillance is indicated. Transformation of the ileal mucosa is rare but surveillance is indicated in cases of unremitting pouchitis, primary sclerosing cholangitis, and colonic dysplasia in the original specimen.

Haemorrhoidectomy

Types
- open haemorrhoidectomy (Milligan-Morgan).
- closed haemorrhoidectomy (Fergusson).
- stapled haemorrhoidopexy.

Indications
- prolapsing haemorrhoids (third/fourth degree)
- non-responsive to other treatments such as sclerotherapy or banding.

Complications
- bleeding – reactionary; secondary.
- pain
- anal stenosis – prevented by leaving adequate skin bridges between sites of excision
- recurrence – possibly higher after stapled procedure.

Complications of peripheral vascular surgery

Complications of infrainguinal bypass grafting

Infrainguinal bypass is a common operation with approximately 5–6000 performed annually within the UK. Indications for surgery include:
• short-distance claudication
• chronic, severe limb ischaemia with rest pain with or without gangrene/ulceration
• acute lower limb ischaemia.

The level of bypass depends on the extent of the peripheral vascular disease. Infrainguinal reconstruction includes femoral-popliteal (above or below the knee), femoral-crural (tibial or peroneal vessels), and popliteal-crural or -pedal. An autologous long saphenous vein is used as conduit of choice as it is resistant to infection and has superior, long-term patency. It can be used *in situ*, after ligation of tributaries and valve disruption using a valvulotome, or may be reversed. Although there is no significant difference in patency rates between *in situ* and reversed grafts, the latter technique is increasingly used as it allows the graft to be tunnelled and so be protected from skin wound complications. If no suitable short or long saphenous vein is available, arm veins may be harvested and joined end-to-end to achieve the required length. In the absence of autologous vein a prosthetic conduit made of PTFE (polytetrafluoroethylene) or Dacron (polyester) is an alternative.

Early complications (within 30 days of surgery)

General complications

Atherosclerosis is a generalized disorder and commonly affects the coronary and cerebral arteries, in addition to those of the lower limb. Patients with lower limb peripheral vascular disease are usually elderly and have significant co-morbidity, in particular pulmonary and renal insufficiency. Pre-operatively raised troponins, reflecting myocardial injury, are common in patients presenting with acute limb ischaemia and these individuals are at particularly high risk. Acute myocardial infarction (AMI), stroke, and pulmonary complications account for the majority of post-operative deaths. An estimated 30-day mortality of around 2–3% exists for elective surgery within the UK. Overall mortality in patients presenting with acute ischaemia is 9–22%. Embolic occlusion is more dangerous than thrombosis because the cause is related to underlying arrhythmias or AMI.

Specific complications

Wound haematoma

This can result from anastomotic bleeding, bleeding from the graft tunnel, or from inadequately ligated venous tributaries. The majority of haematomas resolve spontaneously but evacuation is recommended if a haematoma becomes infected or compresses the graft with compromise of flow.

Graft thrombosis

Graft thrombosis is the principal cause of graft failure in the early post-operative period, and is usually related to a technical problem with the graft or an 'inappropriate' procedure being performed.

Technical problems:
- Poor quality vein – diseased or small calibre (<3mm).
- Residual valve cusps within an *in situ* venous conduit following inadequate valve stripping with valvulotome.
- Poor anastomotic technique.
- Kinking or compression of the graft.
- Unfortunately, prosthetic graft thrombosis can occur as a primary event with no underlying technical problem due to the inherent thrombogenicity of the synthetic material.

Inappropriate procedure:
- Poor inflow – a significant aortoiliac stenosis merits a procedure to improve inflow prior to bypass (i.e. angioplasty, stent, bypass graft).
- Poor run-off – poor outflow from graft adversely affects patency.

Graft thrombosis results in lower limb ischaemia, which may threaten limb viability. Beware of a falsely reassuring hand-held Doppler signal as fresh thrombus within an occluded graft may oscillate to produce a signal. Ischaemia may be more profound than the pre-operative state because collaterals are damaged during bypass surgery. Urgent return to theatre for graft thrombectomy is required. On-table thrombolysis may be used and a completion angiogram taken before definitive correction of any technical graft problem (e.g. vein patch angioplasty or graft replacement). The urgency of surgery is high in venous conduits that rely on graft flow for their own metabolic needs. Delay beyond 6 hours results in such endothelial damage that graft salvage or prolonged patency is unlikely and graft replacement is required. After 28 days, percutaneous catheter thrombolysis is an option followed by correction of any predisposing underlying technical problem. In the absence of an underlying graft defect, consideration should be given to warfarinization.

Consequences of reperfusion

Reperfusion of ischaemic limbs may result in local and systemic complications.

Local manifestations and compartment syndrome:

This results from reperfusion-triggered inflammation within the limb and is most likely to complicate revascularization for acute ischaemia. It is of particular concern if the viability of the lower limb was threatened with signs of advanced ischaemia being present (i.e. paraesthesia, muscle weakness, and muscle tenderness). Reperfusion of ischaemic muscle triggers a cascade of inflammatory metabolic events that cause capillary leak and swelling and a rise in the intracompartmental pressure (normally <30mmHg in a normotensive patient). The consequent reduction in transcapillary diffusion causes ischaemia at a cellular level. Venous outflow is also obstructed, causing oedema and a further rise in interstitial pressure. A vicious cycle is thus established with progressive swelling, rising intracompartmental pressure, and cellular ischaemia. In the terminal phase, compartmental pressures can exceed systolic blood pressure, peripheral pulses are lost, and limb loss is the likely outcome.

Pain, which is disproportionate to physical signs, is the key to early diagnosis. Muscle tenderness, pain on passive extension, and hypoaesthesia in the distribution of the peripheral nerves running through the compartment support the diagnosis. In the leg, the anterior compartment is most susceptible and early signs include paraesthesia in the first web space and an inability to dorsiflex the foot as a result of deep peroneal nerve ischaemia. The presence of foot pulses does not exclude the diagnosis; by the time these are lost, the chances of limb salvage are poor.

An intracompartmental pressure of >30–50mmHg, measured by a pressure transducer and needle, is diagnostic of compartment syndrome and immediate four-compartment (anterior, lateral, superficial, and deep posterior) fasciotomies should be performed. Treatment delay can lead to irreversible nerve damage and muscle necrosis with subsequent healing by fibrosis resulting in Volkmann's ischaemic contracture.

Systemic manifestations:
These arise due to release of anaerobic metabolites into the systemic circulation. Metabolic acidosis and hyperkalaemia are the most immediate consequences and may result in myocardial depression and fatal arrhythmias. Skeletal muscle rhabdomyolysis results in myoglobinuria, which is a potent cause of acute renal failure. The proinflammatory mediators (cytokines, free radicals, prostaglandins, kinins, nitric oxide, activated leucocytes, etc.) generated within the reperfused limb also pass into the systemic circulation and may induce systemic inflammatory response syndrome (SIRS) that may progress to multiple organ dysfunction syndrome (MODS) (☐ see Chapter 2, Infection, p.29).

Management of reperfusion sequelae requires good general post-operative care with particular attention paid to:
• High index of suspicion for compartment syndrome.
• Electrolyte balance, especially treatment of hyperkalaemia. May also involve specific treatment of myoglobinuria:
  • Correction of hypovolaemia (injured muscle sequestrates massive amounts of fluid). Fluid replacement to increase urine output to 1ml/kg/hr.
  • Facilitate clearance of haem proteins from circulation – alkalinization of urine using sodium bicarbonate and acetazolamide.
  • The osmotic diuretic, mannitol, has been recommended.
  • Hypocalcaemia may occur and require replacement infusion.
  • Treatment should be continued until myoglobinuria resolves.
  • Established oliguric renal failure requires formal renal support.

The severity of these events is proportional to the degree and length of limb ischaemia. Consequently, non-viable acutely ischaemic lower limbs (paralysed, insensate with muscle turgor and fixed mottling) should not be reperfused and the patient treated with primary amputation or palliative care.

Surgical site infection
This is most likely to occur in the groin wound in patients who are obese, diabetic, or on corticosteroids. This is a particularly dangerous situation in the presence of prosthetic graft material, which is highly susceptible to infection. Meticillin resistant *Staphylococcus aureus* (MRSA) is an increasing cause of post-operative wound and graft infections. Methods to reduce the risk of MRSA infection include:
• Scrupulous ward hygiene.
• Pre-operative patient screening with skin and nasal eradication treatment, e.g. nasal mupirocin and antiseptic (triclosan or chlorhexidine) baths.
• Short pre-operative stay to avoid colonization.
• Separate pre- and post-operative wards/bays.
• Prophylactic antibiotics.

Patients with established surgical site infection should be started on intravenous antibiotics, guided by microbiological culture results, and the wound re-dressed regularly and closely observed. Every effort should be made to ensure adequate nutrition, including the use of nutritional supplements. For patients who die, the presence of MRSA should be recorded on the death certificate.

Graft infection
Although graft infection can present in the early post-operative period, it usually presents between 1 and 6 months post-operatively.

Skin flap necrosis
This can occur if the skin flaps are undermined when harvesting the vein. It can also follow infection.

Skin flares
An untied tributary of the long saphenous vein used as an *in situ* graft may result in an arteriovenous fistula. As the fistula matures and flow increases, the skin becomes reddened and eventually necroses. Fistulas can be identified by a duplex ultrasound scan and their position marked on the skin for ligation under local anaesthesia.

Lymphocele formation
Damage to the afferent lymphatics or lymph nodes during groin dissection may result in a local collection of lymph (lymphocele). If aspirated they tend to re-accumulate and risk superadded infection. Lymphatic leaks through the wound can be managed by placing a stoma bag over the fistulous opening. With patience, 90% resolve spontaneously, although this may take many months. Persistent cases may be re-explored with ligation of leaking lymphatics, if identified, or a sartorius muscle transposition flap may be undertaken.

Intermediate complications (between 1 and 12 months after surgery)

These principally consist of three problems that may result in graft failure: graft stenosis, graft infection, and false aneurysm.

Graft stenosis

Approximately 20–30% of infrainguinal grafts develop a stenosis within the first 12 months of surgery. Although they are often asymptomatic, those that are haemodynamically significant may result in graft thrombosis.

Vein grafts

Peri-operative manipulation of a vein graft results in endothelial loss, which may only partially recover. Damage during surgery, and exposure to arterial pressure, results in the development of myointimal hyperplasia. This occurs between 1 and 24 months post-operatively and is characterized by smooth muscle migration from media to intima, smooth muscle proliferation, and the deposition of extracellular matrix. Focal accumulations may occur and are equally distributed at the proximal and distal anastomoses and in the main body of the graft. The causes or mechanisms governing the development of vein graft stenoses are not understood but are likely to relate to both local and systemic factors:

Local factors:
• Mechanical trauma to endothelium during surgery – includes clamp damage, rough handling, and excessive distension of reversed saphenous vein. During *in situ* bypass grafting, the passage of the valvulotome produces endothelial damage.
• Prolonged warm ischaemic time injuring endothelium.
• Use of poor quality vein or diseased vein (peri-adventitial fibrosis, varicosities, venous blebs), small-calibre vein (<3mm), or composite vein. Sites of valve disruption have shown no correlation with stenosis sites.
• Low shear stress – the development of turbulent flow and vortices in peri-anastomotic areas are associated with areas of graft and native artery that are exposed to low shear stress in which myointimal hyperplasia appears to be promoted.

Systemic factors:
• Elevated plasma fibrinogen, fibrinopeptides, Von Willebrand's factor, lipoprotein A, and cigarette smoking are associated with the development of graft stenosis.
• Aberrant vascular smooth muscle response, assayed in cell culture, has been postulated as a factor.

Prosthetic grafts

Smooth muscle and endothelial cells only migrate 1–2cm from the native artery into the ends of the graft. Complete endothelization within prosthetic grafts does not take place in humans; they become lined with a 'neointima' of proteinaceous material composed mainly of fibrin. In the absence of an endothelial monolayer, the luminal surface is thrombogenic and primary thrombosis can occur below the threshold thrombotic velocity even in the absence of a stenosis. Patients with a history of DVT are at increased risk of prosthetic graft thrombosis and anticoagulation may be indicated. In contrast to venous conduits, stenoses within the body of prosthetic grafts are rare but like vein grafts the peri-anastomotic region may be compromised by myointimal hyperplasia. If a Miller cuff has been fashioned at the distal anastomosis, the myointimal hyperplasia tends to occur at the PTFE-cuff boundary, rather than the cuff-native artery transition. Should the graft thrombose, the presence of the cuff is thought to 'protect' the arterial run-off vessels from occlusion.

Duplex surveillance
Because of the 20–30% risk of stenosis within 12 months, many vascular centres undertake a duplex surveillance programme. Scans are performed at intervals (e.g. 1, 3, 6, 9, and 12 months) post-operatively. Detection of a significant stenosis allows a relatively simple intervention in the form of angioplasty, open patch angioplasty, or an interposition graft to prevent graft failure. Graft failure carries a 50% risk of limb loss with consequent financial cost and loss in quality of life for the patient. Duplex surveillance has been shown to improve the assisted primary patency rates of vein grafts, but this does not necessarily correlate with limb salvage or quality of life. The benefit of surveillance has been questioned but remains routine practice.

Treatment of graft stenosis
Stenoses within the body and peri-anastomotic regions of a graft are generally treated by balloon angioplasty in the first instance. If this fails, surgery in the form of patch angioplasty or interposition grafting is required to correct the stenosis. Angioplasty is usually avoided within the first 28 days after surgery.

Graft infection
Prosthetic graft infection is a well-recognized and feared complication of vascular surgery, with an overall incidence of around 2% (ranging between 1% and 6% in published series) for prosthetic grafts. More recently, MRSA has been identified as a causative agent in secondary haemorrhage from vein grafts. Graft infection commonly presents with localized signs of cellulitis, a sero-purulent discharge or sinus formation, or non-specific systemic manifestations including pyrexia and general malaise. The patient often has sepsis or bacteraemia with a raised neutrophil count and inflammatory markers. Anastomotic false aneurysms are associated with infection and haemorrhage may occur. Mycotic aneurysms of native vessels, septic emboli, or other forms of metastatic infection are less common sequelae. Vein grafts are more resistant to infection, although *in situ* grafts are at risk if the overlying skin breaks down. Vein graft infection tends to present with anastomotic secondary haemorrhage, which can be life-threatening. Infection usually takes place at the time of graft implantation, although any subsequent source of bacteraemia is a potential risk. The most commonly isolated pathogenic organism is *Staphylococcus aureus*, but *Staphylococcus epidermidis*, pseudomonads, *Escherichia coli*, and *Klebsiella* and *Salmonella* spp. can also be isolated. One worrying trend over the past few years is the emergence of MRSA as a common pathogen in graft infection. The proportion of graft infections caused by MRSA is increasing, with some centres reporting as much as a 2–40% increase over the past 5 years.

Treatment of secondary haemorrhage requires pressure over the bleeding point with simultaneous resuscitation and urgent transfer of the patient to theatre for graft ligation, when the native artery is oversewn or vein patched and the surrounding area debrided. Distal revascularization may be attempted using vein, but only through a non-infected site to a more distal patent vessel. In those patients with a non-viable leg, primary amputation may need to be considered to preserve life in catastrophic haemorrhage.

False aneurysm formation

False aneurysm formation is a recognized complication of vascular surgery with an overall incidence of 2–3% after femoral anastomosis (including aortofemoral grafts). Although false aneurysms may occur through acquired defects in the body of prosthetic grafts, they are much more likely to result from anastomotic dehiscence related to the use of prosthetic material, infection, delayed fracture of suture material, and/or poor surgical technique. They may be detected incidentally during follow-up examinations or the patient may present with a painless or painful groin swelling and occasionally with haemorrhage. Duplex ultrasound usually confirms the diagnosis and arteriography is usually needed to define the local vascular anatomy prior to surgical repair. Surgical options include direct graft replacement or patching of the defect.

Late complications (12 months after surgery)

Disease progression

Extension of the atherosclerotic disease in either the inflow or run-off to an infrainguinal graft is the commonest cause of graft failure in this period. It typically occurs after 2 years. Angioplasty or surgery may be used to maintain the patency of the graft.

False aneurysm

Prosthetic grafts may degenerate and develop a false aneurysm around the body of the graft but more commonly these occur at the anastomosis (📖 see above).

True aneurysms

Aneurysmal dilatation of the body of vein grafts has been reported. These are likely to result from transmural ischaemia or trauma incurred at the time of vein harvesting. They have the potential to rupture, thrombose, or embolize with subsequent graft failure. The best treatment for true aneurysms is repair using an interposition vein graft.

Accelerated atherosclerosis

This has been demonstrated in up to 15% of femoral-popliteal vein grafts and characteristically occurs after 3–5 years. It can be distinguished from 'spontaneous' atherosclerosis by its greater cellularity and lipid content. It is a potential source of graft failure.

Outcome

Following infrainguinal reconstruction, outcome can be measured in terms of graft patency, limb salvage in the critically ischaemic, and quality of life. In addition to the development of graft stenoses, many other local factors influence primary graft patency including the level of distal anastomosis, patency of distal run-off, indication for bypass (claudicants can expect better patency rates than the critically ischaemic), ankle brachial-pressure index (ABPI), and the quality of the vessel used for the distal anastomosis. Patency of below-knee bypass is strongly influenced by the type of bypass conduit, with PTFE performing least well. Many explanations for this have been proposed and include compliance mismatch between graft and native artery, iatrogenic injury from anastomotic suturing, and low shear stress at the 'heel' and 'toe' of the distal anastomosis inducing myointimal hyperplasia. Consensus report results for 5-year patency rates are shown in the table below:

Femoral-popliteal bypass	Claudication	Critical ischaemia
Vein	80%	66%
Above-knee PTFE	75%	47%
Below-knee PTFE	65%	65%

Complications of open abdominal aortic surgery

Abdominal aortic reconstruction is undertaken for both aneurysmal and occlusive disease.

Complications of elective abdominal aortic aneurysm surgery

An artery is often defined as aneurysmal when there is a 50% increase in the diameter of its wall, or more pragmatically when the diameter of the aorta exceeds 3cm. Degenerative abdominal aortic aneurysms (AAA) primarily affect elderly men (male: female, 5:1) and have a 5% prevalence in males between the ages of 65 and 74 years. They involve the suprarenal aorta in 5% of cases and 5% are associated with a peri-aortic/retroperitoneal inflammatory reaction that may expand to encase adjacent structures, complicating surgery.

Elective repair for large aneurysms is undertaken when the risk of death from rupture outweighs the risks of elective surgery. In the UK, in a patient of 'average fitness', intervention is usually considered when the maximal diameter reaches 5.5cm. The annual risk of rupture of a 4–5.5cm AAA is approximately 1% but increases rapidly with increasing size such that at 6cm the annual risk of rupture is around 10%. Patients with AAA <5.5cm should undergo periodic duplex ultrasound surveillance. Less common indications for intervention include:

- Rapid expansion – >0.5cm in 6 months.
- Symptomatic aneurysms – painful and considered to have high risk of rupture.
- Required for concurrent repair of thoracic aortic or iliac aneurysms.

Currently two forms of surgical intervention are potentially possible:

- Conventional open repair – transperitoneal (most common) or extraperitoneal approach to the abdominal aorta and replacement of the aneurysmal segment with a prosthetic graft.
- Endovascular aneurysm repair (EVAR) – the aneurysm wall is excluded from the circulation by a stent graft.

Early complications of open AAA repair

Mortality

The 30-day mortality for elective aneurysm repair in contemporary randomized trials is 5–6% but in centres treating patients at higher risk this is likely to be an underestimation.

Although AAAs are not caused by atherosclerosis, the risk factors for AAA development overlap those of atherosclerosis (i.e. male, hypertension, smoking); consequently smoking-related co-morbidity is common and about 25% of patients have associated generalized atherosclerotic disease. Cardiac events account for 70% of all fatalities in the early post-operative period. Risk to the individual patient rises sharply with age or the presence of ischaemic heart disease, chronic obstructive pulmonary disease (COPD), and renal impairment. The decision to operate is therefore based on the patient's physiological versus chronological age and investigations such as cardio-pulmonary exercise testing are increasingly used as a guide. Mortality is largely related to aortic cross-clamping and the trans-peritoneal approach to the aorta. Aortic cross-clamping is associated with a rise in left ventricular end-diastolic pressure causing subendocardial ischaemia. This can precipitate arrhythmias or progress to AMI. Prolonged clamping may result in significant ischaemia-reperfusion sequelae. The transperitoneal approach itself is associated with post-operative wound pain, cardiorespiratory depression, and gastrointestinal dysfunction. There is increasing evidence that mortality rates are more favourable after a range of vascular surgical operations in centres performing a high volume of cases. This is due to a range of factors including surgeon expertise and the availability of the complex care these patients require (ICU, renal support, etc.).

Specific complications

Damage of adjacent structures

These are more likely during inflammatory AAA repair due to involvement of neighbouring structures in the peri-aortitis.

- Enteric injury – the fourth part of the duodenum may be damaged during dissection of the AAA neck with a subsequent risk of graft infection or an aortoduodenal fistula. During a transperitoneal approach, inadvertent enterotomy may occur during division of dense adhesions from previous surgery.
- Damage to the left renal vein – can complicate dissection of aneurysm neck. It may be intentionally divided during repair of juxtarenal aneurysms. Collateral venous drainage usually prevents renal venous infarction but reduced renal function following ligation has been reported.
- Damage to the left ureter – may result in urinoma, urinary fistula formation, and ureteric stricture. During inflammatory AAA repair, identification of the ureters may be aided by insertion of ureteric stents.

Primary haemorrhage

Excessive intra-operative bleeding is a hazard even in elective repair and significant volumes of blood can be quickly lost from brisk back bleeding from the inferior mesenteric and lumbar arteries. Other sources of loss include an aortocaval fistula, anastomotic bleeding, and inadvertent damage to aortic branches or the iliac and left renal (especially if retroaortic) veins. Patients taking a combination of aspirin and clopidogrel may be particularly problematic.

Reactionary haemorrhage

Bleeding in the immediate post-operative period can be a result of technical problems (e.g. anastomotic, lumbar, and inferior mesenteric arteries) or coagulopathy. Coagulopathic bleeding problems are well recognized even after the repair of elective infrarenal aneurysms. Volume-expansion products, massive blood transfusion, acidosis, anticoagulant therapy, cell salvage, and prolonged clamp times have all been implicated. Hypothermia has been shown to inhibit the coagulatory cascade, activate the fibrinolytic cascade, and induce platelet dysfunction.

Haematomas are a potential source of infection, have been implicated in the development of multi-organ failure, and their reabsorption can cause derangement of liver function tests and clinical jaundice. Closure of the walls of the aortic sac and peritoneum over the aortic graft aims to provide a degree of tamponade and minimize haematoma formation.

Acute ischaemic colitis

The incidence of left-sided colonic ischaemia is 2% after elective aortic surgery. This can rise, however, up to 12% following emergency aneurysm repair. The blood supply to the left colon is from branches of the inferior mesenteric artery (IMA). Collateral supply is from the middle colic branch of the superior mesenteric artery and from the internal iliac artery via the middle and inferior rectal arteries. If the collateral supply is poor then ligation of the IMA during reconstruction can result in colonic ischaemia. In practice, if the colon looks dusky and ischaemic during surgery then the IMA should be re-implanted. Profound ischaemia results in colonic infarction with perforation/faecal peritonitis. Lesser degrees of reduced perfusion may induce ischaemic colitis, which presents with pyrexia and bloody diarrhoea. Ischaemia confers a 40–50% mortality, which rises to over 90% if the ischaemia is transmural. Sigmoid tonometry has been advocated as a method of early detection of colonic ischaemia, but remains a research tool. Mild degrees of ischaemic colitis may be managed conservatively if the patient continues to improve. However, if progressive ischaemia is suspected a laparotomy and Hartmann's procedure should be performed.

Distal embolization

During elective repair, the iliac arteries are often clamped before the proximal clamp is applied to avoid distal embolization of atheromatous plaque or thrombus. Large emboli can result in acute lower limb ischaemia. When the clamps are released the common femoral arteries in the groin may be compressed to divert any emboli into the internal iliac system, which has lesser clinical consequence. 'Trash foot' occurs when numerous small emboli lodge in the microcirculation. Mild cases may be recognized by multiple small cutaneous infarcts to the feet but ischaemia may be profound and lead to limb loss.

Rare complications

Graft occlusion

Thrombosis of the graft in the early post-operative period is rare due to high blood flows.

Paraplegia

Spinal cord ischaemia can result from a combination of intra-operative hypotension, prolonged clamp times, over-sewing of lumbar arteries supplying the cord, and ischaemia-reperfusion injury. It complicates only 0.2% of elective abdominal aneurysm repairs but this rises to 2% for emergency repairs.

General complications

Cardiac events

These are responsible for the majority of early post-operative fatalities, due to AMI and arrhythmias as outlined earlier. Pre-existing cardiac disease – including AMI within 3–6 months, unstable angina, complex arrhythmias, or uncontrolled congestive cardiac failure – grossly elevate operative mortality rates and should generally be regarded as contraindications to open surgery. Patients with ischaemic heart disease who have undergone coronary revascularization can expect a normal operative mortality rate. There is now evidence to support the use of β-blockade and statin therapy during the peri-operative period in patients with coronary artery disease and this is used in some centres.

Respiratory failure

The combination of the deleterious effects of general anaesthesia and mechanical ventilation together with post-operative wound pain results in reduced respiratory excursion, mucus plugging, and basal atelectasis with a drop in functional residual capacity. These result in hypoxaemia necessitating oxygen therapy and predispose to pneumonia. Optimal pain control, usually involving epidural anaesthesia, and intensive physiotherapy can minimize or reverse these changes. In addition, the systemic surgical insult together with the effects of reperfusion may result in SIRS that may progress to acute lung injury or even acute respiratory distress syndrome (ARDS). However, the latter more commonly complicates the repair of ruptured AAA.

Cerebrovascular accidents

Intra-operative hypotension in a generalized arteriopath carries a risk of stroke. This can be related to proximal internal carotid artery (ICA) disease or to intracerebral vascular disease. Carotid endarterectomy should only be undertaken in symptomatic patients with a known significant ICA stenosis (i.e. >70%).

Complications relating to the transperitoneal approach

- Ileus – excessive handling, cooling, and desiccation of the intestines as well as leakage of blood within the peritoneal cavity can all cause a delay in the return of gastric, colonic, and small intestinal function. The use of a self-retaining retractor may well avoid some of these problems, especially if the bowel is kept within the abdominal cavity. Gastroparesis, small-bowel ileus, and colonic pseudo-obstruction can all complicate AAA surgery.
- Hypothermia – this is common following aneurysm repair. Prophylactic measures such as the use of warmed infusions and warming blankets and mattresses should be employed. Hypothermia is a significant cause of post-operative coagulopathy.
- Acute pancreatitis – this is a rare consequence of blunt injury to the pancreas (e.g. retractor-related) during mobilization of the aneurysm neck.

Wound complications

A full-length, midline incision or transverse incision is used to gain access to the infrarenal aorta. Superficial and deep SSIs and full-thickness wound dehiscence are well-documented complications in the early post-operative period. The use of a transverse abdominal incision may be associated with less post-operative wound pain and fewer pulmonary complications, and a reduced incidence of incisional herniation. For those patients undergoing aortobifemoral reconstruction, groin wound infection and breakdown may occur, as well as the formation of lymphoceles.

Deep venous thrombosis

Prophylactic doses of subcutaneous low molecular weight heparin are given in the evening, thus avoiding any problems with epidural insertion on the morning of surgery. Many surgeons avoid the use of intra-operative anti-thromboembolism disease (TED) stockings to avoid increasing lower limb ischaemia during aortic cross clamping. They are generally recommended post-operatively but should be avoided in patients with significant peripheral arterial disease.

Intermediate and late complications

Graft infection

Graft infection has an incidence of 1–3% and a mortality rate of 50%. Infections may occur at the time of surgery, through haematogenous spread, or from extension from adjacent structures. Grafts may erode into adjacent viscera and an aorto-duodenal fistula between the proximal anastomosis and the fourth part of the duodenum is the most common. These may present insidiously with anaemia, pyrexia, and raised inflammatory markers or acutely with catastrophic upper gastrointestinal bleeding (haematemesis and/or melaena). Any patient with haematemesis after an AAA repair must be assumed to have an aorto-duodenal fistula until proven otherwise. Fistulation into the colon is less common and presents in a similar way with lower gastrointestinal bleeding. Repair involves removal of the contaminated/infected graft, aortic closure, and revascularization of the lower limbs by either axillo-bifemoral bypass using prosthetic graft, *in situ* reconstruction with rifampicin-bonded graft, or increasingly *in situ* reconstruction with superficial femoral vein.

Graft occlusion

Patency rates for suprainguinal reconstruction are excellent and exceed 90% at 5 years. Anastomotic myointimal hyperplasia and progressive atherosclerotic disease may occur and result in thrombosis.

Anastomotic false aneurysm

This affects up to 3% of aortic reconstructions and in particular the femoral anastomoses of aorto-bifemoral grafts.

Erectile dysfunction

Sexual dysfunction can occur as a result of damage to the pre-aortic nervi erigentes during dissection of the aneurysm sac.

Extraperitoneal approach

The infrarenal aorta can be exposed using a retroperitoneal approach, which has the potential advantages of less intra-operative fluid loss, reduced post-operative ileus, less haemodynamic stress, reduced post-operative wound pain, and subsequent pulmonary complications. However, access to the right iliac arteries may not be as good as the more commonly utilized transperitoneal approach.

Complications of emergency AAA surgery

Emergency repair is undertaken for patients with a ruptured AAA. This should be distinguished from patients undergoing 'urgent' operations who present with pain considered to be due to the AAA but who have no leak detected on CT scan or at operation. Although such patients are at a lower risk than true ruptures, they still have a higher operative mortality rate (around 10%) than true elective repairs.

The complications of emergency surgery are those of elective surgery but are more common. Certain areas are worthy of particular note:

• Mortality – the overall mortality of patients with ruptured AAA is 80–90%. Around 50% die before reaching hospital and of those surviving to surgery, the 30-day mortality rate is 40–50%.

• Intra-operative haemorrhage – technical problems in gaining prompt control of the AAA neck can lead to rapid exsanguination and death on the operating table. The use of a cell-salvage system provides an immediate source of transfusion and may reduce the need for homologous blood. The causes of coagulopathy outlined earlier are both more common and more extreme after emergency repair. As a result, post-operative reactive haemorrhage is more frequent and it is common for patients on arrival in the intensive care unit to have significantly deranged haemostasis such as thrombocytopenia and/or disseminated intravascular coagulation.

• Following a technically successful repair the morbidity and mortality rates are high. The combined insult of hypotension, massive blood transfusion, ischaemia-reperfusion injury, and extravasation of blood into the retroperitoneum or peritoneal cavity triggers a cascade of proinflammatory events such as neutrophil activation and the release of inflammatory mediators (cytokines, prostaglandins, free radicals, kinins, nitric oxide, bacterial endotoxin, etc.) (📖 see Chapter 2, Infection, p.29). This body-wide inflammatory response may be apparent clinically through the development of SIRS. The addition of infectious complications may fulfil the definition of sepsis. Previously overwhelmed anti-inflammatory processes may restore homeostasis with recovery of the patient, but all too often the proinflammatory reactions persist and the patient continues to decline with the development of MODS. This carries a poor prognosis with 40%, 60%, and 98% mortality for one-, two-, and three-organ system failure, respectively.

Manifestations of MODS
(📖 See also Chapter 2, SRS, sepsis, MODS, and organ failure, p.46.)

Respiratory failure
ARDS is the pulmonary manifestation of MODS and is characterized by profound hypoxaemia, non-cardiogenic pulmonary oedema, reduced pulmonary compliance, and ventilation–perfusion mismatch. Standard intermittent positive-pressure ventilation may not be adequate to maintain oxygenation, so that pressure-controlled ventilation, inverse inspiratory: expiratory ratio ventilation, prone positioning, or nitric oxide therapy may be required. Hospital or ventilator-associated pneumonia, barotrauma, and oxygen toxicity may also contribute to respiratory failure.

Cardiovascular failure
Various types of shock may occur post-operatively, including hypovolaemic, cardiogenic, and septic. After adequate volume replacement, inotropes or vasopressors are often required as determined by invasive cardiovascular monitoring.

Renal failure
Some 70% of all patients undergoing emergency AAA repair develop acute renal impairment. This is often due to a combination of factors:
- Prerenal – intra-operative hypovolaemic shock or post-operative septic shock can result in renal hypoperfusion and acute tubular necrosis. Inotropes and vasopressors may further reduce renal perfusion. Surgical factors may contribute, including a supra- or juxtarenal clamp site and ligation of the left renal vein when gaining proximal AAA control.
- Renal – nephrotoxic drugs (aminoglycosides, non-steroidal anti-inflammatory drugs), haemoglobinuria, myoglobulinuria, and renal artery stenosis can all add to the renal insult.

Disseminated intravascular coagulation (DIC)
Volume-expansion products, massive blood transfusion, hypothermia, acidosis, anticoagulants, and a suprarenal clamp site are all implicated in the development of DIC. It is characterized by a consumption coagulopathy with platelet aggregation and activation of the coagulation and fibrinolytic cascades. The end result is microvascular thrombosis, resulting in end-organ ischaemia and contributing to MODS, and enhanced fibrinolytic activity resulting in uncontrolled bleeding. Treatment requires correction of the cause if possible and administration of blood products that may include packed red cells, platelets, fresh-frozen plasma, cryoprecipitate and/or factor VII concentrates. Haematological advice should be sought.

Gastrointestinal failure
Shunting of blood away from the gut in SIRS can damage the integrity of the gut's mucosal barrier, allowing the translocation of bacteria and endotoxins into the systemic circulation. These may promote the development of SIRS/MODS. Stress ulceration is another consequence of reduced blood flow to the gut. Early enteral feeding may reduce these complications, as well as providing nutritional support for patients' increased metabolic requirements.

Complications of endovascular aneurysm repair (EVAR)

Endovascular repair of any aneurysm consists of the deployment of a stent graft within the vessel lumen that effectively 'relines' the artery. If successful, the blood trapped within the sac thromboses, excluding the aneurysm from the rest of the circulation. With time, as the sac contents organize and contract, the aneurysm diameter decreases. This principle may be used in the treatment of aneurysms throughout the body but the term endovascular aneurysm repair (EVAR) generally refers to the treatment of AAA and was first reported in 1991.

AAA may be treated with simple tube or aorto-uni-iliac devices (with the contralateral iliac artery occluded and perfusion restored with a femoro-femoral bypass) but the great majority of cases require a modular bifurcated device. These are usually inserted via the common femoral arteries with the main body of the graft deployed from one side, which extends from the aneurysm neck to the ipsilateral iliac artery. The main body has a short side limb that must then be cannulated from the contralateral femoral artery to allow the deployment of a second stent graft to complete the bifurcated repair. General or regional anaesthesia is typical but femoral insertion under local anaesthesia is possible. EVAR is not possible for AAA with short, angulated, or diseased necks, or if the iliac arteries are very tortuous, narrow, or diseased.

If the femoral or external iliac arteries are too narrow or diseased, the grafts may occasionally be deployed via a prosthetic conduit anastomosed to an iliac artery. With thorough planning, technical failure requiring conversion to open repair is rare in contemporary series (1%).

Early complications

Mortality

As stent grafts are deployed intraluminally, the transperitoneal approach to the aorta and aortic cross-clamping are avoided, thus reducing the physiological insult to the patient. Reduced morbidity and mortality rates, reduced post-operative pain, and reduced hospital stay are potential benefits of this approach.

The 30-day mortality after EVAR in patients considered fit enough to undergo open AAA repair is between 1.2 and 1.7%; roughly one-third of the open surgical risk. This procedure-related benefit in mortality persists to at least four years. In patients considered too unfit to tolerate open repair, the 30-day mortality is 9% and intervention in these patients is unlikely to be better than observation alone due to their high background risk of death from stroke, myocardial infarction, or cancer.

Endoleak

This is persistent blood flow into the aortic sac after stent graft deployment. It is classified by the leak origin. They can also be classified into primary endoleaks if present at the time of stenting, or secondary if they occur thereafter.

Classification of endoleaks:

Type I: Arterial attachment site leak
A   Proximal end of graft
B   Distal end of graft
C   Iliac occluder (if aorto-uni-iliac stent graft)

Type II: Aortic branch leaks (e.g. lumbar, inferior mesenteric, median sacral, accessory renal, internal iliac)
A   Simple (from only 1 branch)
B   Complex (>1 branch)

Type III: Defect in graft
A   Leak from junctions in modular stent graft
B   Fabric disruption (hole in side of stent graft)

Type IV: Graft porosity allowing flow through the graft wall (<30 days after placement)

Type V: Endotension (see Endotension, p. 223)

Primary type I and III endoleaks need to be corrected before the patient leaves theatre by additional or extension stent grafts, as they are highly unlikely to resolve spontaneously. Primary type II and IV endoleaks can be observed initially as most resolve.

Renal artery occlusion

This is a rare but potential risk of EVAR and is caused by the proximal part of the stent impinging on the renal artery ostia. No adverse effects on renal function result if the uncovered portion (the metal struts used to anchor the graft) is deployed across the origins of the renal arteries, although the long-term effect of this is unknown.

Damage to native iliac arteries during deployment

The iliac arteries must be of reasonable calibre (>8mm) and relatively non-tortuous to allow successful stent deployment. Deployment carries a risk of intimal dissection and flaps, embolization of atheromatous plaque, thrombosis, rupture, and false aneurysm formation.

Distal embolization of atheromatous plaque

This can occur during stent deployment and may require a femoral embolectomy.

Microembolization

Microembolization may occur resulting in 'trash phenomena' to the feet. Massive microembolization resulting from endoluminal manipulation within the aneurysm sac has been reported and can involve the renal, visceral, and lower limb arteries. It is associated with SIRS and MODS and carries a poor prognosis.

Stent migration

Inadequate fixation of the proximal stent graft can allow early migration and the development of a type I endoleak. In addition, as the stent graft slips inferiorly, it may kink and thrombose or sections may dislocate causing a type III endoleak.

Other complications

Renal impairment

Occurs in 25% of patients. May occur through the usual mechanisms of injury (e.g. hypotension) but may also result from iodinated contrast, renal artery emboli, or stent graft deployment across renal arteries' origins.

Back pain

Common following stent deployment and presumed to be related to arterial stretch by the stent graft.

Groin wound complications

This is of particular significance if an aorto-uni-iliac stent has been used with a femoro-femoral crossover graft, which is at risk of infection as it lies within the subcutaneous tissues.

Post-operative pyrexia

Manipulations within the aneurysm sac releasing proinflammatory cytokines is the postulated mechanism behind the low grade pyrexia (37–38°C) that may follow EVAR. It settles within a few days and requires no specific treatment other than the exclusion of infective causes.

Intermediate and late complications of EVAR

The lower peri-operative mortality of EVAR is offset by the uncertain long-term performance. In contrast to open repair, regular surveillance with either serial CT scans or plain abdominal radiographs in combination with duplex ultrasound are required to monitor sac diameter, detect endoleak, and exclude stent migration. Re-intervention rates of 20% over 4 years have been reported but these may fall as the benign nature of most type II endoleaks is realized and as stent graft design improves.

Graft thrombosis

A successfully treated AAA reduces in diameter and shortens with time. Even in the absence of migration, this can result in kinking of the graft and possibly thrombosis. In addition, limb dislodgement may occur with the risk of developing type III endoleak. Limb occlusion may also occur from progression of atherosclerotic disease in the native iliac or femoral arteries.

Endoleaks

Secondary endoleaks, not visible on early peri-operative imaging, may appear after a period of time. Type I and III endoleaks are usually associated with high pressure within the sac. If untreated, these are likely to result in sac enlargement with the risk of rupture or neck dilatation and stent graft migration. As with primary leaks, these may be treated with a balloon expandable stent to reappose stent graft and arterial wall or with the insertion of further stent grafts. Both primary and secondary type II endoleaks can usually be observed as long as they are not associated with sac enlargement. Troublesome type II leaks may be percutaneously embolized. If unsuccessful, laparoscopic clipping is well described but if not technically possible, conversion to open surgery may be necessary with all its attendant risks.

Endotension (also called type V endoleak)

With successful EVAR, the pressure within the AAA sac between the arterial wall and the stent graft should fall. Endotension, in its strictest definition, describes the situation when the pressure remains or becomes elevated within the sac without detection of an endoleak. Postulated mechanisms include an undetectable or intermittent endoleak, transmitted pressure through the graft, and/or high osmotic pressure within the sac that draws in water. It is relatively rare but if associated with an expanding sac diameter there is a risk of stent migration or type I endoleak. The most appropriate treatment is debated but ranges from observation through to laparoscopic division of aortic branches suspected of type II endoleak and decompression of the sac into the peritoneum.

Stent migration

Ongoing expansion of the aortic neck due to endoleak or stent graft undersizing can allow late migration, precipitating further endoleak, graft thrombosis, or disconnection of the graft limbs.

Femoral false aneurysm

Can complicate the transfemoral approach required for stent deployment.

Complications of surgery for aorto-iliac occlusive disease

Reconstruction for aorto-iliac disease can be anatomical or extra-anatomical and generally carries higher rates of morbidity and mortality than interventional radiological techniques so should be reserved for when the latter is not feasible or durable. Such reconstruction is largely performed for critical ischaemia, but can be considered in the short-distance claudicant who is fit.

Anatomical

Aortobifemoral bypass

This can be performed for aortic occlusive disease or bilateral iliac disease. A transperitoneal approach is needed requiring aortic cross-clamping and so morbidity and mortality are parallel with elective AAA repair. The 5% mortality rate rises in the presence of cardiorespiratory or renal disease. However, long-term results are excellent with a 90% 5-year patency.

Ilio-femoral bypass

This can be used for unilateral iliac occlusion. It can be performed as a unilateral procedure or as a crossover. It avoids the use of a transperitoneal approach and has a 3% mortality rate. Long-term results are also good with around 80% patent at 5 years.

Extra-anatomical

Extra-anatomical reconstruction may be considered in the presence of intraperitoneal sepsis or for a patient with significant medical co-morbidity (i.e. severe cardiorespiratory or renal impairment) requiring aorto-iliac reconstruction. The avoidance of aortic cross-clamping and a transperitoneal approach to the aorta reduces operative morbidity and mortality. However, patency rates are less favourable.

Axillo-bifemoral bypass

Axillo-bifemoral bypass can be used for aortic occlusion, bilateral iliac segment disease, or following the removal of an infected aortic graft. Mortality lies at around 3%. As this bypass requires the use of long lengths of subcutaneously placed prosthetic graft, patency rates are poor at between 58 and 93% at 1 year. Complications are similar to other arterial reconstructions (e.g. infection, pseudoaneurysm, etc.) but brachial plexus injury or upper limb embolization may also occur.

Femoro-femoral crossover

Used for unilateral iliac occlusion as an alternative to aorto-iliac reconstruction or for perfusion of the contralateral leg after deployment of an aorto-uni-iliac stent graft. Mortality is around 2% and patency rates of up to 70% at 5 years are possible.

Complications of thoracoabdominal aneurysm repair

Aneurysms involving the descending thoracic and abdominal aorta are traditionally classified as thoracoabdominal aneurysms (TAA). The Crawford classification is as follows:

• Type I: descending thoracic aorta to proximal abdominal aorta (up to coeliac axis)
• Type II: descending thoracic aorta to abdominal aortic bifurcation
• Type III: mid-descending thoracic aorta to abdominal aortic bifurcation
• Type IV: from level of diaphragm to abdominal aortic bifurcation
• Type V: mid-descending thoracic aorta to proximal abdominal aorta.

TAAs are usually due to degenerative disease or dilatation of the wall of the false lumen of a chronic dissection. Back pain is more commonly present than in AAA and acute or worsening pain may precede rupture or intramural dissection. The natural history of TAA is less well documented than that of AAA. The annual rupture risk at 6cm diameter is approximately 4% and increases rapidly with size so that the risk is 43% at 7cm.

There are three potential methods of repair:
• open surgery
• hybrid repair
• branched stent grafts.

Open repair

For open surgical repair the patient is positioned on their right side and the aorta is accessed through a midline abdominal incision extended through the costal margin and along the 7/8th rib for the lower thoracic aorta or 4/5th rib for the upper. The abdominal aorta is approached retroperitoneally following medial visceral rotation of the colon, spleen, and pancreas. A prosthetic graft is used to replace the aneurysmal aorta with an inlay technique. Intercostal and visceral (renal, coeliac, and superior mesenteric) arteries require re-implantation. Operative morbidity is high and mortality ranges from 10 to 35%. The majority of early post-operative deaths are due to cardiac dysfunction and coagulopathy, whereas late deaths are largely related to the development of MODS. Complications are similar to those encountered during AAA surgery. There are, however, some specific points to be aware of.

Bleeding and coagulopathy

Reactive haemorrhage is a major problem following TAA repair and can be due to technical problems or coagulopathy. Of all patients undergoing thoracoabdominal aneurysm repair, 8% require emergency re-exploration and these account for 26% of early post-operative deaths in this subgroup. Prolonged supracoeliac clamp times are implicated in the development of DIC, and it has been shown on an animal model that the development of DIC is related to occlusion of the superior mesenteric artery (versus coeliac). Ischaemia-reperfusion has been shown to alter small-bowel permeability with loss of the mucosal barrier. Bacterial and endotoxin translocation, acidosis, and hyperkalaemia within the mesenteric effluent have all been implicated in the development of DIC but the exact mechanism remains unclear. This ischaemia-reperfusion injury is also strongly implicated in the development of MODS.

Paraplegia

Following open TAA repair, the incidence of paraplegia from spinal cord ischaemia was around 10% but is nearer 2% in expert hands. Division of intercostal or upper lumbar vessels, which may supply the artery of Adamkiewicz, can result in spinal cord injury. Other factors include the extent of the aneurysm (highest in Crawford type II), clamp times, hypotension, and intercostal reattachment. To minimize paraplegia risk, reconstruction should be performed as quickly as possible (i.e. the 'clamp and go' technique) or sequential clamping may be employed. More recent developments for spinal cord protection include CSF drainage, hypothermia, partial left heart bypass, selective visceral artery perfusion, and circulatory hypothermic arrest.

Respiratory failure

Respiratory failure is a major source of morbidity post-operatively with an incidence of over 20%. The insertion of a double-lumen endotracheal tube is required to allow collapse of the left lung to facilitate aneurysm repair. Pulmonary collapse and post-operative pain following combined thoracotomy and laparotomy can result in atelectasis and sputum retention with consequent infection. Post-operatively, these patients are managed on the intensive care unit where prophylactic thoracic epidural, chest physiotherapy, and oxygen therapy are routinely used. A mini-tracheostomy may be inserted and suction employed in those with sputum retention. Prolonged post-operative ventilation may require tracheostomy to facilitate weaning.

Visceral ischaemia-reperfusion injury

The use of a supracoeliac clamp site means that most intra-abdominal viscera are subject to an ischaemia-reperfusion insult and this is implicated in the pathogenesis of spinal cord injury, acute renal failure, DIC, and SIRS/MODS.

Hybrid repair

This initially involves the extra-anatomical vascularization of the renal, coeliac, and superior mesenteric arteries with either venous or prosthetic grafts. The origins of these key branches are then ligated. A stent graft is then deployed to exclude the aneurysm and its branches (renal, mesenteric, intercostal, etc.) from the circulation. For type I and II TAA the take-off zone may need to include the aortic arch. The left subclavian artery origin can usually be safely covered by the proximal graft if the vertebral artery is not dominant or the internal thoracic artery has not been utilized for previous CABG. The left carotid origin may also be covered but requires prior carotid carotid bypass to maintain cerebral perfusion. Despite no attempt at maintaining intercostal perfusion, paraplegia rates appear to be considerably less than in open surgery. The advantage of this technique is the avoidance of the risks of thoracotomy, but type I endoleak is a common problem and mortality remains substantial at around 13%.

Branched stent grafts

Custom-made modular stent grafts allow 'relining' of the TAA while maintaining renal and mesenteric perfusion. Operative mortality appears lower than with open or hybrid repair but the procedure is technically challenging, the financial expense is considerable, and the long-term results are unknown.

Complications of carotid endarterectomy (CEA)

Stroke is the third commonest cause of death in the UK, with an annual incidence of 2 per 1000 population. Eighty per cent of strokes are ischaemic in origin and around 50% of these have significant internal carotid artery (ICA) disease. Meta-analysis of large randomized controlled trials have demonstrated a clear benefit in long-term stroke reduction using carotid endarterectomy plus best medical treatment versus best medical treatment alone in patients with carotid territory symptoms (transient ischaemic attack including amaurosis fugax or non-disabling ischaemic stroke) and a >70% ICA stenosis (the number needed to treat to prevent one stroke is 6.25). However, to achieve such risk reduction, surgical complications must be minimized such that the combined peri-operative stroke and mortality rate should be below 6% and stroke rate below 3–5%. In the UK, carotid surgery is performed under either general or local anaesthesia. Most CEAs are performed for symptomatic carotid disease but there is some evidence for treating certain patients with asymptomatic disease and those undergoing coronary artery bypass surgery.

Early complications

Mortality

The 30-day mortality rate for CEA is around 1–2%. Perhaps surprisingly, myocardial infarction and arrhythmias account for most peri-operative deaths.

Stroke

The overall stroke rate in the early post-operative period ranges from 2.4 to 6.9% in reported series. The majority of all early post-operative strokes (2–3%) are due to intra-operative emboli. Early stroke can be classified as operative if the patient awakens from general anaesthesia with a new neurological deficit. These are usually caused by emboli dislodged during dissection of the carotid arteries, cross-clamping, shunting, and restoration of blood flow. Surgical technique can clearly affect this and care must be taken to minimize the risks by carefully ensuring a complete endarterectomy, tacking down the distal intima, irrigating with heparinized saline to remove particulate debris, back bleeding the ICA first to remove air and debris, and restoring flow initially into the external carotid artery.

Intra-operative strokes

Intra-operative cerebral hypoperfusion can result in cerebral ischaemia and irreversible neurological deficit. Patients with a pre-existing stroke or those with a haemodynamically significant (>50% stenosis) contralateral ICA disease are particularly at risk from fluctuations in cerebral perfusion pressure. The use of a Javid, Sundht, or Pruit shunt, from the common carotid to internal carotid artery, can protect against ischaemia but may dislodge emboli during their insertion. Shunt use varies widely between surgeons and may be guided by the use of monitoring techniques that assess the adequacy of cerebral perfusion. These include stump pressure (ICA pressure after common and external carotid vascular clamps are applied), transcranial Doppler, near infra-red spectroscopy, electro-encephalography, and somatosensory-evoked potentials. All these methods have significant false negative and positive rates. The most sensitive means of evaluating ischaemia directly is to perform CEA under local anaesthetic and insert a shunt if the patient develops neurological symptoms.

Post-operative strokes

These usually occur within 6h of surgery. They are often related to thrombosis and/or embolism from the endarterectomy site. Arterial thrombotic occlusion can be confirmed on duplex and merits re-operation with thrombectomy as this may improve the neurological deficit. The use of a carotid patch, instead of primary closure of the carotid artery, may reduce the risk of thrombotic stroke. Haemorrhagic stroke may also occur and is related to aspirin, heparin, and uncontrolled hypertension.

Blood pressure changes

The aetiology of blood pressure changes around the time of carotid surgery is not completely understood. Intra-operative bradycardia and hypotension are likely to arise as a consequence of stimulation of the carotid sinus. Stimulation during surgery can produce reflex bradycardia and hypotension and for this reason the nerve to the carotid sinus (a branch of IX) should be blocked by local anaesthetic infiltration if there are problems during the procedure.

Post-operative hypertension

This is a major problem with a reported incidence of up to 66%. It may be related to devascularization of the carotid sinus nerve or to effects of the local anaesthetic wearing off. It is associated with myocardial infarction and the development of the hyperperfusion syndrome (see below), and for these reasons it is vital that blood pressure is well controlled.

Hyperperfusion syndrome

Increased cerebral perfusion to the ipsilateral cortex is well documented following CEA and may be caused by a loss of cerebral autoregulation. The cerebral hyperperfusion syndrome is associated with uncontrolled post-operative hypertension. In extreme circumstances it can result in seizures, confusion, and cerebral haemorrhage.

Bleeding and haematoma

The use of aspirin and systemic heparin reduce stroke but do result in an increased risk of wound haematoma. Many surgeons use a small, sealed suction drain to prevent this.

False aneurysm formation

This can complicate haematoma formation if suture line bleeding continues. The incidence ranges from 0.1 to 0.6%.

Infection
Wound infection following carotid surgery is rare (0.1%). If a synthetic carotid patch is used this may become infected with potential secondary haemorrhage or false aneurysm formation.

Venous carotid patch dehiscence
This occurs in up to 0.5% of patients, resulting in potentially catastrophic secondary haemorrhage. A Dacron patch is used by most surgeons.

Cranial nerve injuries
These are relatively common with an incidence of 2–7% and include:
- Recurrent laryngeal branch of the vagus nerve (X): 1–25%. It runs in the tracheo-oesophageal groove. Injury results in an overtly hoarse voice.
- Superior laryngeal branch of vagus nerve (X): unknown true incidence. Runs in carotid sheath posterior to ICA and ECA. Dysfunction of the external laryngeal branch results in reduced voice quality.
- Hypoglossal nerve (XII): 1–13.5%. This nerve crosses anteriorly to the ICA and ECA, 2–4cm above the carotid bifurcation, and injury results in deviation of the tongue towards the side of the injury.
- Marginal mandibular branch of the facial nerve (VII): 0.5–15%. Runs inferior and parallel to the ramus of the mandible. May be damaged by a skin incision along the anterior border of sternomastoid that extends up to the angle of the mandible or from excessive retraction on to the mandible.
- Great auricular and transverse cervical nerves. These are commonly divided by the incision along the anterior border of sternomastoid. Patients should be warned to expect paraesthesia in the distribution of these nerves. Men particularly need to be warned because of the risk of shaving injuries!

Immediate and late complications

Carotid re-stenosis
The overall risk of stroke relating to an internal carotid endarterectomy site is 1% per annum. The incidence of carotid re-stenosis (>50%) lies around 13%, and is due to myointimal hyperplasia in the shorter term and progressive atherosclerosis in the longer term. It is more common in women, and there is some evidence to suggest that patching the carotid artery in women may reduce this incidence. The majority of patients are asymptomatic and for this reason duplex surveillance is not routinely employed during the follow-up period. Re-operation is only necessary for recurrent symptoms and is needed in only 1–3.6% of all patients.

Complications after cardiothoracic surgery

Commonest early cardiac complications and treatment

Atrial fibrillation (📖 Arrhythmias and pacing p. 248)
- Give 10–20mmol K^+ via central line to optimize serum K^+ at 4.5–5.0mmol/l.
- Give 20mmol Mg^+ empirically via central line if none given post-operatively.
- Give 300mg amiodarone IV over 1hr in patients with good left ventricular function, followed by 900mg amiodarone IV over next 23hr.
- In patients with poor left ventricular function give digoxin in 125μg increments IV every 20min until rate controlled, up to max. of 1500μg in 24hr.
- Consider synchronized DC cardioversion for unstable patients (📖 Arrhythmias and pacing p. 248).

Bleeding (📖 Bleeding p. 238)
- If bleeding is >400ml in 30min, or patient is haemodynamically unstable, they may need emergency re-exploration. Obtain help.
- Give gelofusine to optimize CVP 10–14 and systolic BP 80–100mmHg.
- Order further 4 units of blood, 2 units FFP, and 2 units platelets.
- Request clotting screen, full blood count, and chest X-ray.
- Transfuse to achieve Hb >8.0g/dl, platelets >100 × 10^9/l, APTT <40.
- Give empirical protamine 25mg IV and consider aprotinin (📖 Bleeding p. 238).

Profound hypotension (📖 Low BP after cardiac surgery p. 240)
- Obtain immediate help.
- Quickly assess pulse, rhythm, rate, CVP, O_2 saturation, and bleeding.
- Defibrillate VF or pulseless VT, treat AF as above.
- Treat bradycardia with atropine 0.3mg IV or consider pacing (📖 Arrhythmias and pacing p. 248).
- Give gelofusine to raise CVP to 12–16mmHg, place bed head down.
- If cardiac tamponade suspected (📖 Bleeding p. 238) prepare for re-sternotomy.
- If patient is warm and vasodilated, draw up 10μg of metaraminol into 10ml of saline, give 1ml through a central line, and flush.
- If patient is still profoundly hypotensive give 1ml 1:10 000 adrenaline IV.

Poor gases
- If O_2 saturation is <85% and falling, obtain immediate help.
- Increase FiO_2 to 100% temporarily and check the pulse oximeter.
- Look at expansion, auscultate the chest, check PaO_2.
- If you suspect a tension pneumothorax treat immediately.
- Suction ET tube, check that patient is not biting on it.
- Check that the drain tubing is patent and drains are on suction.
- Treat bronchospasm with a salbutamol 5mg nebulizer.
- Disconnect from the ventilator and hand-ventilate the patient.
- Obtain a chest X-ray; look for pneumothorax, haemothorax, atelectasis, ET tube position, and lobar collapse, and treat accordingly.

Poor urine output (□ Common renal complications p. 254)
- Check that Foley catheter is patent.
- If the patient is hypotensive treat this first (□ Low BP after cardiac surgery p. 240).
- Give a fluid challenge of gelofusine to raise the CVP to 14mmHg.
- If the patient is well perfused and the CVP is >14mmHg, give 20mg furosemide IV and repeat if indicated.

Normal post-operative course

Cardiac patients

First 6 hours

- Inotropic support usually needs to be increased during the first 6 hours.
- Pacing may be required (□ Arrhythmias and pacing p. 248).
- Many patients can be extubated within 6 hours.
- A diuresis of at least 1ml/kg/hr should be expected.
- Mediastinal drainage should decrease steadily.
- Insulin requirements increase; aim to keep blood glucose at 5–8mmol/l.
- Continue prophylactic antibiotics for three doses in 24 hours.
- Aspirin 75mg once daily should be started orally but pre-operative anti-anginals can be discontinued.

Day 1

- Inotropes are weaned.
- Most patients are extubated.
- Chest drains are removed after 3 hours of consecutive zero drainage.
- Post-drain removal chest X-ray is taken.
- The patient is transferred from ICU to HDU, and mobilized.
- Routine oral medication is commenced:
  - aspirin 75mg once daily
  - LMW heparin, e.g. clexane 40mg subcutaneously, once a day
  - furosemide 40mg once daily
  - pre-operative statin
  - ACE inhibitor and/or beta blocker if tolerated
  - paracetamol 1g 6-hourly
  - lactulose 10ml twice daily, senna two tablets
- Patients who require formal anticoagulation are started on warfarin.
- Patients should be eating and drinking.

Day 2

- Monitoring lines (arterial, CVP, and urinary catheters) are removed.
- The patient is transferred from HDU to the ward.
- PCA should be discontinued.
- Insulin sliding scales are discontinued and normal anti-hyperglycaemic regimens commenced if the patient is eating and drinking.

Day 3

- Anticoagulation should be therapeutic for mechanical valves; start IV heparin or therapeutic dose of LMWH if this is not the case.
- If there are no contraindications (e.g. heart block, bradycardias, INR>3.0) remove temporary pacing wires.

Day 4

- Patients should complete a satisfactory stairs assessment with a physiotherapist.
- All blood results and imaging should be returning to normal values.
- Adequate pain control should be possible with regular paracetamol.

Day 5–7
- The patient should be ready for discharge home.
- Weight should be back to baseline and diuretics may be discontinued in the patient with good LV function.

Routine tests
Protocols vary but this is a common standard:

Blood tests
FBC, clotting, U&Es on day 1, day 2, day 3, day 5, and day 7.

ECG
1–2 hours post-op, 12 hours post-op, and day 2 post-operatively.

Chest X-rays
Daily if chest drains are present on suction, immediately post-drain removal, and day 2, 4, and 7 thereafter.

Trans-thoracic echo
Day 5 for valve surgery patients, particularly mitral valve repairs.

Thoracic patients
- Epidurals should be continued for 3–4 days if possible; effective pain control helps optimize lung function. The urinary catheter should remain in place while the patient has an epidural.
- Drug chart should contain:
  - LMWH, e.g. clexane 40mg subcutaneously once daily
  - saline nebulizers 5ml 6-hourly
  - COPD/asthma: salbutamol 5mg and 250mg nebulized atrovent
  - analgesia, e.g. paracetamol 1g 6-hourly (IV more effective than rectal or oral) and opiate analgesia, e.g. oral tramadol 1g 6-hourly if required
  - prophylactic antibiotics, e.g. cefuroxime 1.5g IV, three doses in 24 hours
- While the patient has drains, request and review daily CXRs.
- Mediastinoscopy patients can normally go home on first post-operative day.
- Other patients can usually go home once all drains are removed and CXR is satisfactory.

Cardiac surgery complications

Table 11.1 Complications of anaesthesia

Procedure	Complication
Induction	Haemodynamic instability, myocardial ischaemia, malignant hyperpyrexia, allergic reactions
Intubation	Loss of airway control, aspiration, damage to teeth/crowns, damage to oropharynx, damage to vocal cords, malposition of ET tube
Ventilation	Atelectasis, air trapping, chest infection
Radial and femoral catheters	Peripheral ischaemia, superficial sepsis, haematoma, local neuropathy
Central venous line	Pneumothorax, carotid artery puncture, brachial plexus injury, haemothorax, haematoma, arrhythmias, malplacement, kinking, loss of guide wire into heart
PA catheter	As for central line, also: pulmonary artery rupture, complete heart block, tricuspid valve damage, balloon rupture, thrombus formation
TOE	Damage to oropharynx, oesophageal rupture

Table 11.2 Complications of bypass

System	Complications
Cannulation	Atheromatous emboli (CVA), aortic dissection, peripheral ischaemia (femoral cannulation), selective perfusion head and neck arteries due to malplacement of cannula, damage to right atrium, IVC and SVC tear, damage to coronary sinus, damage to RCA and SA node, haemodynamic instability, massive air embolus
Cardiovascular	Massive fluid retention, peripheral oedema, decreased myocardial compliance, myocardial stunning, ischaemia-reperfusion injury
Respiratory	Perivascular oedema, reduction in effects of surfactant, decrease in FRC, and compliance, atelectasis, increased physiological shunts, ARDS
Renal	Acute renal failure, decreased renal perfusion, sodium and water retention, haemoglobinuria
Hepatobiliary	Jaundice, fulminant hepatic failure, acute pancreatitis
Gastrointestinal	Gastritis, peptic ulceration, mesenteric ischaemia, increased permeability to endotoxins
Nervous system	CVA, cognitive deficit
Haematological	Microemboli, activation coagulation and complement cascades, DVT and PE are unusual

Table 11.3 Complications of specific cardiac operations

Operation	Complication
Median sternotomy	Re-sternotomy for bleeding, sternal SSI, pseudoarthrosis, dehiscence, brachial plexus injury, pain, keloid scar
Re-sternotomy	Trauma to right ventricle or aorta and catastrophic haemorrhage, injury to patent grafts causing intractable VF
Thoracotomy	Re-thoracotomy for bleeding, SSI, seroma, damage to nerve to serratus anterior, loss of mobility, chest infection, haemothorax, prolonged air leak
Cardiotomy	AF, cardiac tamponade, pericardial effusion, aortic dissection, CVA, phrenic nerve injury, mediastinitis
CABG	Graft occlusion, steal syndromes, ischaemia, leg vein harvest site SSI, oedema from long saphenous vein graft (LSVG) harvest, pleural effusion on side of IMA harvest, hand ischaemia and neuropraxia if radial artery harvest
AVR	CVA, heart block requiring permanent pacemaker, paraprosthetic leak, prosthetic valve endocarditis, prosthesis failure
MVR	CVA, heart block, inadvertent occlusion of coronary artery or coronary sinus, AV dehiscence, paraprosthetic leak, prosthetic endocarditis, valve thrombosis
Thoracic aorta repair	CVA, paraplegia from spinal ischaemia, peripheral limb and end organ ischaemia

Consent

The following complications should be specifically described when obtaining informed consent from patients for cardiac surgery:
- Death (calculate percentage risk from Euroscore).
- Stroke (2–3% for coronary artery bypass, 5% for calcified aortic valve surgery, 5–10% for prior history of CVA or concomitant carotid artery surgery).
- Re-sternotomy for bleeding (2–3% for routine cases, increased risk in patients still on aspirin and clopidogrel).
- Arrhythmias 30%.
- Permanent pacemaker (2–3% for aortic valve replacement).
- Deep sternal wound infection (0.5% in routine cases, 1–3% in diabetics, active smokers, and obese patients).
- Superficial wound infections (10%).
- Chest infections (10% in routine cases, 20% in active smokers).
- Peptic ulcer disease (1–2% in routine cases with no previous history).
- Acute renal failure requiring dialysis (1% in cases with no previous history of renal impairment).
- Prosthetic endocarditis (1–2%).
- Prosthesis failure (☐ Complications of valve surgery p. 250).
- Paraplegia in thoracic aortic surgery.

Bleeding

Excessive bleeding is bleeding that falls outside the 'normal' pattern of bleeding post-cardiotomy (see box below). **Call for senior help if the patient is haemodynamically compromised.**

> **'Normal' bleeding**
>
> Mediastinal bleeding is normally greatest in the hours immediately following theatre, tailing off to near zero over the course of the following 6–12 hours. While bleeding varies depending on a number of peri-operative factors, acceptable rates of bleeding are **approximately**:
> - less than 300ml/hour for 1 hour
> - less than 200ml/hour for 2 consecutive hours
> - less than 100ml/hour for 3 consecutive hours.
>
> The trend should be decreasing.

Think about
- Is the patient haemodynamically compromised?
- Does the patient need re-sternotomy to sort out a surgical problem?
- Is the bleeding due to coagulopathy?

Ask about
- Blood pressure, pulse, and CVP.
- The **exact** amount of bleeding in the last hour.
- The amount of volume replacement needed.
- Fall in Hb (this is estimated regularly in the blood gases).
- Most recent APTT, APTR, or INR, platelets, fibrinogen, heparin levels.
- Whether the patient has been sat up or rolled; this may cause an old collection of blood to suddenly drain, simulating active bleeding.
- Whether the patient was on aspirin or clopidogrel until surgery.

Look for
- **Cardiac tamponade is a life-threatening emergency. It is an indication for urgent re-sternotomy (☐ Bleeding p. 238). Call for senior help.**
- Blood rising rapidly up the drainage tubing when you lift it up.
- Bright red blood in the drainage tubing suggesting an arterial bleed.
- Bleeding cannula sites suggesting coagulopathy.

Investigations
- APTT, APTR, platelets, fibrinogen levels, heparin levels.
- Chest X-ray (blood may be collecting in the pleura).

Management
- **If bleeding approaches 500ml in 30 minutes, or the patient is haemodynamically unstable, call for senior help and prepare for emergency re-sternotomy (☐ see box p. 239).**

Emergency re-sternotomy: call for senior help

Indications

1. Incipient or actual cardiac arrest due to cardiac tamponade or torrential haemorrhage; **do on ITU if no time to transfer patient.**

2. Excessive bleeding: re-exploration is indicated for excessive bleeding that persists after coagulopathy has been corrected: theatres.

- **Think!** Do you need a perfusionist? Ask someone to phone the surgical consultant responsible for the patient.
- While the anaesthetist sedates the patient, prep and drape.
- Open the wound down to the sternum with a knife.
- Cut the sternal wires with a wire cutter, and if there is no wire cutter use a heavy needle holder to twist wires until they fracture.
- Pull **all** the wires out; wire fragments can lacerate the heart.
- Gently lever the sternum open with your fingers.
- Place the sternal retractor and carefully expose the heart.
- You should see an immediate improvement in filling and perfusion pressures if there was tamponade.

- Give blood, or gelofusine if no blood available, to maintain MAP 70–75mmHg, and CVP 8–10.
- Put the bed flat or head down if you have trouble achieving these parameters.
- If you do not have recent clotting results:
  - order 4–6 units of blood and 2 units of FFP
  - ask for platelets if the patient was on clopidogrel or aspirin until surgery
  - give 25mg protamine empirically; if this was well tolerated in theatre it should be well tolerated in ICU
  - if the patient was on aspirin or clopidogrel pre-operatively consider giving tranexamic acid 2g, but discuss this with your senior.
- If you do have clotting results:
  - order 4–6 units of blood and give to maintain Hb >8.0g/dl
  - give platelets to maintain platelet count >100⁹/l (1U increases platelets by about 10⁹/l in a 70kg adult)
  - give protamine to correct elevated APTT or APTR
  - give FFP to correct elevated APTT or APTR (roughly 5–10ml/kg will be issued)
  - give cryoprecipitate to achieve fibrinogen 1–2mg/l (10 bags will raise fibrinogen by about 0.6mg/l).
- Avoid giving large volumes of cold fluid; use infusion warmers.
- Warm the patient to 37°C; hypothermia suppresses coagulation mechanism and platelet function.
- Control hypertension with adequate sedation and ↑GTN, and control shivering with 25mg pethidine IM or IV.
- Avoid the use of colloid volume expanders unless blood products are unavailable and the patient is hypovolaemic.
- Withhold post-operative aspirin and any anticoagulants.
- Ensure patency of chest drains by milking them regularly.

Low BP after cardiac surgery

Normally aim for a systolic BP 110–130mmHg, or MAP of 70–75mmHg. Some patients need higher and some lower pressures than this; if the patient is passing >1ml/kg/hour of urine and is not acidotic, their blood pressure is probably adequate.

Causes of ↓BP after cardiac surgery

Nine commonest causes:
- Patient is vasodilated – reduce GTN, think about noradrenaline.
- Patient is hypovolaemic – give fluid and assess bleeding
  (□ Bleeding p. 238)
- Temporarily impaired LV – start inotropes
- Arrhythmia – treat aggressively (□ Arrhythmias and pacing p. 248)
- Sedation – give careful fluid bolus and consider metaraminol.
- Cardiac tamponade – call for immediate senior help
- Postural – patient has been sat up – give fluids.
- **Not** hypotension – normal BP for patient! Check pre-op BP.
- **Not** hypotension – artifact: check non-invasive BP manually.

Other causes
- Pump failure:
  • poor LV pre-op, RV dysfunction
  • hypoxia, acidosis, hypercarbia, hypoglycaemia, hyperkalaemia
  • arrhythmias, myocardial ischaemia
  • drugs – amiodarone, beta blockers, propofol, fentanyl, epidural
- Hypovolaemia:
  • actual – haemorrhage, polyuria, inadequate volume replacement
  • relative – sepsis, vasodilatation (propofol, GTN), epidural anaesthesia, anaphylactic reactions
- Mechanical causes:
  • intracardiac – valve thrombosis, acute regurgitation, PE
  • extracardiac – cardiac tamponade, tension pneumothorax

Think about
- Is the patient haemodynamically compromised?
- Is there an acute cause?

Ask about
- **Exact** blood pressure, pulse rate and rhythm, and CVP.
- Dizziness and chest pain if the patient is awake.
- Rate of bleeding if the patient has chest drains.
- Amount of volume replacement required.
- Amount of inotrope infusions.
- Recent changes such as removal of pacing wires, new drug regimens.
- Pyrexia, abdominal symptoms, blood sugar.

Look for

- **Evidence of poor tissue perfusion**: cool, clammy peripheries, ↓urine output, ↑Creatinine, confusion, myocardial ischaemia, metabolic acidosis.
- **Causes:**
- **Cardiac tamponade:**
  - ↑CVP or JVP, ↓BP, ↑pulse (if not beta-blocked)
  - excessive widening of the mediastinum on CXR
  - tachycardia and dysrhythmias, including VF and EMD
  - ECHO may show clot in the pericardium and RV diastolic collapse.

  Impaired LV:
  - ↑CVP or JVP, ↓BP, ↑pulse (if not beta-blocked)
  - ↓BP with fluid challenge
  - history of poor LV pre-op.

  Hypovolaemia:
  - causes: surgical bleeding, polyuria, GI bleed
  - ↓CVP (<8mmHg) or JVP, ↑HR
  - reduced skin turgor, dry mucous membranes, patient thirsty
  - overall negative fluid balance.

  Peripheral vasodilatation:
  - causes: GTN, propofol, sepsis, ACE-inhibitors, epidurals
  - patient peripheries feel warm, palpable peripheral pulses.

  Other causes:
  - arrhythmias, changes in inotropes and antihypertensives
  - systemic problems (GI bleed, tension pneumothorax, hypoglycaemia, sepsis)
  - myocardial ischaemia (angina, ST segment changes).

Investigations

- Usually cause is apparent from focused history and examination.
- ECG, CXR, arterial blood gases for PaO_2, $PaCO_2$, Hb, K^+, glucose.

Management

- Treat obvious specific causes: **immediately life-threatening causes are:**
  - **Cardiac tamponade** – definitive treatment emergency requiring re-sternotomy: fluids, inotropes, and pressors are temporary measures.
  - **Arrhythmias** – VF, VT, asystole, loss of pacing, heart block (📖 see Arrhythmias and pacing p. 248).
  - **Massive haemorrhage** (📖 see Bleeding p. 238).
  - **Tension pneumothorax**: 14 gauge cannula second intercostals space in mid-clavicular line, definitive management is a chest drain.
- Treat hypovolaemia:
  - Give colloid to achieve CVP 12–16mmHg or systolic BP >100mmHg.
  - Lie the patient down; if necessary put the bed head down.
  - Treat bleeding (📖 see Bleeding p. 238).
- Treat peripheral vasodilatation:
  - Reduce GTN, remove warming blankets.
  - Dilute 10mg metaraminol in 10ml N saline, give ½ml IV and flush.
  - Consider noradrenaline infusion.

- Treat poor LV:
  - Correct hypoxia, hyperkalaemia, and acidosis.
  - Treat hypoglycaemia.
  - Stop recent infusions that may cause ↓LV (amiodarone, propofol).
  - Start small dose of dopamine or adrenaline.
  - Treat myocardial ischaemia by starting GTN.
  - Discuss with senior as patient may need re-sternotomy or intra-aortic balloon pump (📖 see Chest pain after cardiac surgery p. 244).

Chest pain after cardiac surgery

Chest pain is very common after cardiothoracic surgery, but it normally reflects the effects of a median sternotomy, rib retraction, and drains. Taking a careful pain history should help differentiate between the causes of chest discomfort listed in the box below. **Wound pain is usually sharp or sore, and worse with deep breathing or coughing, or palpation.**

Causes of post-operative chest pain

Dull, central ache
- Myocardial ischaemia (usually brought on by exertion); ECG changes usually suggest the source of the problem:
  - V1–V4: LAD territory – problem with LIMA
  - I, II, aVF: inferior wall – problem with vein graft to PDA or RCA
  - V3–V6 – possibly problem with vein graft to OM/intermediate.
- Cardiac tamponade.
- Pericarditis (classically soreness rather than ache).
- Peptic ulcer disease, oesophagitis, rarely pancreatitis.

Pain on movement
- Musculoskeletal pain, wound infection, unstable sternum.
- Chest drains.

Pleuritic pain
- Chest infection.
- Pneumothorax.
- Haemothorax, pleural effusion, empyema.
- Chest drain *in situ*.
- Pulmonary embolism.

Think about
- Is this normal wound pain or does it reflect serious problems?

Ask about
- Whether the patient is haemodynamically unstable.
- Whether pain is worse with breathing deeply or coughing.
- Whether pain is sharp, sore, dull, or heavy.
- Whether pain is like angina before the operation.
- What brought the pain on and how long the pain has lasted.
- Whether there are associated symptoms such as dyspnoea or nausea.

Look for
- Hypotension, tachycardia, and tachypnoea.
- Evidence of infection: pyrexia, cellulitis, or pus.
- Level of epidural cover in thoracic patients; if your touch feels the same bilaterally in the incision dermatomes the block is ineffective.
- Sternal 'click' (palpable movement of the sternal edges on coughing in patient with a median sternotomy incision; suggests an unstable sternum).
- Recent reduction in analgesia, or failure to take regular analgesia.

Investigation
- Troponin to exclude MI (TropT >3.4μg/l more than 48 hours post-CABG has a 90% sensitivity and almost 95% specificity for MI).
- WCC and CRP for suspected infection, wound swabs.
- ECG.
- Trans-thoracic ECHO if cardiac tamponade is suspected.
- Chest X-ray.

Management
'Normal' wound pain
- Reassure the patient that their operation has not 'gone wrong'.
- Remember that regular analgesia is usually more effective than 'on demand'.
- Avoid NSAIDs in asthmatics, patients with renal impairment, patients with peptic ulcer disease, and elderly patients. If you have to prescribe them, limit to 48 hours and prescribe omeprazole 20mg once daily.
- Remember the analgesic ladder and escalate appropriately:
  - paracetamol 1g orally 6-hourly, PR or (most effective) IV
  - codydramol two tablets orally 6-hourly
  - paracetamol 1g orally or PR 6-hourly and tramadol 100mg orally 6-hourly
  - paracetamol 1g orally or PR 6-hourly and tramadol 100mg orally 6-hourly and ibuprofen 200–400mg orally as required for breakthrough pain (max. 6-hourly)
  - paracetamol 1g orally or PR 6-hourly and morphine PCA or infusion.
- Ask an anaesthetist to review the epidural if the block is inadequate.

Wound problems
- Unstable sternum may reflect underlying wound infection:
  - swab the wound and start empirical antibiotics (e.g. ciprofloxacin 500mg bd)
  - give analgesia as above; a 'cough-lock' sometimes helps
  - discuss with senior cover; the definitive management is re-sternotomy.
- Treat wound infection aggressively: mediastinitis and broncho-pleural fistulas are potential complications with high mortality:
  - infected wounds should be swabbed and empirical antibiotics started (e.g. IV cefuroxime 1.5g and metronidazole 500mg 8-hourly)
  - consider a vacuum pump dressing (negative pressure therapy) or surgical debridement if there is frank pus; discuss with senior help.

Myocardial ischaemia
- Uncommon but serious complication post-cardiac or thoracic surgery:
  - sit the patient up, give 6–8l O_2 by face mask
  - give 75mg aspirin
  - give 40mg clexane SC daily.

- discuss with senior cover immediately and cardiology registrar; intra-aortic balloon pump, coronary angiography, or re-sternotomy may be indicated in patients post-coronary artery bypass grafting.
  - An intra-aortic balloon pump is a sausage-shaped balloon inserted into the aorta via the femoral artery. It inflates during diastole and deflates during systole. This reduces the work of the ventricle and improves coronary perfusion, reducing myocardial ischaemia. Limb ischaemia is one complication.

Arrhythmias and pacing

Common arrhythmias post-operatively are:
- atrial fibrillation and atrial flutter
- atrial ectopics
- ventricular ectopics and ventricular tachycardias
- sinus tachycardia
- junctional bradycardias and tachycardias
- bradycardias
- heart block

Over one-third of patients experience these arrhythmias post-operatively after cardiothoracic surgery. They are rarely benign; complications include major haemodynamic compromise, as well as stroke and other embolic complications.

VF, VT, PEA, and asystole in cardiac surgery patients

Use the ALS algorithm **and** talk to senior cover, because the following adjuncts **must** be considered as they are potentially life-saving measures:
- In bradycardia, asystole, and PEA, connect temporary pacing wires to a pacing box and pace.
- **Emergency re-sternotomy** to correct underlying problem, e.g. graft occlusion, tamponade; allow internal cardiac massage or addition of pacing wires.

Think about
- Is the patient haemodynamically compromised? **Needs immediate definitive management.**
- Is this a sign of a serious underlying surgical problem?

Ask about
- If patient is symptomatic, including unresponsive, chest pain – **needs immediate definitive management**.
- Blood pressure, pulse rate.
- K^+.
- Oxygen saturation, PaO_2.

Look for
- Pre-operative anti-arrhythmics (particularly beta blockers) not recommenced.
- ECG changes suggesting myocardial ischaemia.
- Temporary pacing wires.

Investigation
- K^+, Mg^{2+}
- pH, $PaCO_2$, PaO_2
- 12-lead ECG

Management
- Ask nurses to place patient on a monitor.
- If haemodynamically unstable go straight to **definitive management**
- Aim for serum K^+ 4.5–5.0:
  - give 10–40mmol KCl in 100ml 5% dextrose via CVP line over 20 minutes (fastest)
  - or 40mmol KCl in 1l 5% dextrose or normal saline via peripheral line over 8 hours
  - or three tablets Sando-K 8-hourly for 48 hours
- Hyperkalaemia is not usually a problem; if serum K^+ >6.0 give 50ml 50% dextrose with 15 units Actrapid insulin over 20 minutes, check BMs, and repeat if necessary.
- Aim for serum Mg^{2+} of 1.0:
  - give 2.5–5g $MgSO_4$ via central line over 20 minutes.
- Correct hypoxia and hypercarbia.

Definitive management
Atrial fibrillation and flutter
- Amiodarone for cardioversion (avoid in patients with poor LV):
  - loading via central line: 300mg IV over 1hr, then 900mg over 23hrs
  - loading orally: 400mg 8-hourly for 24hrs
  - maintenance: 200mg 8-hourly oral 1 week, 200mg bd PO 1 week, 200mg od 6 weeks.
- Digoxin for rate control (better than amiodarone in poor LV):
  - loading via central line: 125mg over 20 minutes, repeated up to a maximum of 1250mg, or until rate control achieved
  - maintenance: 62.5–250mg orally od titrated to digoxin levels.
- DC cardioversion for persistent or compromising AF – patient should be sedated with anaesthetic assistance; give synchronized DC shocks of 50J, then 100J, then 200J, then 360J until sinus rhythm restored. If unsure ask senior cover or cardiology for assistance.

Bradycardia
- Pacing if epicardial wires are present (📖 see Pacing after cardiac surgery).
- Atropine 300–900µg IV.
- Adrenaline ½ml of 1:10 000 IV, consider isoprenaline infusion.

Pacing after cardiac surgery

- Temporary pacing wires are commonly attached to the epicardium and brought out to the skin after cardiac surgery, especially AVR.
- Wires may be attached to the right ventricle or right atrium.
- You can therefore pace the ventricles or the atria.
- To pace you must know whether the wires are atrial or ventricular; connect a pair of wires to a pacing box, usually via a pacing lead.
- The safest mode of pacing is demand (DDD) where the box will not pace the heart unless it senses no activity, at a rate of 60–90, 5–10mV.
- If patient loses pacing and cardiac output **get immediate help**, **check all connections** and **start basic life support**.

Complications of valve surgery

Table 11.4 Overview of the complications of valve surgery

Complication	Mechanical valve	Bioprosthetic valve
Infective endocarditis	0.5% within 30 days, 2% at 5 years	0.2% within 30 days, 2% at 5 years
Prosthesis failure	Negligible	Aortic 30% at 15 years, mitral 60% at 15 years
Bleeding problems	7% of patients have a major bleeding episode p.a. Mortality 1.3% p.a. Thrombosis: 95% of cases	If on aspirin patients over 65yrs have 5-year 0.2–0.4% incidence of GI bleeding Thrombosis: 5% of cases
Heart block	13% transient, 2% permanent Uncommon in MVR	13% transient, 2% permanent Uncommon in MVR
CVA and death	CVA higher. Survival same. No difference	CVA lower. Survival same. No difference

Infective endocarditis

Infective endocarditis complicates 0.2–0.5% of mechanical valve replacements within 30 days of surgery, 2% at 5 years, and 1% per annum thereafter. The figures for tissue valves are similar, but slightly less at 30 days.

- Blood cultures should be taken in any valve patient with a temperature greater than 36.5°C more than 3 days post-operatively.
- Standard advice regarding antibiotic prophylaxis for invasive procedures should be adhered to from day 1 after surgery, not just following discharge. Bladder catheterization should be covered by one dose of gentamicin 120mg IM, for example.
- Any potential source of bacteraemia should be treated aggressively; infective endocarditis can result from venflon cellulitis, superficial SSIs, urinary and respiratory tract infections, and most commonly infections related to arterial and central venous catheters.

Paraprosthetic leak

Incidental paraprosthetic leaks occur in about 5–10% of aortic valve replacements and 10–20% of mitral valve replacements. Paraprosthetic leaks within 30 days of surgery are usually either the result of the sewing ring being poorly seated within a calcified, irregular annulus, or the result of a suture cutting out of the annulus. Wash jets, the regurgitant jets typical of the valve mechanism, may be mistaken for paravalvular leaks.

- Late paravalvular leaks are usually associated with endocarditis, in which case they almost inevitably require surgical repair after treatment with antibiotics.
- High velocity paravalvular leaks may cause haemolysis severe enough to be an indication for valve replacement.
- If neither haemolysis nor infective endocarditis is present, the management of the paravalvular leak depends on the degree of

haemodynamic compromise; small leaks that do not progress can be treated conservatively for many years.

Prosthesis failure

Structural problems not associated with thrombosis, endocarditis, haemo-lysis, or haemorrhage may necessitate valve replacement.

- Structural failure of mechanical valves is rare; the few valves that have had a higher than expected incidence of problems, such as the silver-coated sewing ring of the Silzone valve, have been withdrawn.
- 70% of patients with aortic bioprostheses are free from structural failure at 5 years, compared to only 40% for mitral bioprostheses.
- Patients are reviewed yearly, either by the cardiologists or by the cardiothoracic surgeons, with a transthoracic echo to identify and monitor valve failure.
- The indications for surgery for structural failure of a bioprosthesis are the same as for regurgitant lesions of native valves.

Valve thrombosis

- Valve thrombosis is rare in the appropriately anticoagulated patient.
- The incidence is the same in patients with tissue valves as it is in appropriately anticoagulated patients with mechanical valves: 0.2–5.7% per patient per year.
- The cause of valve thrombosis is most commonly inadequate anticoagulation because of poor compliance, changes in other medication, and illness; 95% of cases of valve thrombosis therefore occur in mechanical valves.
- Mechanical mitral valves are affected in over 60% of cases and mechanical aortic valves affected in 30% of cases.
- Smaller diameter aortic valves are affected more commonly than larger valves.
- Patients with prosthetic valve thrombosis may present with pulmonary oedema, poor peripheral perfusion, and systemic embolization; acute haemodynamic compromise is more common.
- Thrombi less than 5mm that are not obstructing the valve orifice or mechanism may be treated with formal anticoagulation alone, but larger thrombi require thrombolysis, which is replacing surgery as a means of treatment.

Complete heart block

About 15% of patients undergoing isolated mitral or aortic valve replace-ment suffer transient heart block post-operatively, and so most surgeons routinely place temporary epicardial pacing wires.

- Heart block normally settles after 3 to 4 days as haematoma and oedema resolve; persistence beyond this should be discussed with a cardiologist in case a permanent pacemaker is indicated.
- About 2% of aortic valve surgery patients require permanent pacemaker insertion; this is a day case procedure and should not delay discharge, but may be postponed until the INR is <1.5.
- The pre-operative risk factors for PPM are not well defined but probably include pre-operative heart block and heavily calcified valves.

Respiratory complications

Chest infection

The reported incidence of pneumonia after cardiac surgery varies from 2–20%. The variation in incidence reflects variation in diagnostic criteria.

Diagnosis

A history of cough with purulent sputum or purulent secretions aspirated from the ET tube suggest chest infection. Pyrexia, bronchial breath sounds, reduced air entry, leucocyte neutrophilia, raised CRP, and signs of consolidation on chest X-ray confirm the diagnosis. Culture of sputum may yield sensitivities of causative organisms. In the dyspnoeic, hypoxic patient perform arterial blood gases to guide immediate management.

Management

There is no good evidence that prophylactic physiotherapy helps to prevent chest infection after surgery. The single most important intervention is to prevent patients with active chest infections undergoing surgery; any elective patient with a current cough (dry or productive), temperature, clinical signs of chest infection, neutrophilia, or a suspicious chest X-ray should be deferred for a fortnight and then reassessed. Other risk factors include active smokers, or those who have stopped smoking within the last 6 weeks, patients with COPD or obesity, patients requiring prolonged ventilation, and patients who aspirate, particularly those recovering from stroke.

- Physiotherapy helps the patient with a cough to expectorate sputum and prevent mucus plugging.
- Effective analgesia is important to allow patients to cough.
- Definitive treatment is antibiotics; empirical antibiotic cover varies between institutions but oral ciprofloxacin 250mg twice daily provides good Gram negative and positive cover until organism sensitivities are known.
- Suspected aspiration pneumonia should be treated with IV cefuroxime 1g and metronidazole 500mg 8-hourly.
- If the patient requires oxygen (PaO_2 <8.0kPa on room air), humidifying it reduces the risk of mucus plugs and makes secretions easier to shift.
- CPAP can be used to improve basal collapse.
- The hypoxic, tachypnoeic, tiring patient on maximal respiratory support should be reviewed urgently by an anaesthetist.

Pulmonary embolism

Post-operative pulmonary embolism is rare (less than 0.5% of cases) because bypass results in a residual heparin effect, haemodilution, thrombocytopaenia, and platelet dysfunction, and low molecular weight heparin and TED stockings are increasingly widely used. Off-pump cases receive a large dose of heparin intra-operatively as well as DVT prophylaxis. (☐ Diagnosis and management is discussed in more detail on pp.121–122)

Vocal cord problems

The incidence after cardiac surgery is probably about 1–2%. Patients present with hoarseness, breathlessness, and difficulty phonating and expectorating. These patients should be seen by an ENT surgeon.

Exacerbation of COPD

The incidence of moderate to severe COPD in cardiac surgical patients is about 5%.

- Most studies show that mild to moderate COPD is not associated with a significant increase in post-operative complications, mortality, or length of stay.
- Severe COPD and pre-operative steroid use has an associated mortality of up to 20% following cardiac surgery, with significantly poorer medium- and long-term outcomes.
- Ensure that all patients on pre-operative beta-agonist inhalers are routinely prescribed regular post-operative nebulizers (saline 5ml, salbutamol 2.5–5mg, and becotide 500μg 8-hourly as required).
- Beta blockers may be safely recommenced, but beware of starting beta blockers for the first time in patients with asthma or severe COPD.
- In hypoxic patients with COPD, give maximal oxygen by CPAP if necessary and monitor blood gases; do **not** restrict oxygen for fear of reducing hypoxic respiratory drive, as cardiac arrest is a far more important complication than problems due to hypercapnia.

Pleural effusion

Up to 40% of patients undergoing cardiac surgery develop pleural effusions, which may be unilateral or bilateral. IMA harvesting is associated with a higher rate of ipsilateral pleural effusions: up to 75% of patients are affected. It is unclear if pleurotomy at the time of IMA harvest or taking pedicled rather than skeletonized IMA increase the risk of pleural effusion.

Diagnosis

Dyspnoea, pleuritic chest pain, decreased air entry, dullness to percussion, and ↑CRP and WCC suggest a pleural effusion. It may be difficult to distinguish between consolidation and effusion on a chest X-ray, but a meniscus is suggestive of pleural effusion and an air-fluid level diagnostic of a hydropneumothorax. If in doubt ultrasound will quantify the size of the effusion and locate a safe area and direction for drainage.

Management

- Small pleural effusions can be treated with increasing diuretic therapy (furosemide 40–80mg once daily).
- Large pleural effusions (more than 3–4cm deep on ultrasound) should be drained with a pigtail catheter if late, or a formal chest drain if early and likely to be predominantly blood and clots.
- Leave the drain in until less than 100ml drains in 24 hours.

Phrenic nerve paresis

Electrophysiological testing demonstrates unilateral phrenic nerve damage in a quarter of cardiac surgical patients, and bilateral damage in about 1%. Although direct trauma, particularly during IMA harvest, devascularization, traction from the sternal retractor, and diabetic neuropathy have all been suggested as causes, the single most important factor is probably cold injury from slush placed in the pericardial cradle for topical cooling. Unilateral injury is of limited importance.

Common renal complications

Acute renal failure

📖 The aetiology, diagnosis, and management of renal failure on ITU are described on p.260. Patients who have returned to the ward, with elevated creatinine and urea, should be weighed daily and have daily serum urea and electrolytes. If renal markers deteriorate:
- Consider inserting a urinary catheter and commence a strict fluid balance chart.
- Recheck the drug chart for nephrotoxic medication and stop ACE-inhibitors, NSAIDs, and antibiotics such as teicoplanin and gentamicin.
- Actively look for and exclude relative hypotension, hypovolaemia, sepsis, and delayed cardiac tamponade as reversible causes.
- If the patient is hypovolaemic, stop diuretic therapy and hydrate carefully.
- Ask yourself if the patient needs readmission to HDU for central venous monitoring and inotropic support.

Refractory peripheral oedema

Most patients have a capillary leak syndrome after cardiopulmonary bypass and retain fluid. In most patients this corrects with a large diuresis, encouraged with loop diuretics, over the first few days post-operatively, but in a minority significant fluid overload persists. If patient weight remains >3kg above pre-operative weight:
- Check serum electrolytes and treat appropriately.
- Check albumin – if it is low it may take days to weeks to correct even with nutritional supplements.
- If oedema is refractory to furosemide after an increase to 80mg orally twice a day, consider a stat dose of oral daily bumetanide (2mg) or metolazone (5mg), which may be repeated if creatinine is not elevated.
- Spironolactone 25–50mg orally once daily is a potassium-sparing diuretic that is effective for management of ascites and pleural effusion.
- Consider a fluid restriction to 1500ml per 24 hours.
- Treat symptomatically with TED stockings and elevation of legs.
- Consider an echo to rule out tamponade or heart failure. Unilateral peripheral oedema may be caused by DVT, cellulitis, extravasation of IV fluids, stroke, haematoma, and saphenous vein harvest.

Hypokalaemia

Hypokalaemia (K^+ <4.0) is common and, as it predisposes patients to arrhythmias such as AF and digoxin toxicity, it should be treated. Hypokalaemia is normally caused by diuretic therapy, insulin sliding scales, diarrhoea and vomiting, steroids, and poor nutrition. Acute severe hypokalaemia (K^+ <3.0) in post-operative cardiac patients may result in life-threatening arrhythmias. It can be recognized by small or inverted T waves, depressed ST segments, and prolonged PR interval and U waves on the ECG.
- Educate the patient about which foods are rich in potassium (bananas, prunes, apricots, tomatoes, orange juice) and ensure availability.

- Change furosemide to co-amilofruse 5/40 or 2.5/20, which contains frusemide (either 40mg or 20mg) and amiloride (5mg or 2.5mg), and is a potassium-sparing thiazide diuretic.
- Add oral potassium supplements up to 160mmol daily (one tablet of Sando-K contains 20 mmol of K^+; one tablet of Slow-K, which is better tolerated by most patients, contains 12.5mmol KCl).
- If a central line is in place give 20mmol KCl in 50–100ml of 5% dextrose over 20 minutes to 1 hour.
- If it is necessary to use a peripheral line place a maximum of 40mmol of potassium in 1l 5% dextrose running at a maximum of 125ml/hour.
- Monitor K^+ daily and avoid discharging the patient home on a combination of potassium supplements and potassium-sparing drugs, as rebound hyperkalaemia is a risk.

Hyperkalaemia

Hyperkalaemia (K^+ > 5.0mmol/l) is seen in the setting of renal failure, tissue necrosis, and potassium-sparing diuretics and supplements. Acute hyperkalaemia (K^+ > 6.0mmol/l) can cause life-threatening ventricular arrhythmias. ECG changes that herald myocardial dysfunction are flattened P waves, wide QRS complexes, tenting of T waves, and in peri-arrest hyperkalaemia, a sine wave appearance.

- Treat the patient with ECG changes as an emergency.
- Treat the underlying cause.
- Give 50ml of 50% dextrose containing 15 units of Actrapid insulin as an infusion over 10 to 20 minutes, repeating as necessary and monitoring blood sugars after each infusion.
- Give 10ml calcium gluconate 10% IV over 2 minutes, and repeat.
- Calcium resonium enema binds K^+ and removes it from the body.
- Dialysis should be urgently considered in patients with refractory hyperkalaemia despite these measures, and irrespective of renal function.

Hyponatraemia

Hyponatraemia (Na^+ <125mmol/l) occurs in water overload where patients have been given 5% dextrose fluid maintenance over long periods rather than normal saline, and as a result of diuretic therapy, diarrhoea and vomiting, renal failure, cardiac and liver failure, and SIADH (syndrome of inappropriate ADH secretion). Profound hyponatraemia leads to confusion and fits as a result of potentially life-threatening cerebral oedema. Assess the patient for dehydration or oedema, and measure urine osmolality and urinary sodium. SIADH is diagnosed by finding concentrated urine (sodium >20mmol/l) in the setting of hyponatraemia or hypo-osmolar plasma (<260mmol/kg) and low serum cortisol levels without oedema or hypovolaemia.

- If the patient is oedematous, restrict daily fluid intake initially to 1.5–1.0l.
- Stop thiazide diuretics, but continue loop diuretics.
- If dehydrated give 1l normal saline IV over 8–12 hours, or 1.8% saline.
- SIADH occurs in 1–2% of cardiac surgery patients as a result of increased secretion of vasopressin (or antidiuretic hormone) and should be treated by a combination of fluid restriction for several days and loop diuretics; sodium supplements may also help.

Gastrointestinal symptoms

Abdominal pain

Causes of abdominal pain in cardiac patients

- constipation or paralytic ileus
- wound pain or muscular pain from coughing
- myocardial ischaemia or lower lobe pneumonia
- peptic ulceration
- pancreatitis
- gall bladder pathology including cholecystitis and biliary colic
- small and large bowel obstruction
- ischaemic bowel
- perforated viscus, including pre-operative diverticular disease.

Distinguishing between peritonitis and colicky pain is particularly difficult in elderly, sedated, or confused patients following cardiac surgery. Classic signs of peritonitis and localizing signs are frequently not present despite major intra-abdominal pathology. Take a full history, note recent drug regimes, examine the patient, and request full blood count, U&Es, LFTs, amylase, CRP, blood gases, and abdominal plain and erect chest X-rays in the first instance. Stool and blood cultures should be taken when there is diarrhoea.

Constipation

Failure to pass stool by day 4 post-operatively is not uncommon. Constipation may be caused by reluctance to use a bed pan, lack of privacy, immobility, pain on straining from wounds or anal fissures, dehydration, poor nutrition, inadequate dietary fibre, opiate analgesia, iron supplements, tricyclic antidepressants, and spinal anaesthesia. Treatments are:

- Bulking agents such as increasing dietary fibre with bran or dried fruit or methylcellulose, all of which increase stool bulk and decrease transit time.
- Stool softeners such as liquid paraffin, glycerine suppositories (1 to 2) or phosphate enemas (1 to 2) once daily.
- Osmotic agents such as lactulose or oral magnesium hydroxide should be taken with plenty of oral fluids.
- Stimulants such as senna, bisacodyl, sodium docusate, or co-danthramer, which should not be used in the long term as tolerance develops.

Diarrhoea

Liquid stools may be caused by pre-operative conditions such as inflammatory bowel disease or irritable bowel, or acute GI pathology including ischaemic bowel and GI bleeding, but is more commonly due to inappropriate prescribing of laxatives, antibiotic therapy, digoxin, and cimetidine. Pseudomembranous colitis is caused by overgrowth of *Clostridium difficile* following antibiotic therapy, particularly with cephalosporins; send stools for culture and treat positive *C. diff* toxin diarrhoea with either oral metronidazole or oral vancomycin.

Nausea and vomiting

This affects up to 75% of patients after cardiac surgery. It predisposes to increased bleeding, incisional hernias, aspiration pneumonia, reduced absorption of oral medication, impaired nutrition, and metabolic abnormalities such as hypokalaemia. Causes include:

- Bypass, prolonged surgery, anaesthetic agents (e.g. etomidate, ketamine, N_2O), intra-operative and post-operative opioids, spinal anaesthesia, and gastric dilatation from ineffective bag and mask ventilation or CPAP.
- Post-operative ileus, bowel obstruction, constipation, gastric reflux, peptic ulceration or bleeding, medications including many antibiotics, NSAIDs, opiates, statins, pancreatitis, sepsis, and hyponatraemia.

Paralytic ileus

Paralytic ileus occurs in about 1–5% of patients after cardiac surgery. It may share features with small bowel obstruction, including nausea, vomiting, constipation, and dilated loops of gas-filled bowel on an abdominal plain X-ray, but with absent or reduced bowel sounds, little pain, and they may be passing flatus.

- Possible causes include gastric distension from ineffective bag and mask ventilation or CPAP, splanchnic and mesenteric ischaemia, venous congestion, pseudomembranous colitis, drugs (particularly opiates), and other GI pathology including peptic ulceration, cholecystitis, and pancreatitis.
- Pass an NGT to decompress the stomach and consider a flatus tube.
- Stop opiates and contributing drugs.
- Put the patient on nil by mouth and give normal saline 80–125ml/hour IV.
- Prolonged ileus and pseudo-obstruction may necessitate colonoscopy.
- Mobilizing the patient may help.

Gastrointestinal complications

Serious gastrointestinal complications occur in about 2% of patients following cardiac surgery. A previous history of abdominal pathology, age, length of bypass, and poor cardiac output are all probable risk factors. The diagnosis is more difficult in post-operative, sedated, confused, and elderly patients, but the management is much the same as in non-surgical patients. Half of these patients proceed to abdominal surgery where the mortality is as high as 20%.

Upper gastrointestinal bleeding

Upper GI bleeding is most commonly caused by peptic ulcer disease, followed by gastritis, oesophageal varices, oesophageal tears, and occasionally trauma to the oesophagus or oropharynx from intubation with NG tubes and trans-oesophageal Doppler probes. Risk of bleeding after cardiac surgery is increased by the stress of major surgery, anticoagulation, NSAIDs, coagulopathy, and splanchnic hypoperfusion.

Lower gastrointestinal bleeding

Lower GI bleeding is characterized by fresh rectal bleeding, but may require passage of an NGT or even OGD to exclude an upper GI source. Common causes are mesenteric ischaemia, infective colitis including C. *difficile*, angiodysplasia (Heyde's syndrome when associated with aortic stenosis), and diverticulitis. Mesenteric angiography may be necessary to identify the lesion before surgical resection.

Mesenteric ischaemia

Mesenteric ischaemia may be caused by global hypoperfusion due to low cardiac output states, sepsis, hypovolaemia, atherosclerotic embolism, thromboembolism, DIC, or HITT. It presents on the ITU as sepsis, worsening metabolic acidosis, failure to absorb NG feeds, and abdominal distension. Extubated patients may complain of severe abdominal pain, nausea, and vomiting. Diarrhoea, which may initially be bloody, is often present. Bowel sounds are absent. Peritonism is a late sign suggesting perforation. Diagnosis on clinical grounds is difficult in the paralysed and ventilated patient. Contrast CT or angiography are useful. Definitive management is laparotomy and resection of ischaemic segments with or without primary anastomoses. Not infrequently, infracted areas of bowel are so widespread that surgery is 'open and close' only.

Bowel obstruction

Small and large bowel obstruction post-cardiac surgery is most commonly due to adhesions from previous surgery, followed by incarceration of hernias (inguinal, femoral, epigastric, incisional). Rare causes include occult carcinoma and pseudo-obstruction. Small bowel obstruction, which requires urgent general surgical review and surgery if not resolved within 24–48 hours, is characterized by colicky abdominal pain, nausea, vomiting, and distended loops of small bowel on plain abdominal X-ray (central, valvulae conniventes across the entire lumen of bowel, which measure >6cm in diameter). Large bowel obstruction can usually be managed conservatively for longer.

Pancreatitis

A transient small rise in serum amylase is seen in over one-third of patients; pancreatitis occurs in 1–3%. It is caused by splanchnic hypoperfusion, but systemic emboli, prolonged use of vasopressors, and activation of inflammatory pathways on bypass also contribute. Pre-operative factors such as steroid use, gall stones, alcohol abuse, and hyperlipidaemia are less important. Any patient with abdominal pain should have a serum amylase check. Complications of pancreatitis include shock, ARDS, renal failure, $\downarrow Ca^{2+}$, and DIC. Management is conservative.

Cholecystitis

This has an incidence of up to 1 in 200 after cardiac surgery, with patients presenting up to 2 weeks after surgery with fever, nausea, and abdominal pain. Diagnosis is by ultrasound, and treatment is medical (IV fluids, NBM, and antibiotics). The aetiology is ischaemic injury and cholecystectomy or percutaneous drainage may be indicated.

Hepatobiliary complications

Hepatic failure

Approximately 25% of patients develop mild hepatic dysfunction after cardiac surgery with a transient rise in liver enzymes and bilirubin. Fulminant hepatic failure, which complicates less than 0.1% of cardiac surgery patients with no known pre-operative hepatic dysfunction, has a mortality of about 80%.

Aetiology

- *Pre-operative dysfunction*: hepatitis, cirrhosis, biliary obstruction.
- *Haemolysis*: blood transfusion, haematoma, paravalvular leak, glucose 6-phosphate dehydrogenase deficiency, prolonged bypass, excessive use of pump suckers.
- *Hepatocellular injury*: exacerbation of pre-operative disease, low cardiac output states, splanchnic ischaemia, prolonged high dose adrenaline (causes splanchnic hypoperfusion), right heart failure, hepatotoxic drugs (paracetamol, halothane, anti-retrovirals).
- *Cholestasis*: intra-hepatic (hepatitis, hepatocellular necrosis, cholestasis, parenteral nutrition, sepsis, drugs including opiates) and extra-hepatic (biliary tract obstruction).

Diagnosis

Fulminant hepatic failure is acute hepatic failure occurring within 8 weeks of exposure to the insult, and complicated by hepatic encephalopathy. In addition to increases (in the high thousands) in AST, ALP, LDH , and several-fold increases in gamma-GT and bilirubin, features of hepatic failure include:

- jaundice (secondary to conjugated hyperbilirubinaemia)
- hepatic encephalopathy
- coagulopathy (secondary decreased clotting factor production)
- ascites
- sepsis, including increased susceptibility to fungal infections
- acid-base disturbance: commonly metabolic acidosis due to ↑lactate
- metabolic derangements: commonly ↓Na
- hypoglycaemia due to glycogen depletion
- cerebral oedema and raised intracranial pressure
- hepatorenal and hepatopulmonary failure
- reduced systemic vascular resistance
- arrhythmias including VF.

Management

Modest elevations in liver enzymes and bilirubin are usually transient and benign; no action other than reducing hepatotoxic medication is usually required. Management of fulminant hepatic failure is mostly supportive:

- Check blood glucose frequently and replace as indicated.
- Treat cerebral oedema with mannitol.
- Renal failure requires dialysis.
- Cardiovascular support requires PA catheter insertion and inotropes.
- Give empirical antibiotic prophylaxis.

Hepatorenal failure

Hepatocellular failure is commonly complicated by renal failure. This is attributed to:

- ↑peripheral vasodilatation
- ↑renal vasoconstriction
- resulting in ↓glomerular filtration rate and oliguria.

If there is no clear primary cause of renal failure, this is called hepatorenal syndrome. Evidence from transplantation suggests that the renal failure is entirely secondary to liver failure as the renal failure improves both after liver transplantation, and after transplantation of the affected kidney into an individual without liver dysfunction. The renal dysfunction is proportional to the severity of hepatocellular failure, and acute tubular necrosis may supervene. Therapy is supportive: careful management of filling and systemic vascular resistance. Dialysis may be required for refractory acidosis, hyperkalaemia, and fluid overload.

Hepatopulmonary syndrome

Hepatocellular failure is less commonly complicated by hypoxaemia, as a result of abnormal ventilation-perfusion ratios and diffusion capacity. This is attributable to:

- ↑intrapulmonary vasodilatation
- ↓PVR
- failure of oxygen to diffuse as readily into the centre of dilated vessels
- ↑cardiac output limiting the time for gas exchange.

Stroke after cardiac surgery

The incidence of stroke after cardiac surgery is about 2%. This is the same for off-pump surgery. Patients with one or more risk factors have a much higher incidence of stroke, which affects consent and operative planning.

Risk factors for stroke after cardiac surgery

- increasing age (>80 years risk of CVA 5–10%)
- diabetes
- previous history of stroke or TIA (increases risk threefold)
- carotid artery atherosclerosis
- peri-operative hypotension
- calcified ascending aorta
- calcified aortic valve
- left-sided mural thrombus
- cardiotomy
- long duration of CPB
- post-operative AF
- failure to give anti-platelet therapy post-operatively.

Aetiology

Embolic
- microemboli, debris from operative field
- mural thrombus
- debris from valve excision, particularly calcified aortic valve
- septic emboli from endocarditis
- trauma to aorta from cannulation and clamping
- air embolism
- carotid atheroma.

Haemorrhagic
- heparinization on bypass
- post-operative warfarinization.

Cerebral hypoperfusion or hypoxia
- carotid and vertebral artery stenosis, dissection
- hypotension
- circulatory arrest (long period or insufficient cooling)
- raised ICP
- profound hypoxia before, during, or after bypass for >3 minutes.

Clinical features

Most neurological deficits are apparent once sedation has been weaned (i.e. within 24 hours), but one-third of strokes occur several days post-operatively. Any deficit resolving within 24 hours is called a transient ischaemic attack (TIA). Clinical features include:
- Failure to regain consciousness once sedation has been weaned.
- Hemiplegia (middle cerebral artery or total carotid artery occlusion).
- Initial areflexia becoming hyperreflexia and rigidity after a few days.
- Aphasia, dysarthria, ataxia (gait or truncal), inadequate gag reflex.

- Visual deficits, unilateral neglect, confusion.
- Persistent, marked hypertension.
- Hypercapnia.

Diagnosis

The aim is to establish a definitive diagnosis, establish a cause to guide appropriate secondary prevention, and establish a baseline of function to help plan long-term rehabilitation, or withdrawal of therapy.

- Carry out a full neurological examination (cognitive function, cranial nerves, and tone, power, reflexes, and sensation in all four limbs).
- Modern contrast head CT will show infarcts within 2 hours (older scanners may not pick up lesions until they are 2–3 days old). You must distinguish between haemorrhagic and ischaemic CVAs (1 in 10 are hemorrhagic). MRI is necessary to image brainstem lesions.

Prevention

Carotid endarterectomy

The single most important pre-operative intervention is identifying significant carotid artery disease. All patients with a previous history of stroke or TIA or with a carotid bruit should undergo duplex ultrasonography of their carotids. Some surgeons duplex all patients over the age of 80, and all patients with other severe extra-cardiac arteriopathy.

Performing carotid endarterectomy before cardiac surgery has a peri-operative risk of MI of 5–7%, and if carotid endarterectomy is left until after cardiac surgery the risk of peri-operative CVA is 5–7% performing cardiac and carotid together is associated with worse outcomes.

Operative technique during cardiac surgery

- Selection of cannulation sites can be guided by intra-operative ultrasound of the ascending aorta, which identifies diseased plaques at risk of embolization, and is much more accurate than digital palpation.
- Meticulous removal of debris from the operative field in open heart (especially aortic valve) surgery, exclusion of air from all arterial lines, and thorough de-airing are key parts of stroke prevention.
- 'No touch' technique in coronary artery bypass grafting.
- Systemic cooling provides some additional cerebral protection.
- Limiting use of pump suction reduces microemboli.

Post-operative measures

Aspirin (and clopidogrel after CEA) and blood pressure control.

Neurological complications

Confusion

Confusion after cardiac surgery is common. It is often obvious, with a disoriented, uncooperative, or hallucinating patient. Frequently, confusion is not overt, consisting of inactivity, quietness, slowed thinking, and labile mood, and it is only spotted by relatives or nursing staff. Actively assess whether the patient is oriented in time, person, and place. Perform a quick mental state examination if you are still unsure.

Common causes of confusion

- medication (particularly benzodiazepines, opiates, anticonvulsants)
- stroke
- hypoxia, hypercapnia
- shock
- 'post-pump' (micro air emboli)
- sepsis
- alcohol withdrawal
- metabolic disturbances ($\downarrow$glucose, Na^+, pH; $\uparrow Ca^{2+}$, Cr, urea, bilirubin)
- post-ictal
- pre-operative dementia.

Management

- If the patient's behaviour poses a physical danger to themselves or others, it may be necessary to sedate as first-line management; haloperidol 2.5mg may be given up to a total of 10mg in 24 hours orally, IM, or IV, but if the patient remains disturbed 2.5–5mg of midazolam should be given IV and the patient placed under close observation.
- Beware of sedating the hypoxic or hypotensive patient as this may trigger a cardiorespiratory arrest.
- Assess and treat hypoxia.
- Reassess the drug chart; stop opiates and benzodiazapines.
- Correct metabolic abnormalities.
- Alcohol withdrawal is diagnosed from a history of chronically high alcohol consumption, often with raised gamma-GT, combined with psychomotor agitation post-operatively. It can be treated with either diazepam, haloperidol, or by allowing the patient either dehydrogenated alcohol or 1 unit orally.
- Perform a neurological examination to look for focal neurological deficit and consider head CT to exclude stroke.
- Reassure patient and relatives; confusion is common, almost always reversible, and it is not a sign that the patient is 'going mad'.

Seizures

Seizures may be generalized (loss of consciousness with or without tonic-clonic features, absence seizures, atonia) or partial (localized to part of one hemisphere). Causes of seizures include:

- Physical: stroke, intracranial bleed, cerebral air emboli, septic emboli.
- Metabolic: withdrawal of alcohol, anticonvulsants, or benzodiazepines; $\downarrow\uparrow$glucose, Na^+, pH, Ca^{2+}, $\uparrow$Creatinine, urea, bilirubin; tricyclic antidepressants; lignocaine toxicity.

Management

Status epilepticus is any seizure lasting >30 minutes, or repeated seizures without intervening consciousness. Treat by securing the airway, give oxygen, suction if required, give diazepam 10mg IV over 2 minutes, and then 5mg/minute until seizures stop or respiratory depression occurs, then start phenytoin 15mg/kg IV up to 50mg per minute if seizures continue. Most seizures are self-limiting; start regular phenytoin as prophylaxis and look for an underlying cause.

Peripheral nerve injuries

Brachial plexus injury

This is caused indirectly by sternal retraction, and directly by trauma when placing central lines. It presents as paraesthesia and weakness in the C8–T1, and if severe C6–C7. Formal diagnosis is by electromyogram (EMG) studies. It can be avoided by placing the sternal retractor as caudally as possible and opening it slowly. Treatment is physiotherapy, with referral to a pain service for chronic pain unresponsive to analgesia.

Horner's syndrome

Ptosis, miosis, anhydrosis, and enophthalmos resulting from damage to the sympathetic nerve supply to the eye at any stage from its journey from the central nuclei and spinal cord to post-ganglionic fibres via the stellate ganglion. Inadvertent damage during central line placement, carotid endarterectomy, harvest of the very proximal IMA, and stroke may cause this syndrome. Treatment is symptomatic.

Recurrent laryngeal nerve palsy

This may occur as a result of IMA harvesting, trauma to the arch of the aorta, e.g. from cannulating, trauma to the nerve in the neck from internal jugular vein cannulation, pressure injury from a malpositioned endotracheal cuff, and cold injury. It presents as hoarseness and breathlessness after extubation. Patients should be seen by an ENT surgeon.

Phrenic nerve palsy

This is discussed on p. 232.

Sympathetic dystrophy (radial and saphanous nerve)

Injury to these nerves when harvesting conduit usually results in paraesthesia (over the anatomical snuff box in radial nerve injury and over the medial malleolus and ankle in saphenous nerve injury). Occasionally this is associated with increasing pain, swelling, and trophic changes (hair loss, shiny skin). Sympathetic dystrophy is difficult to treat; it may respond to NSAIDs such as ibuprofen, regular analgesia, or amitryptiline for intractable neuropathic pain.

Ulnar nerve injury

Failure to protect the arms with padding intra-operatively may lead to ulnar nerve paresis from pressure injury to the ulnar nerve as it passes round the medial epicondyle of the elbow.

Surgical site infection

(📖 see Chapter 2)

Deep sternal wound infection (DSWI)

Definition of deep sternal wound infection

The North American Center for Disease Control and Prevention defines this as infection involving tissue deep to the subcutaneous layers **and** positive cultures, macroscopic or histological evidence, symptoms, or pus.

The incidence of deep sternal wound infection is reported at 0.5–5%. As up to 75% of wound infections present after discharge from hospital, the incidence is frequently underreported. Risk factors include:
- *Pre-operative*: age, diabetes, obesity, smoking, steroid therapy, COPD.
- *Operative*: paramedian sternotomy, bilateral pedicled mammary artery harvest, prolonged surgery, poor surgical technique (including excessive bone wax and cautery to the periosteum, inaccurate placement of sternal wires, poor aseptic technique).
- *Post-operative*: re-sternotomy for bleeding, multiple transfusions, mediastinal bleeding, prolonged ventilation, impaired nutrition.

Diagnosis
- Fever, leucocytosis, positive blood cultures.
- Sternal 'click' (ask the patient to cough or turn their head left and right while feeling for movement in the sternum).
- Serous or purulent discharge from the wound.
- Wound dehiscence.
- Pericardial effusion on CT chest or ECHO.
- Chest X-ray may show fractured or migrating sternal wires.
- CT may show evidence of non-union, pus, and osteomyelitis.

Prevention
- *Pre-operative*: weight reduction in obese patients, reducing steroid therapy, optimizing respiratory function, screening for and treating MRSA.
- *Operative*: meticulous aseptic and operative technique. Separate leg and sternal wound instruments (sharing increases the incidence of *E. coli* sternal wound infection). Appropriate antibiotic prophylaxis.
- *Post-operative*: wash hands between examining each patient (alcohol rinse has been shown to be more effective than soap and water at reducing cross infection).

Management
- A cough lock may reduce pain and reduce the impact of dehiscence.
- Antibiotics.
- Negative pressure wound (vacuum assisted closure) dressing.
- Surgical debridement and rewiring may be necessary.

Rewiring for sternal wound infection

This is never undertaken lightly. Patients may have multiple organ dysfunction as a result of sepsis, tissues are friable, and surgery often takes place at a time when adhesions are maximal (4–6 weeks post-operatively). The principles are the same as for an elective re-sternotomy (📖 Bleeding p.238). Ensure that the patient has appropriate antibiotics on induction. Devitalized tissue is debrided back to bleeding margins, including the sternal edges, which need to be undermined sufficiently to place sternal wires. All pus is evacuated from the pericardium, paying great care to anastomotic lines, any of which may be involved in infection. Send pus and bone for culture to guide treatment and detect osteomyelitis. Where there is a lot of infected material it is reasonable to place a VAC dressing between the sternal edges, and return for closure in a few days time once the wound is clean. Where primary closure cannot be achieved due to multiple extensive debridements, options include pectoralis major advancement flaps, transrectus abdominus muscle (TRAM) flaps, and (rarely) omental flaps. Plastic surgeons should be involved for the last two, and in some practices are involved from initial presentation. There are many alternative primary closures, though none have been proved superior:

• standard closure
• antiseptic washout
• Robicek closure
• sternal bands
• irrigation systems.

Superficial sternal wound infection

The incidence of superficial sternal wound infection is about 3–10%, superficial saphenous vein harvest site infection up to 25%, and superficial radial wound harvest site infection about 5%. Diagnosis is usually based on presence of local cellulitis or discharge. Swab the wound and take blood cultures if pyrexial. Management includes:

• antibiotics
• incision and drainage of pus
• negative pressure dressing (vacuum assisted closure) for deep wounds with large amounts of pus
• monitoring for any signs of deep sternal wound infection.

Wound complications

Sternal instability and sterile dehiscence

Sterile sternal instability and dehiscence is usually due to poor surgical technique, or 'cheese-wiring' of sternal wires through a soft, osteoporotic sternum. The incidence is 1–2%. The patient complains of excessive chostochondral pain and 'clicking' on movement and instability may be palpated when the patient coughs. These may be managed either conservatively with prophylactic antibiotics and support dressings, or with elective sternal rewiring. If it does not become infected, an unstable sternum eventually forms a cartilaginous flexible union or pseudoarthrosis. An unstable sternum is a risk factor for prolonged ventilation and chest infections in the post-operative period.

Sternal dehiscence

Sternal dehiscence presents similarly to abdominal wound dehiscence:
- serosanguinous discharge from the wound on day 3–5 post-operatively
- ↑WCC
- sudden opening up of wound on coughing or straining.

Return the patient back to bed, reassure them, cover the wound with sterile saline-soaked gauze, give the patient 2.5mg IM morphine, with nil by mouth. Take microbiology swabs. Most patients should be taken back to theatre for debridement and re-wiring. Occasionally, for example where wires have cheese-wired through soft sternums, patients are managed conservatively with negative pressure (vacuum assisted closure) dressings and cough-locks.

Hypertrophic and keloid scars

Midline incisions have a tendency to form raised red hypertrophic scars. Keloid scars (where the lumpy scar tissue exceeds the margin of the scar) are common in patients of African descent. There is no known way of avoiding these unsightly scars, apart from attempting to minimize the length of the sternotomy incision, or considering submammary incisions.

Sternal wires

Sometimes patients complain of prominent sternal wires. This is commonest in very thin patients. If the sternum is stable, the sternal wires may be removed. This should be done under general anaesthetic with appropriate monitoring; even a simple removal of sternal wires can turn into an unexpected re-sternotomy. If the patient is unhappy with just one or two wires, make sure you mark them with the patient pre-operatively. These can be removed through stab incisions.

Table 11.5 Complications of thoracotomy incisions

Incision	Complications
All major thoracic incisions	Immediate: respiratory compromise, trauma to underlying viscera and neurovascular structures (usually from poor patient positioning on table or over-retraction)
	Early: major haemorrhage requiring resternotomy/rethoracotomy, superficial wound infection
	Late: chronic pain syndromes, scarring
Median sternotomy	Immediate: brachial plexus, phrenic nerve injury
	Early: deep sternal wound infection, mediastinitis, sternal dehiscence
	Late: chronic osteomyelitis, sternal instability, incisional hernia, prominent sternal wires requiring removal, keloid, hypertrophic scarring
Posterolateral thoracotomy	Immediate: major air leak, pneumothorax, brachial plexus and peripheral nerve injury
	Early: prolonged air leak, effusion, deep wound infection, empyema
	Late: seroma, chronic pain, paraesthesia, herniation lung
Anterior thoracotomy	Immediate: respiratory compromise
	Early: wound infection, empyema
	Late: chronic pain, paraesthesia
Thoracoabdominal	Immediate: respiratory compromise
	Early: wound infection, empyema
	Late: chronic pain, paraesthesia, incisional hernia
Mediastinoscopy	Immediate: injury to neck vessels, thyroid, trachea, laryngeal nerve palsy, wound infection
VATS	Immediate: trauma to intercostal neurovascular bundle, underlying lung injury, brachial plexus injury, major air leak, conversion to conventional thoracotomy
	Early: wound infection
	Late: port site recurrence, port site herniation
Redo incision	As for individual incision with greatly increased risk of trauma to underlying structures and major haemorrhage

Haematological complications
(📖 see Chapter 6)

Heparin-induced thrombocytopaenia (HIT)
HIT occurs in about 5% of patients receiving heparin (5.5% of patients on bovine heparin, 1.0% with porcine heparin). It is characterized by formation of complement-mediated heparin-dependent IgG platelet antibody. It occurs 5–10 days after initiation of heparin therapy, or after the first dose of heparin in patients with previous exposure to heparin within the last 3 months.

Diagnosis
- Decrease in platelet count by over 30% to 150 × 10⁹/l, or by over 50%, **and** positive serology for HIT antibodies.
- Heparin induced thrombocytopaenia and thrombosis (HITT) occurs in about 20% of patients with HIT, is characterized by major thrombotic episodes, and has a mortality of about 30%.
- Patients may show tachyphylaxis to heparin, as well as bleeding complications.

Treatment
- Discontinue all heparin therapy, including heparinized saline flushes.
- If it is at all possible, delay any surgery requiring bypass until HIT antibodies are undetectable, and then follow standard heparinization, but do not use heparin in the post-operative period.
- If it is impossible to delay bypass surgery then danaparoid and iloprost are alternatives to heparin with the major disadvantages that they cannot be reversed after bypass, and require specialized assays.
- Hirudin, iloprost, danaparoid, and warfarin are alternative anticoagulants to heparin in the post-operative period.

Disseminated intravascular coagulation (DIC)
DIC is extremely rare during bypass but may occur post-operatively as a complication of sepsis, transfusion reaction, drug reaction, transplant rejection, and aortic aneurysm surgery. It is characterized by widespread activation of coagulation, resulting in the formation of intravascular fibrin, fibrin degradation products, consumption of platelets and clotting factors, and ultimately thrombotic occlusion of vessels. Patients may present with bleeding from indwelling venous lines, wounds, and minor abrasions.

Diagnosis
- There is no single diagnostic test. The following findings suggest DIC:
- sudden fall in platelet count to <100 × 10⁹/l
- bleeding and/or thrombotic complications
- ↑APTT, PT, INR
- ↑fibrin degradation products (D-dimers)
- ↓fibrinogen in severe DIC.

Management
The key is to treat the underlying disorder. Bleeding patients should receive FFP, platelets, blood, and cryoprecipitate as indicated by coagulation screens. Patients with thrombosis should be heparinized.

Excessive warfarinization

Management depends on whether the patient is bleeding, and why they are warfarinized:

- If the INR is <5.0 and the patient is not bleeding, simply omit warfarin and recheck INR daily, restarting warfarin once the INR is within target range.
- If the INR is >5.0 give 10mg vitamin K orally.
- If the patient is bleeding give FFP and up to 5mg vitamin K orally.
- If the patient has a mechanical valve the risk of thromboembolic events when anticoagulation is reversed is about 0.016% per day; anticoagulation with heparin or warfarin should be recommenced within 1–2 weeks once any bleeding complications have resolved.

General thoracic complications

Intrapleural space

Key facts

- Intrapleural spaces develop when the lung fails to fill the pleural cavity after collapse or resection in approximately one-third of pulmonary resections.
- The intrapleural space is normally obliterated by re-expansion of the remaining lung, mediastinal shift post-pneumonectomy, narrowing of the intercostal spaces, and elevation of the ipsilateral hemidiaphragm.
- Failure to obliterate the pleural space is due to poor compliance of the residual lung (due to atelectasis or consolidation, or incomplete removal of cortex during decortication for empyema), persistent air leaks, and occasionally mediastinal fibrosis.
- Around two-thirds undergo spontaneous resolution, and half of the remainder resolve with insertion of an intercostal drain. The rest persist, with half of them becoming infected, resulting in an empyema.

Clinical features and treatment

- Indistinguishable on CXR from a pneumothorax.
- Pleural spaces can be prevented by placement of large-gauge pleural drains at apex and base of the lung to drain fluid and air.
- In extensive resections where it is anticipated that a pleural space is more likely, some surgeons perform a phrenic nerve crush to elevate the ipsilateral hemidiaphragm at the expense of its function.
- Thoracoplasty, where a subperiosteal resection of the first two to three ribs is performed, reduces the apical pleural space.
- In pneumoperitoneum, which is not widely performed, up to 1500ml of air are insufflated into the peritoneum to elevate the diaphragm, obliterating the pleural space.
- Treatment of post-operative pleural space includes encouraging lung expansion using physiotherapy and early mobilization, and generation of non-invasive mechanical and physiological positive pressure using continuous positive airway pressure.
- Prevention of mucus retention is the key; oxygen should be humidified wherever possible, saline as well as bronchodilator nebulizers given regularly, and adequate analgesia and chest physiotherapy employed to maximize cough effectiveness.
- Intercostal drains are routinely placed on low pressure suction at −3 to −5kPa. If there is no air leak and the lung is fully inflated. This is discontinued after 48 hours prior to drain removal. However, if the lung fails to re-expand fully, thoracic suction may be increased slowly up to −10kPa.
- Persistent pleural spaces may be treated conservatively if small and not associated with air leaks or infection.
- Large persistent pleural spaces are followed up with serial chest X-rays; elective thoracoplasty is now not commonly performed for these.

Surgical emphysema

Key facts

- This is the presence of subcutaneous air.
- Air usually enters the soft tissues through a wound, usually from a major intrathoracic air leak, or occasionally entrained from outside the chest wall.

Clinical features and treatment

- Swelling that is 'crunchy' to touch and on auscultation.
- Swelling may be localized to drain or wound site, but in severe cases it extends rapidly across the trunk and over the neck, face, and both limbs.
- The patient may be unable to open his/her eyes because of palpebral swelling, and the voice has a characteristic nasal sound because of swelling of the soft tissues of the pharynx, which is occasionally severe enough to compromise the upper airway.
- Establish the airway, locate the source of the leak, and treat it.
- Obtain CXR to look for pneumothorax; insert chest-tube immediately if you suspect tension pneumothorax.
- On CXR subcutaneous emphysema outlines muscle and fascial layers.
- With appropriate insertion of an intercostal drain, surgical emphysema normally resolves over the course of 5–10 days.

Chylothorax

Key facts

- Chylothorax complicates <0.5% of lung resections for bronchogenic carcinoma, and up to 3% of oesophagectomies.
- It is commoner after pneumonectomy than after lobectomy.
- It is usually due to intra-operative injury to the thoracic duct/ tributaries.
- Resection of large proximal tumours, extensive lymphadenectomy and dissection, and redo-surgery all increase the risk of injury.

Clinical features

- Injury may be noticed intra-operatively (milky fluid accumulates in the field) and should be repaired or both ends of the duct ligated.
- Post-op persistent serosanguinous pleural drainage >500ml per day suggests a chylous leak. If the patient is NBM, fluid may be clear.
- Drain fluid triglyceride >110mg/dl is diagnostic.

Treatment

- Management is initially conservative. Large-gauge intercostal drains are mandatory for effective drainage of the pleural space.
- Place patient on a no-fat medium-chain triglyceride diet.
- Conservative management is successful in half of cases in 10 to 14 days.
- A chyle leak refractory to conservative management should be ligated or repaired surgically as it predisposes to infection, as well as having an adverse impact on nutritional status.
- The standard approach is ligation of the thoracic duct near the diaphragm, which can be carried out via a low left or right thoracotomy or a laparotomy. VATS approaches are used increasingly frequently.

Lung resection

Death and recurrence
- Mortality 1.2–1.5% for lobectomy and 3.2–10% for pneumonectomy.
- Age >65 and ischemic heart disease are risk factors for mortality.
- Causes of operative death include respiratory failure and pneumonia, bronchopleural fistula, cardiac failure, and occasionally haemorrhage.
- Five-year survival is 60–70% for patients undergoing resection of stage 1 adenocarcinoma, 50% for stage IIa, and 25% for stage IIb.
- Patients with recurrent disease have a median survival of 18 months.

Bronchopleural fistula (BPF)
Key facts
- A large communication between the bronchi and pleural space, usually with empyema as the bronchi are colonized with bacteria. Mortality is up to 30%.
- The incidence of BPF after resection for lung malignancy is 1–5%.
- Pre-operative risk factors include advanced age, malnutrition, steroids, and neo-adjuvant radiotherapy. Intra-operative risk factors include devascularized stump or anastomosis, and incomplete resection margins.
- Post-operative risk factors include wound infection.
- Pedicled flaps of pericardial or pleural fat, or intercostal muscle applied to the bronchial stump or anastomosis, can help prevent suture line breakdown and formation of a BPF in high-risk cases.

Clinical features
- Classically BPF presents 7–10 days post-op, rarely months post-op.
- Features include:
  - Fever, purulent cough that may be worse when lying on the contralateral side, persistent large or worsening air leak and/or pleural collection, and occasionally subcutaneous emphysema.
  - Inflammatory markers are raised, and chest radiography shows a collection, often with a fluid level.
  - Following pneumonectomy, a **decrease in the fluid level** as a result of air entering the pleural space and some fluid leaving it via the bronchial tree (rather than the steady increase normally observed post-operatively) is pathognomonic of a BPF.
- Bronchoscopy may identify large fistulas, or dehiscence of the anastomosis. Small fistulas or leaks may only be detectable as local movement of secretions, or a small area of inflammation or granulation.

Treatment
- Intercostal drain (which needs radiological guidance if lung adhesions are likely) to drain the empyema, address the air leak, reduce sepsis, and most importantly prevent further aspiration of pus into the bronchial tree.
- One-third of small, early fistulas not due to residual local tumour and occurring in well patients close spontaneously with an intercostal drain.
- Large fistulas, those associated with incomplete resection margins, wound infection, and large air leaks, and those not responding to conservative management require surgical repair – options include:
  - thoracotomy, decortication, drainage empyema, repair of fistula

- completion pneumonectomy may be unavoidable
- myoplasty and thoracoplasty to obliterate the space
- muscle and tissue flaps to wrap around the anastomosis
- VATS repair may be an option in small, early BPFs
- Claggett technique involves irrigating the pleural space with antibiotics, packing the space with sterile gauze to encourage granulation tissue, and resecting a rib space leaving an open thoracostomy.

Prolonged air leak

Key facts

- Prolonged air leak is defined as one lasting >7 days post-operatively.
- Clinically the underwater seal bubbles continuously; if the air leak is small the underwater seal only bubbles on coughing.
- Small air leaks normally close spontaneously 2–5 days post-op.
- Large air leaks due to problems at the bronchial stump or anastomosis, trauma to the bronchial tree, bullae, or large surface area of raw lung parenchyma (e.g. after redo-thoracotomy or decortication) are normally persistent and if identified intra-operatively need definitive management.

Treatment

- Obtain a CXR and check for pneumothorax in patients with new air leak.
- Post-operatively air leaks are treated by encouraging lung expansion as apposition of lung surfaces reduces air leaks (increasing suction, chest physiotherapy, incentive spirometry, early mobilization, etc).
- Always check for obvious extra-pleural sources of air leak, including drain site, drain position, all drain connections, underwater seal, and suction.
- Pulling the drain back a few centimetres and/or reducing suction may help if the drain is lying directly over the source of the air leak.
- Additional drains may be placed under radiological guidance.
- Talc slurry pleurodesis is employed for patients with persistent air leaks considered too frail to tolerate further surgery; a suspension of talc, local anaesthetic, and saline is injected using aseptic technique into the intercostal drain to encourage the lung to adhese to the chest wall.
- Keep the drain, trim, and replace underwater seal with a one-way Heimlich flutter valve if the pleural space does not increase off suction – carries an increased risk of empyema, but air leak may resolve.

Complications of bronchial and tracheal resections

- Sleeve resections have an operative mortality approaching 7.5%.
- Local recurrence is as high as 10%.
- Ischaemia or dehiscence of the bronchial anastomosis leading to bronchopleural fistula affects 3–5% of patients; investigate bronchoscopically.
- Any failure of the anastomosis requires re-exploration and repair.
- Excessive granulation tissue may form at the site of the anastomosis; this may be removed bronchoscopically. Anastomotic strictures may respond to bronchoscopic dilatation with solid bougies or balloon dilators.
- Completion pneumonectomy may be the only treatment option.

Oesophagectomy (📖 see Chapter 9, p.159)

Death and recurrence
- Mortality rates are 0–17.3% and very unit/surgeon dependent.
- Risks for mortality include: low functional ability pre-op; pulmonary, cardiac, or hepatic dysfunction; and tumour location.
- The commonest cause of operative death is sepsis, normally from anastomotic failure, followed by respiratory failure and MI.
- Recurrence rate after macroscopically curative resection is approximately 50% at 5 years, with over 80% of recurrences occurring within 24 months of surgery, and 60% of recurrence occurring in patients with stage 3 and 4 disease.
- Where there is recurrence within 2 years, 50% survival is <9 months.

Anastomotic leak
Key facts
- Anastomotic leak is the single largest cause of post-operative mortality.
- The primary aetiology is ischaemia from inadequate preservation of local and regional blood supply during mobilization.
- The site of the anastomosis, which may be cervical or thoracic, dictates the likelihood of dehiscence, the presentation, and the morbidity.
  - intrathoracic anastomoses have a dehiscence rate of approximately 10%, compared to closer to 20% for cervical anastomoses
  - the mortality associated with leakage from intrathoracic anastomoses is as high as 75% compared to 20–30% for cervical dehiscence.

Clinical features
- Contained thoracic leaks are usually heralded by a pleural effusion or pneumothorax associated with sepsis.
- Cervical leaks present with cellulitis and surgical emphysema.
- Both types may present as septic shock associated with purulent drainage in the first 48 hours post-operatively.
- Leaks may be clinically silent, and identified on routine contrast studies.
- Request gastrograffin contrast studies and CT.

Treatment
- Small anastomotic leaks may heal spontaneously if the lung is completely expanded (effectively buttressing the anastomosis) and there is no distal obstruction, and insertion of an intercostal drain may be all that is required.
- Persistent leaks are managed by direct repair or with pedicled flaps via thoracotomy for thorascopic approaches.
- The wound should be reopened; leaks contained within the neck fascial compartments may be treated conservatively, but if there is mediastinitis, surgical exploration, debridement, and repair are indicated.
- If conduit ischaemia is followed by gastric necrosis, surgical exploration, resection of ischaemic stomach, and stoma formation is the only option for treatment and mortality is high.
- Percutaneous drainage and TPN may be used in clinically silent leaks.

Anastomotic strictures

Key facts
- Anastomotic strictures occur in up to 20% of oesophagectomies.
- Early strictures are due to inflammatory changes from wound healing.
- Late strictures are usually related to local cancer recurrence or chronic reflux oesophagitis.

Clinical features and treatment
- Strictures present with progressive dysphagia ± odynophagia.
- Investigation of early strictures centres on defining the anatomy.
- Detection of anastomotic recurrence in late strictures needs gastrografin swallow, contrast enhanced CT, and oesophagoscopy with biopsy to identify cancer recurrence.
- Most strictures respond to dilatation, which is associated with a rate of oesophageal perforation of less than 5%.
- Resection is an option for persistent strictures in otherwise fit individuals without evidence of recurrence.

Functional disorders

Dumping syndromes
- There are two types of 'dumping' syndrome:
  - Early dumping results from rapid transit of high molecular weight solids into the jejunum resulting in hyperglycaemia, and transit of water down the osmotic gradient into the bowel lumen. Early dumping affects up to 20% of patients and presents with nausea, vomiting, diarrhoea, faintness, and dyspnoea within minutes of ingesting a meal.
  - Late dumping is caused by reactive hypoglycaemia. Patients present with dizziness, breathlessness, and nausea 1 to 3 hours post-prandially.
- Both dumping syndromes may improve with time. Eating smaller meals more frequently, avoidance of dairy products and high carbohydrate meals, avoiding excessive fluid intake with meals, and anti-diarrhoeal agents are all helpful.

Delayed gastric emptying
- Delayed gastric emptying may be due to vagal denervation, torsion, and compression, the pressure difference between the intrathoracic neo-stomach and the abdominal duodenum, or mucosal oedema.
- These patients are at risk of regurgitation, reflux, and aspiration pneumonia acutely, and stricture formation and malnutrition in the longer term.
- Erythromycin improves gastric emptying.
- Gastric outlet obstruction may require pyloroplasty.

Mediastinal surgery

Resection of anterior mediastinal masses

- Resection of thymoma and other invasive mediastinal masses may result in damage to either phrenic nerve, the left recurrent laryngeal nerve, chylothorax, and major vascular structures.
- In thymectomy for myasthenia gravis, up to 50% of patients will be in remission 20 years following surgery (compared to 20% 1 year post-operatively), and up to 90% will be in partial remission.
- Respiratory failure post-operatively is the next single most important complication, affecting up to 5% of patients who may be electively ventilated post-operatively in order to avoid this complication.
- Careful pre-operative planning, including optimizing medical therapy, plasmapheresis, careful titration of anaesthetic agents, and avoidance of neuromuscular blockade, is the key.
- Post-operative respiratory failure is managed with re-intubation and ventilation.

Mediastinoscopy and mediastinotomy

- The morbidity and mortality of mediastinoscopy is low, with complication in less than 2% of patients.
- The most important complication is haemorrhage, usually resulting from blunt dissection or inadvertent biopsy of a major vascular structure such as the aorta, pulmonary trunk, superior vena cava, azygous vein, or innominate artery.
- Small tears and venous bleeding can normally be controlled by direct packing and pressure.
- Significant damage to vascular structures requires emergency thoracotomy or sternotomy and surgical repair.
- Rarely, tears in the pulmonary trunk or posterior aorta may be inaccessible without cardiopulmonary bypass, and damage to the distal right or left pulmonary artery may be impossible to address without pneumonectomy.
- Atherosclerotic embolization from the aortic arch or ischaemia from compression of the innominate artery may rarely cause stroke.
- Oesophageal or bronchial perforation, which are uncommon complications, may not be recognized intra-operatively; they may present after the patient has been discharged home, with sepsis, pleural effusion, or surgical emphysema. Both injuries require surgical repair either at the time of surgery if recognized intra-operatively, or post-operatively.

Acknowledgement
Some of the material for this chapter was adapted from Chikwe, Beddow, Glenville (2006) *Cardiothoracic Surgery*, Oxford University Press, Oxford.

Complications of abdominal transplant surgery

Kidney transplantation

Over the last 40 years kidney transplantation has evolved from an 'experimental' therapy to the gold standard treatment for most patients with end-stage renal failure. Transplantation is beneficial in terms of life expectancy, quality of life, and cost when compared to both haemodialysis and peritoneal dialysis. The main limitations to transplantation are a lack of suitable organs either from cadaveric or living donors. The outcomes expected are excellent with 1-year patient and graft survival rates of over 90%. Despite this the procedure is associated with recognized complications in the immediate, early, and late post-operative periods.

Immediate complications

Patients undergoing transplantation are at significant peri-operative risk as they have, by definition, significant life-threatening co-morbidity. This may be the causative factor for their renal failure, examples being diabetes or hypertension, or there may be associated diseases such as ischaemic heart disease or rheumatological and vasculitic conditions. The associated drug treatments may also pose specific complications and risks. It is perhaps not surprising that death with a functioning graft is the commonest cause of graft loss in the early post-operative period. Graft-specific complications occurring within the immediate post-operative period (first 24 hours) are shown in the box on the next page and discussed in detail below.

Hyperacute/accelerated acute rejection

Hyperacute and accelerated acute rejection is mediated by preformed anti-donor antibodies. This is extremely rare and may reflect issues with mismatching of blood type or the presence of preformed anti-HLA antibodies in sensitized patients. The pathogenesis of this type of rejection is that rapid complement activation results in intravascular thrombosis and graft destruction within a short time. Prevention is by accurate pre-transplant cross matching and desensitization of patients with pre-formed antibodies.

Post-operative complications

Immediate (0–24 hours)
- hyperacute/accelerated acute rejection
- polyuria/oliguria/anuria
- hypovolaemia
- haemorrhage
- renal artery/renal vein thrombosis
- ureteric leak/obstruction.

Early (24 hours to 14 days)
- delayed graft function (DGF)
- calcineurin inhibitor (CNI) toxicity
- rejection
- lymphocele
- infection
- wound complications

Late (2 weeks onwards)
- infection
- renal artery stenosis
- late acute rejection
- chronic allograft nephropathy
- post-transplant lymphoproliferative disorders (PTLD) and malignancy
- metabolic, e.g. tertiary hyperparathyroidism, post-transplant diabetes mellitus (PTDM).

Polyuria/oliguria/anuria
Immediately post-transplant patients may have varying degrees of renal function. This is multi-factorial and may reflect their pre-transplant renal function and their peri-operative fluid balance. The use of intra-operative diuretics (mannitol or frusemide) may drive the transplanted kidney as well as native kidneys and polyuria can be dramatic. If significant polyuria occurs metabolic complications can arise, particularly with respect to calcium and magnesium, and subsequent sequelae may be precipitated. Hypovolaemia may also occur if fluid replacement is inadequate.

Approximately one-third of patients are oliguric or anuric and although this is not accurately predictable, the risk of slow or delayed graft function (DGF) is increased with kidneys from older donors and with longer cold ischaemia times. It is rare in live donor renal transplants and this reflects the pathogenesis, which is multi-factorial but related to acute tubular injury (ATN) associated with ischaemia during the organ retrieval process, cold storage, and subsequent ischaemia-reperfusion. Other contributing factors occur such as the events leading to brain stem death, the 'autonomic storm', and to donor instability.

Diagnosis is by exclusion of other causes of oliguria and good perfusion on duplex ultrasound.

Treatment is by fluid optimization and dialysis when required. Pharmacological manipulation is often practised in patients with DGF although the evidence for this practice is limited.

Haemorrhage

Haemorrhage should always be considered if the patient is hypovolaemic. As with any vascular procedure, peri- and post-operative bleeding can occur. Despite the relative coagulopathy associated with poor platelet function in uraemia and the use of heparin in haemodialysis patients, the incidence of haemorrhage in transplantation is low and can often be managed conservatively as the usual cause of bleeding is from small vessels rather than the anastomosis. Late haemorrhage can occur from mycotic aneurysms of the anastomosis but this is fortunately rare.

Hypotension not responding to fluids and oliguria should raise the suspicion of bleeding and drains should be closely monitored (although a blocked drain does not exclude bleeding!). An ultrasound scan should be performed to exclude a haematoma and if this is causing compression of the vessels or ureter it should be drained either operatively or percutaneously.

Renal artery/renal vein thrombosis

Vascular thrombosis is the main cause of graft loss in the first few days, although the incidence is less than 5%. Both are usually due to technical issues at the time of surgery (multiple, short, or damaged vessels) although patients with thrombophilia are also at increased risk.

The diagnosis should always be suspected in patients with oliguria or anuria and a functioning transplant. It may be associated with haematuria and pain over the transplant. Rarely if a total venous occlusion occurs the kidney may split, resulting in significant haemorrhage.

The diagnosis is by duplex ultrasound scan. Lack of flow in the vessels is an ominous sign and despite reports of grafts being salvaged it is almost always associated with graft loss and an early transplant nephrectomy is required at the time of exploration.

Ureteric leak or obstruction

The transplanted ureter is deprived of its segmental blood supply and relies solely on the main renal vessels. Injury to lower polar arteries devascularizes the ureter and renders the ureteroneocystostomy (UNC) ischaemic. This results in a urine leak if the anastomosis becomes disrupted and usually presents in the first few days post-transplant. This is diagnosed when urine is revealed through the drain (compare drain fluid with serum level creatinine to be certain), or a collection is seen around the kidney on ultrasound scan. Treatment is conservative with percutaneous drainage and prolonged catheterization. The disruption, if incomplete, may respond to a ureteral stent placed either ante or retrogradely. Obstruction usually implies a mechanical cause and a blocked catheter and extrinsic cause should be excluded first. Stenosis of the UNC usually occurs later unless a technical mishap arises. This presents with pain, transplant dysfunction, and oliguria, and on ultrasound a hydronephrosis is present. Again, percutaneous drainage and stenting is the mainstay of treatment. Few patients require surgical revision but this is usually performed by anastomosis onto the ipsilateral native ureter. The routine use of prophylactic stents is controversial although it may reduce the urinary complication rate.

Early complications

Calcineurin inhibitor (CNI) toxicity

Standard immunosuppressive regimens rely on the use of CNIs, namely ciclosporin or tacrolimus. Both agents are associated with nephrotoxic side effects. High plasma levels of either drug are associated with nephrotoxicity and inhibit renal function. The diagnosis is made on plasma levels as both drugs require close therapeutic monitoring due to their unpredictable pharmacodynamics. Biopsy shows characteristic changes associated with CNI toxicity. Treatment is based on dose reduction until therapeutic targets are achieved. As these drugs have many interactions, other drugs should also be reviewed.

Acute rejection

Acute allograft rejection represents a specific immunopathological process and represents T cell and/or antibody-mediated processes. It characteristically occurs after the first post-transplant week and may occur at any time after, although 90% of episodes occur in the first 3 months. It is recognized by transplant dysfunction and should be suspected when the creatinine rises on sequential days. The diagnosis rests on histological confirmation and different classes of rejection are described. Treatment requires escalation of immunosuppression, usually in the form of pulsed steroids (typically 3 days of high-dose prednisolone) although other protocols exist.

The majority of episodes are fully reversed with treatment.

Lymphocele

Serous fluid may collect in the space around the kidney and is termed a lymphocele. The source of the fluid may be from the transplanted kidney or the iliac perivascular lymphatics. It is important to distinguish a lymphocele from a urine leak by biochemistry (lymphocele will be plasma-creatinine equivalent) and diagnosis and drainage can be done by ultrasound guidance. Small lymphoceles may be treated conservatively but larger ones, and those not resolving with percutaneous drainage, may require operative drainage in the form of peritoneal fenestration, which can be open or laparoscopic.

Infection

Transplant patients have the risk of post-operative infections (chest, UTI, wound) as all post-operative patients do, but additionally have the side effects of immunosuppression. The risk of opportunistic infections is increased, with fungal (*Candida*, *Aspergillus*) and viral infections being of particular concern. Prophylactic antibiotics and antifungal agents are given routinely. Other infections of concern in renal patients are Cytomegalovirus (CMV), *Pneumocystis carinii*, and tuberculosis, for which prophylaxis is given to those at risk.

Wound complications

Transplant patients have multiple risk factors for impaired healing and the rates of wound infection and hernias are higher in transplanted patients.

Late complications

Renal artery stenosis

This is generally a late complication of renal transplant. It may present with gradually deteriorating renal function and drug-resistant hypertension. Duplex ultrasound, MR angiogram, or contrast angiographic studies confirm the diagnosis. The aetiology is unknown although it is more common in end-to-end anastomosis and may represent intimal hyperplasia. Management is with percutaneous trans-luminal angioplasty if technically feasible. If this is not possible, open surgical repair is needed but is associated with graft loss rates as high as 30%.

Malignancy

Immunosuppression is associated with an increased incidence of lympho-proliferative diseases (lymphoma) and also solid organ malignancy. The drugs used for immunosuppression remove normal immunosurveillance and allow mutagenesis to proceed, particularly in viral-induced malignancies (e.g. lymphomas and Epstein-Barr virus). Skin tumours are also a problem in immunosuppressed patients and protective measures against sun damage should be advised.

Liver transplantation

Many of the complications of kidney transplantation are applicable to liver transplantation – particularly those related to immunosuppression. The liver transplant recipient is similarly at high risk with the presence of jaundice, portal hypertension, clotting disorders, and metabolic disturbances associated with liver failure. Haemorrhage is a particular risk in these patients.

The consequences of complications after liver transplantation are amplified as an equivalent organ support option (haemodialysis) does not exist.

Primary graft non-function

The most serious complication of liver transplant is primary non-function and this generally requires urgent re-transplantation. Risk factors include being older, more unstable cardiovascular donors, and longer ischaemic times (>6 hours). However, the only uniform predictor of poor outcome and exclusion criteria for a donor organ is fatty infiltration. Organ donor shortages and a patient's deterioration may require the use of more 'marginal' donors. Primary non-function presents with progressive aminotransferase elevation, hypoglycaemia, renal failure, metabolic acidosis, coagulopathy, and mental confusion.

Renal failure

Many patients following liver transplant require renal support. The pre-operative renal function (hepatorenal syndrome) and operative events (hypotension, IVC clamping, nephrotoxic drugs) all contribute. However, in most patients, with improving clinical condition and fluid optimization, renal function recovers, usually over the first few weeks.

Acute rejection

Liver transplant rejection tends to be cell-mediated and manifests with progressive liver dysfunction. In the early stage it is often asymptomatic, though there may be associated fever. Definitive diagnosis depends on core biopsy, showing evidence of leucocyte infiltration around the blood vessels and bile duct epithelium. Treatment is with pulsed steroids and immunosuppressive manipulation. The vast majority of rejection episodes have little clinical significance (as the liver graft has the ability to regenerate), although refractory rejection results in injury to the biliary epithelium and may proceed to 'vanishing bile ducts' and eventual graft loss.

Non-specific cholestasis

This is a relatively benign condition with an isolated rise in bilirubin and reduced bile output. The transaminases and alkaline phosphatase are relatively normal. Histology shows canalicular bile stasis in the absence of significant inflammation. The cholestasis is self-limiting and resolves within weeks to months after transplant.

Haemorrhage

Bleeding after surgery is suggested by the presence of tachycardia, hypotension, cold peripheries, falling haemoglobin, oliguria, and blood in drain fluid. Minor bleeding may be treated expectantly, but heavier bleeding requires surgical re-exploration. Often the bleeding site is not located, but it may be from an anastomotic site, the gallbladder bed, the cystic artery stump, or a liver laceration. Bleeding may also reflect graft dysfunction but clotting abnormalities must be corrected prior to considering re-operation.

Hepatic artery thrombosis (HAT)

HAT occurs in around 5% of cases and generally reflects technical anastomotic problems. Presentation is variable, with fulminant hepatic failure in approximately half of cases. Bile leaks may occur, classically associated with episodes of bacteraemia or even liver abscess. Other patients may present with biliary strictures. Some patients, mostly children or those with late HAT, are asymptomatic and perfuse their liver on portal venous blood alone. Diagnosis can usually be made on duplex ultrasound study, although CT angio or formal contrast angiography may be used. Surgical exploration, thrombectomy and re-anastomosis may be successful, though re-transplantation is often required.

Portal vein thrombosis

Portal vein thrombosis may occur at any time from immediately postoperatively to months after surgery. Predisposing factors include technical issues (kinking or purse-stringing of the anastomosis) and recipient factors (portal vein thrombosis prior to transplant, hypercoagulable states). Presentation may be with progressive liver dysfunction, or with manifestations of portal hypertension such as ascites and variceal bleeding. Surgical treatment may be successful, particularly when combined with postoperative anticoagulation.

Inferior vena cava (IVC) obstruction

Presentation depends on the site of the occlusion. Obstruction distal to the outflow from the liver graft results in hepatic failure and often death. If the occlusion affects the infra-hepatic IVC, lower body and leg oedema with ascites results. Advances in implantation techniques such as the 'piggyback' technique have reduced many of these issues, although the 'piggyback syndrome' with similar problems is described.

Diagnosis is by duplex scan or angiography. Management may require re-transplant, though thrombolysis, surgical re-exploration, and more recently balloon angioplasty and stenting have been successful.

Bile duct complications

Early bile duct complications are associated with arterial and technical complications and can present as a bile leak or obstruction. Late biliary stenosis following transplant is often anastomosis-related and fibrotic in nature. Management in both cases may be by ERCP and stenting although surgical intervention with Roux-en-Y reconstruction is likely to be required. Biliary sludge can cause anastomotic blockage; ERCP can determine the cause of obstruction.

Recurrent disease

Inflammatory and infective hepatitis can occur in the post-transplant period with original liver diseases, PBC, PSC, and hepatitis C recurring.

Recidivism in alcoholic patients is a significant factor although not all develop recurrent liver disease.

Infection

The infections affecting renal immunosuppressed patients also affect liver transplant patients. Some opportunistic infections can result in liver dysfunction. Herpes simplex hepatitis occurs around 1 month following surgery, and can lead to a devastating necrotic hepatitis and death. It is fortunately uncommon nowadays with the use of prophylactic acyclovir. Adenoviral, herpes zoster, and cytomegalovirus (CMV) hepatitis can likewise give serious hepatitis and usually occur later still, around the second month after transplant. CMV hepatitis is normally milder, often has accompanying leucopenia, thrombocytopenia, and myalgia, and is treated with ganciclovir. Hepatitis B and C can be reactivated in the graft, and usually present later still, up to 6 months after transplant. Hepatitis C infection can be histologically difficult to distinguish from rejection.

Complications of thoracic outlet decompression and thoracoscopic sympathectomy

Complications of thoracic outlet decompression

Thoracic outlet decompression may be performed for thoracic outlet syndrome (TOS) following failure of conservative management. TOS presents with neurogenic symptoms in 95% of cases and arterial or venous in the remaining 5%. Decompression, in the absence of a specific mechanical cause or for venous symptoms, involves first rib resection performed via a transaxillary approach. Alternatively, a supraclavicular approach may be used, which allows excision of a cervical rib, division of fibrous bands, scalenectomy, and treatment of any resultant vascular lesion (e.g. arterial stenosis or aneurysm). This approach provides good exposure in revision surgery. The infraclavicular approach is less popular. The supraclavicular fossa and thoracic outlet contain many vital neurovascular structures and decompression is a technically demanding procedure requiring specialized instruments.

Complications include:

- Pleural tears – these are relatively common, occurring in up to 50% of patients when a supraclavicular approach is made. Pneumothorax can be aspirated with a catheter and the defect sutured if recognized intra-operatively. If not, then post-operative pneumothorax may result in up to 13% of patients. A small pneumothorax may resolve spontaneously but larger ones require a chest drain.
- Haemothorax – occurs in 1% of cases. These should be treated with a chest drain.
- Lymphatic damage – minor lymphatic injury complicates up to 13% of cases and results in small amounts of lymph leakage from the wound or development of a lymphocele. Major lymphatic injury is far less common but can result in a chylous fistula or chylothorax. This includes injury to the thoracic duct on the left side as it turns laterally at the transverse process of C7 to enter the innominate vein.
- Injury to major vessels – occurs in 2% of cases and may involve the subclavian, axillary, internal mammary, or superior intercostal vessels. Uncontrollable haemorrhage using an axillary approach may be difficult to deal with and require conversion to a supraclavicular approach with or without division of the clavicle.
- Nerve injuries – most post-operative nerve injuries are transient neuropraxias due to operative irritation or traction. Nerves at specific risk include:
  - Phrenic nerve – this runs down the anterior border of scalenus anterior. Transient paralysis occurs in up to 8% of patients following a supraclavicular approach, usually manifested as an elevated hemidiaphragm on the post-operative chest radiograph.
  - Long thoracic nerve of Bell (nerve to serratus anterior) – this can be damaged in up to 8% of cases, either via the supraclavicular or transaxillary approach. Winging of the scapula results.
  - Vagus and recurrent laryngeal nerves – these cross anteriorly to the subclavian artery. Damage can result in post-operative problems of deglutination and hoarseness of the voice in up to 2% of patients.

- Intercostobrachial nerve – this can be damaged or may have to be sacrificed during a transaxillary approach. This gives rise to numbness along the medial aspect of the upper arm.
- Brachial plexus – injury to the brachial plexus affects 3% of patients. The trunks and divisions of the brachial plexus are prone to injury as they emerge through the interval between the anterior and middle scalene muscles. Usually this is transient and results in paraesthesia or weakness in the arm.
- Complex regional pain syndrome (📖 see Chapter 16, Complications of orthopaedic surgery, p.319).
- Recurrent symptoms – 90% of procedures result in primary success with an improvement in symptoms. There is a 20% recurrence rate by 18 months and a 30% recurrence in the long term. Re-operation with a different procedure from that used initially carries a 40 to 50% chance of success. Recurrence is usually related to fibrotic scarring at the site of a previous excision impinging on the thoracic outlet.

Complications of thoracoscopic sympathectomy

Thoracic sympathectomy is indicated where ablation of the sympathetic nerve supply to the upper limb is required. Historically it was performed for a wide range of conditions including reflex sympathetic dystrophy, thrombangitis obliterans (Buerger's disease), selected patients with Raynaud's syndrome, and non-reconstructable critical ischaemia of the hand. However, the results were poor and so it is now rarely performed except for patients with disabling palmar and axillary hyperhidrosis or with severe facial flushing who are not controlled with conservative measures.

Open cervical, transaxillary, or trans-thoracic approaches have traditionally been used but these have been superseded by the thoracoscopic approach. One or two ports are inserted intercostally through which a camera and instruments are introduced. The sympathetic chain is divided over the neck of the ribs. Bilateral procedures can be performed at the same sitting and a more rapid recovery is feasible. The operation is performed under general anaesthesia, often with a double-lumen endotracheal tube, and involves the ablation of T2 and T3 sympathetic thoracic ganglia for palmar symptoms with the addition of T4 and maybe T5 if axillary hyperhidrosis is also present. The nerves may be ablated with diathermy, harmonic scalpel, or clips. Axillary hyperhidrosis is increasingly being controlled with recurrent Botox injections with sympathectomy reserved for palmar symptoms.

Intra-operative complications

- Risk of oxygen desaturation with one lung ventilation.

Post-operative complications

- Pneumothorax – this occurs in 5% of patients. Routine chest drainage is not required as inflation of the lung can be directly visualized with the thoracoscope and the wound closed securely. A chest radiograph is taken in the recovery room to exclude this complication. Air leak can occur from inadequate port-site closure or a small puncture to the lung itself. When performing a bilateral procedure, many surgeons insert a drain into the first side to prevent tension pneumothorax during surgery on the contralateral side.
- Surgical emphysema – a small number of patients develop this around the chest wall and neck as a result of air leak.
- Haemothorax – loss of blood into the pleural cavity can occur from damage to the intercostal, pleural, and internal mammary vessels. If not recognized during the procedure, this can result in haemothorax formation and may require a chest tube. Rarely, thoracotomy is required to control significant haemorrhage.
- Pain – many patients experience post-operative periscapular and port-site related pain, which can be reduced by the use of local anaesthetic infiltration at the end of the procedure. The incidence and severity of pain is substantially reduced compared to the open procedure and consequently the respiratory complications of atelectasis and chest infection are reduced.

- Intra-operative damage to intrathoracic structures – injury can occur during the procedure to the lungs, heart, great vessels, etc.
- Horner's syndrome – this occurs in 1% of patients and is due to inadvertent damage to the stellate ganglion. This is usually transient, occurring in 0.5% at 6 weeks and reducing to 0.1% at 6 months.
- Compensatory hyperhidrosis – the most common and debilitating complication. It occurs in almost all patients to some degree. However, if the original hyperhidrosis was severe and the compensatory sweating controllable, the majority of patients are pleased with the overall outcome. It usually involves the trunk but may occur at any site. The aetiology is not clear, but destruction of the T4 ganglion in addition to T2 and T3 is associated with an increased incidence. Similarly, post-gustatory sweating can also occur.
- Hypohidrosis – lack of sweating may result in excessively dry and cracked skin of the palms and axilla. This can be managed with emollients and improves with time.
- Intercostobrachial neuralgia – this can result from damage to the intercostobrachial nerve when the port-site is made in the midaxillary line, fourth intercostal space. This results in paraesthesia or dysaesthesia on the medial aspect of the upper arm.
- Recurrent symptoms – long-term recurrence occurs in around 6% of patients. Re-operation using the thoracoscopic route is usually feasible, although pleural adhesions can hinder the procedure.

Complications of vascular interventional radiology

Vascular interventional radiology

Vascular interventional radiology plays an increasingly common role in the management of patients with vascular disease. Although procedures may be diagnostic or therapeutic, the former are being performed less often as the quality and availability of non-invasive imaging modalities such as computed tomography and magnetic resonance angiography improve.

Diagnostic angiography

Angiography remains the 'gold standard' for obtaining accurate anatomical information about the vascular tree. It also provides information about the direction and rate (subjective) of blood flow. It also allows intraluminal blood pressure to be measured directly across stenoses as a guide to their significance. Although opinions differ, a drop of >20mmHg in peak systolic pressure across a stenosis is commonly regarded as significant and thus warrants intervention.

Intra-arterial digital subtraction arteriography (iaDSA)

The first step in most vascular interventional procedures is vessel puncture and then insertion of a vascular sheath. This is a short plastic tube with a haemostatic valve to prevent back bleeding through which wires, catheters, balloons, and stents can be inserted. For angiography, a catheter is positioned via the sheath into the appropriate artery followed by injection of contrast and acquisition of radiographic images.

Most routine angiography is performed under local anaesthesia via a retrograde (opposite to blood flow) common femoral artery puncture. Alternative access points are the brachial, radial, and popliteal arteries. The incidence of serious complications is around 1%.

Intravenous digital subtraction arteriography (ivDSA)

This is a means of imaging the arterial circulation and avoids the potential complications of direct arterial puncture. It involves positioning a catheter in the right atrium, usually via the common femoral or antecubital veins. A large contrast bolus is administered and images acquired after a delay to allow the contrast to reach the arterial side of the circulation. Image quality, particularly of the distal circulation, is poor because of considerable contrast dilution. The high contrast load may also exacerbate problems of nephrotoxicity and cardiac failure. It was traditionally undertaken in patients with difficult arterial access or as a diagnostic procedure prior to intervention. It has now been superseded by non-invasive imaging modalities such as MR and CT angiography.

Contrast venography

This is now less commonly performed, but still plays a role when duplex ultrasound imaging is insufficient. Ascending venography involves the application of a tourniquet around the ankle to occlude the superficial veins, then injection of contrast into a dorsal vein of the foot. It can be used to demonstrate occlusion of the deep venous system, post-thrombotic stenoses, or perforator incompetence. Descending venography involves the injection of contrast into the femoral vein to look for superficial and deep venous incompetence. Varicography involves injection directly into varicosities to establish the origin of reflux. Complications include local thrombophlebitis, deep venous thrombosis, contrast reactions, and complications arising from the puncture site.

Balloon angioplasty

Percutaneous angioplasty is an established method of treating stenoses/ occlusions within arteries and (less commonly) veins. Arterial angio-plasty is most commonly performed to treat lifestyle-limiting intermittent claudication and critical limb ischaemia. Following vessel catheterization under local anaesthesia, the diseased segment is traversed with a guide-wire under fluoroscopic control. Intraluminal angioplasty involves passing the wire across the stenosis through the arterial lumen. An angioplasty balloon passed over the wire is then inflated causing longitudinal plaque fissuring and consequent luminal gain. Extraluminal or subintimal angio-plasty involves intentionally driving the wire into the arterial wall, crossing the lesion within the wall and then re-entering the lumen more distally. Subsequent balloon inflation effectively results in a controlled arterial dissection with the aim of producing a new 'false lumen' through which the blood will flow.

In general, the more distal the angioplasty within the limb, the worse the primary success rate and the higher the risk of complications. Angioplasty is usually safer than open surgery but still poses a mortality rate of about 1%. The incidence of serious complications lies around 5%.

Vascular stents and stent grafts

Intravascular stents are used for the treatment of stenoses or occlusions in arteries and veins. When stents are deployed without prior balloon angioplasty it is described as primary stenting, e.g. commonly performed for long iliac artery occlusions or for treatment of renal artery stenoses. Secondary stenting is performed following initial angioplasty if the angi-ographic result is poor or pressure gradient too high, or to treat a compli-cation of angioplasty such as flow limiting dissection (see later). Stents are most commonly used in the treatment of arterial lesions but are also used in venous disease, e.g. recanalization of chronically occluded veins after DVT or in relieving malignant vena caval obstruction.

Stents are expandable tubes of metallic mesh, usually inserted via a femoral sheath, and can be divided into two groups. Self-expanding stents are made of Nitinol (nickel-titanium alloy) that has a thermal memory and when released spontaneously expands to a preset diameter at 37°C. The selected stent diameter should be 1–2mm greater than the vessel and the stent continues to expand after its deployment if it has not reached its full size. They are very flexible but may shorten and/or move during deployment, making precise positioning difficult. In contrast, balloon-expandable stents are usually made of stainless steel and require inflation of the balloon within them for expansion. They do not expand beyond the diameter of the balloon and tend to be stiffer with a greater tendency to kink. They were originally preferred over self-expanding stents in applications where precise stent positioning was crucial, e.g. stenting of renal artery ostial stenosis. Modern self-expanding stents do not shorten or shift on deployment to the same degree so this issue is becoming less important.

In comparison, stent grafts (or covered stents) consist of a metallic framework supporting a tube of Dacron (polyester) or PTFE (polytetra-fluoroethylene). They are used when a length of vessel, usually an artery, requires exclusion from the circulation, e.g. treatment of arterial aneurysms or arterial injury, including iatrogenic rupture from overenthusiastic balloon angioplasty. As a result of their greater bulk, they require a greater calibre sheath for the delivery system and thus a larger hole to be made in the artery. Although many applications only require a tubular design, modular bifurcated systems are used in the endovascular repair of abdominal aortic aneurysms.

Haemostasis

The majority of procedures can be performed through a 4–6 French sheath (the number denotes the circumference in mm; when referring to a catheter it is the outer circumference of the tube and when a sheath it is the inner circumference of the tube. Remember that a 4F catheter fits through a 4F sheath). Haemostasis following sheath removal is usually achieved by manual pressure for 10–15 minutes followed by the need to lie supine (and still) for 2–4 hours. Manual haemostasis can be used for sheaths up to 12F but as the diameter increases so does the risk of complications. Several devices are now available (Perclose, StarClose, Angioseal) to close the arterial puncture percutaneously, removing the need for manual pressure and allowing more rapid mobilization. Occasionally these can 'misfire', particularly in a very diseased artery, resulting in a lack of haemostasis or arterial occlusion at the puncture site. Following placement of an Angioseal, repeat ipsilateral puncture is not recommended for 3 months. If arterial occlusion following Angioseal malfunction requires surgical intervention, early clamping of the artery may avoid distal embolization of the foot-plate as the vessels are exposed.

Early complications

All interventional vascular radiological procedures, including angiography, angioplasty, and stenting, involve similar techniques and thus share a number of common complications. Early complications are often manifest immediately, and can be classified as those arising at the arterial puncture site, the intervention site, or remote complications.

Complications at the puncture site

These are the most common of all complications.

Minor bruising

Some cutaneous bruising occurs in most patients and is of no clinical importance.

Haematoma

Usually results from inadequate haemostasis and is usually immediately apparent as a swelling around the puncture site. A haematoma is more likely with big sheaths and in patients who are obese, anticoagulated, thrombocytopaenic, and/or hypertensive. If the groin puncture is 'high' and made in the distal external iliac artery above the inguinal ligament, bleeding may occur into the retroperitoneum and may not be detectable in the groin. The retroperitoneum can accommodate a large volume of blood and the patient presents with all the features of hypovolaemic shock and often only a limited amount of ipsilateral iliac fossa and/or back pain. Conversely, severe pain due to retroperitoneal femoral nerve irritation may occur. Do not be reassured by the lack of a groin haematoma if contacted to see a patient who has a rising pulse rate and is becoming hypotensive, or in apparently disproportionate pain following an arteriogram.

Management

If the patient is shocked, apply pressure to the common femoral/external iliac artery and call for urgent help. As with any acutely ill surgical patient, rapidly assess the airway, breathing, and circulation, establish large calibre IV access, take blood for FBC, U&E, coagulation, and cross match, and administer volume (0.9% saline or colloid; not 5% dextrose) and oxygen. For small haematomas where the bleeding has stopped, ensure that the haematoma is not expanding by drawing a line around its border and observe frequently for an increase in size. If you are in any doubt, obtain an urgent senior opinion. Conservative management (further manual pressure, resuscitation, and correction of anticoagulation) is often all that is required, but the patient should be told that any groin lump may well persist for several months. A few patients have continued uncontrollable bleeding and resuscitation should be continued as the patient is urgently transferred to theatre for exploration.

False aneurysm

A false aneurysm results when there is persistent arterial bleeding from the puncture site into a haematoma and the compressed adjacent tissues form a fibrous sac. The risk factors are the same as for haematomas and they are more common after puncture of the superficial femoral instead of the common femoral artery. Classically, a lump with an expansile pulse is palpable over the punctured artery but the pulsatile nature can be difficult to distinguish from a pulse transmitted through a haematoma. Occasionally there is severe pain due to compression of the adjacent femoral nerve. Ultrasound confirms the diagnosis.

Management

If small, they are likely to spontaneously thrombose (in the absence of systemic anticoagulation) and can be observed with a further scan arranged in a few weeks' time. Larger lesions, and those that continue to expand, may rupture or embolize some of their lining thrombus. If the patient's coagulation is normal, duplex-directed compression and more commonly thrombin injection usually result in false aneurysm thrombosis. Surgery is indicated in patients who fail thrombin injection or those with compression symptoms. At operation, the haematoma is evacuated and the arterial defect repaired.

Local thrombosis

Puncture-site thrombosis usually occurs in arteries with significant plaque at the point of entry. Occlusion may result from a localized dissection (more common with antegrade punctures), thrombosis around a sheath passing through a tight stenosis, after maldeployment of a percutaneous closure device, or after too vigorous compression following sheath removal.

Management

The patient should be reviewed by an experienced vascular surgeon. Immediate intervention is necessary if the limb is acutely ischaemic. If the limb remains adequately perfused, the patient can be observed pending definitive management of the initial problem.

Arteriovenous (AV) fistula formation

Some filling of the venae commitantes can occur after balloon angioplasty and requires no intervention. Rarely, injury to both the artery and the vein may occur at the puncture site and result in an iatrogenic AV fistula. This is more common with punctures into the superficial femoral artery. There is often an arterial bruit and a palpable thrill. The diagnosis is confirmed on ultrasound.

Management

Some resolve spontaneously. Symptomatic or enlarging fistulas require intervention. Treatment options include placing a stent graft across the arterial defect, embolization of the fistulous tract if technically feasible, or surgical exploration.

Femoral nerve injury

This can be caused by the administration of local anaesthetic or by haematoma. The former is very uncommon, but the latter is a cause of significant morbidity and can lead to causalgia lasting many months.

Complications at the intervention site

These may result from wire and catheter manipulations, angioplasty balloon inflation, or stent deployment.

Dissection
The technique of extraluminal/subintimal angioplasty involves the 'controlled' dissection of a vessel to produce a new passage for blood flow. The intimal and medial disruption from luminal angioplasty often results in limited vessel dissection. This will heal in time and is only of consequence if a dissection flap limits blood flow. In addition, the inadvertent subintimal passage of a guide-wire can raise an intimal flap that itself limits flow or precipitates a dissection. As well as obstructing flow, extensive dissections may damage collateral branches, further reducing distal perfusion, and may convert a patient with claudication into a patient with critical ischaemia.

Treatment
Minor, non-flow limiting dissections following angioplasty remodel and require no intervention. Haemodynamically significant dissections may be treated by prolonged (3–5 minutes), low-pressure balloon inflations to encourage the flap to 'stick' against the vessel wall. If this fails, a stent may be deployed to push the flap out of the lumen. If these measures fail and the limb is critically ischaemic, surgical reconstruction will be required.

Vasospasm
Small and medium-sized muscular arteries such as the upper limb and crural vessels are most often affected. Vasospasm may be precipitated by any manipulation of these arteries so may occur if used as a puncture site (upper limb) or as a result of angioplasty (upper limb and crural arteries).

Management
Vasodilators (glyceryl trinitrate and papaverine) are used to prevent and treat spasm. It may also resolve after a few minutes of observation or following gentle inflation of an angioplasty balloon. If there is refractory spasm, the patient should be heparinized to prevent thrombosis. On return to the ward, intravenous prostaglandin (iloprost) or heparin infusion may be a useful adjunct for 24 hours to antagonize spasm and inhibit thrombosis.

Elastic recoil
This is when the angioplasty balloon inflates completely but the stenosis returns on deflation. It is more common when treating eccentric, heavily calcified plaques. Management options are to observe or stent the affected segment.

Guide-wire perforation
Small arterial perforations can occur as a result of guide-wire passage. They often seal if an angioplasty balloon is gently inflated for several minutes at the site of the injury. If this is not successful then stent grafting across the puncture site or open surgical repair is required.

Vessel rupture
Arterial rupture by an angioplasty balloon can result in catastrophic bleeding. The balloon should be gently re-inflated at or just proximal to the site of rupture to minimize bleeding and the patient resuscitated (📖 see earlier section on haematoma). The situation may be salvaged by

covering the site of rupture with a stent graft. If this is not possible, open surgical repair is required as an emergency.

Remote complications

Macroembolization

Thrombosis may occur within and around sheaths and catheters and embolize distally. In addition, atheromatous material may be dislodged from the arterial wall during manipulations, especially after balloon angioplasty. Embolism is reduced by systemic heparinization, primary stenting of high-risk lesions, and regular flushing of sheaths and catheters with heparinized saline. Embolization resulting in distal ischaemia requires treatment. Wide calibre catheters can be advanced to the site of occlusion and the embolus aspirated. Thrombolysis may also be utilized. If this fails, surgical embolectomy may be required.

Microembolization

Microemboli from the surface of an atheromatous plaque or from thrombus lining an aneurysm sac may shower into and sludge up the distal circulation. Involvement of the lower limbs from manipulations in a diseased aorta is the most common cause and may result in 'mottling' (livedo reticularis) visible in the skin and small cutaneous infarcts to the feet ('trash foot'). The ischaemia can be profound causing significant tissue infarction, myoglobinuria with renal dysfunction, and limb loss. Embolic showering into the renal or mesenteric circulation is a rarer but devastating complication.

Management

Peripheral emboli are usually managed conservatively with heparin anticoagulation and prostaglandin infusions to inhibit thrombosis and promote vasodilatation. In some cases a lumbar sympathectomy may be useful to improve skin perfusion and reduce pain. Systemic embolization may be fatal; expert renal management is imperative and signs of bowel ischaemia must not be ignored.

Contrast reactions

Iodinated contrast media can be classified as ionic or non-ionic. The latter are increasingly used as they have a similar osmolality to plasma and have a lower incidence of adverse reactions. This comes at the cost of increased viscosity, which can make injection more difficult, but in practice this is not a significant problem. Approximately 2% of patients exhibit some reaction to iodinated contrast media, with severe reactions to non-ionic agents occurring in 0.04% and very serious reactions in 0.004%. Contrast reactions can be classified as direct or idiosyncratic reactions.

Direct reactions

Due directly to the osmolality and toxicity of the contrast agent. These include a sensation of heat, nausea, and pain. Nephrotoxicity and cardiac ischaemia and dysrhythmias may also occur.

Idiosyncratic reactions
Related to release of vasoactive mediators such as histamine, serotonin, bradykinin, and complement. They vary in severity:
- Mild – metallic taste, nausea, sneezing. Requires reassurance only, no specific treatment needed.
- Intermediate – urticarial rash.
- Severe – vasodilatation, increased capillary permeability, and respiratory smooth muscle contraction results in hypotension, arrhythmias, laryngeal oedema, bronchospasm, pulmonary oedema, etc.
- Death – as a result of the above.

Treatment
The vast majority of severe contrast reactions occur within 20 minutes of contrast administration. All patients should have IV access established before contrast use and resuscitation equipment and drugs should be readily available within the angiography suite. As with any patient who deteriorates rapidly, the airway, breathing, and circulation should be assessed and problems addressed as they are detected. All require oxygen and those with severe reactions may need significant IV volume replacement. Specific treatments include:
- Urticaria – chlorpheniramine 20mg IV. If profound, consider subcutaneous/intramuscular adrenaline (epinephrine), 0.1–0.3ml of 1 in 1000 solution. Repeat as needed.
- Vasovagal syncope – give volume expansion for hypotension and consider atropine 0.6–1.2mg for bradycardia. Repeat, if necessary, after 3–5 minutes, to a 3mg total.
- Bronchospasm – nebulized salbutamol 2.5–5mg and 200mg IV hydrocortisone. If bronchospasm fails to improve, consider subcutaneous/intramuscular adrenaline (0.1–0.3ml of 1 in 1000 solution). If hypotensive, give adrenaline at a greater dose (0.5ml of 1 in 1000 solution) or it can be given intravenously as slowly administered 1ml aliquots of 1 in 10 000 solution.
- Laryngeal oedema and refractory hypotension – IV fluids, chlorpheniramine, hydrocortisone, and adrenaline are required. Senior anaesthetist/intensivist support is required. Intubation or even a surgical airway may be required.

Consider use of H_2-receptor antagonists in addition to H_1-antagonists, e.g. ranitidine 50mg slow IV injection, in severe cases resistant to conventional therapy.

The definitive treatment of all patients with intermediate or severe contrast reactions is on the intensive care unit, where close monitoring can be undertaken and cardiovascular, respiratory, and renal support utilized if necessary.

A history of reaction to iodinated contrast media not surprisingly greatly increases the risk of reaction if exposed again. Therefore, the potential risks of future administration have to be balanced against the benefit in terms of diagnosis and/or treatment. Obviously, if the diagnosis can be achieved by another imaging modality such as ultrasound, MRA, or non-contrast CT, this is preferable. If intervention is still required the alternative contrast agents of gadolinium and carbon dioxide may be adequate. If iodinated contrast use is still justified, premedication with corticosteroids is advocated by some but the evidence is minimal.

Acute renal impairment

Iodinated contrast media are nephrotoxic and contrast nephropathy results in a fall in glomerular filtration rate with a consequent rise in creatinine after the procedure. Serum creatinine usually peaks at 4–7 days then returns to normal but permanent impairment or even end-stage renal failure may occur. Nephropathy risk is increased in older patients (>70 years), those with pre-existing chronic renal impairment (especially if diabetic), congestive cardiac failure, taking nephrotoxic drugs, and with dehydration. Strategies to reduce the severity of nephropathy include: use of alternative tests when possible; 'renal-protection protocols'; using minimal doses of non-ionic, iso-osmolar agents, and using alternative contrast agents such as CO_2. Gadolinium is also nephrotoxic and its administration in patients with renal failure has been associated with nephrogenic systemic fibrosis, so it should be used with care.

Several renal protection protocols are in use but the most important factor is ensuring that the patient is well hydrated by prescribing IV fluids before and after the procedure. Patients with creatinine concentrations above about 180µmol/l may also be prescribed N-acetylcysteine, aminophylline, and/or sodium bicarbonate. However, the evidence for their benefit above good hydration is less strong.

Temporarily withholding nephrotoxic medication such as non-steroidal anti-inflammatory drugs, angiotensin converting enzyme inhibitors, and aminoglycoside antibiotics is prudent.

Lactic acidosis and acute renal failure

Metformin is excreted in the urine and if it accumulates may rarely precipitate lactic acidosis. Current practice is to stop metformin at the time of angiography and for 48 hours post-operatively. It should only be restarted when renal function has been evaluated and found to be normal/recovered.

Intermediate and late complications – after 30 days

Re-stenosis
The tearing of intima and plaque stimulates myointimal hyperplasia, which can result in restenosis causing recurrent symptoms and risk of *in situ* thrombosis. Myointimal hyperplasia also occurs within and at the end of stents and stent grafts. The technical success rate of angioplasty of iliac disease is 90–99% for stenoses and 80–85% for long segment occlusions. Long-term patency rates >70% at 5 years after angioplasty for iliac stenoses can be expected. Stents are often used primarily for iliac occlusions or for stenoses if the result of the initial angioplasty is suboptimal.

Technical success in femoral-popliteal angioplasty is still high at around 95%, but the long-term results are poorer with 5-year patency rates of 55% for stenoses and 42% for occlusions. The use of femoral-popliteal stents is controversial. Initial trial results were disappointing but the use of self-expanding stents is more encouraging. Currently, they are usually reserved for patients with critical limb ischaemia when the initial angioplasty result is poor. If stents are used in the infrainguinal arteries, increased anti-platelet treatment with combined aspirin and clopidogrel for a period of several weeks is usually recommended from evidence extrapolated from coronary intervention. Infrapopliteal angioplasty is also possible but as initial technical success is less sure, complications more likely, and durability limited, it is reserved for limb salvage.

Thrombosis
All metal stents are thrombogenic and thrombosis may occur below the threshold thrombotic velocity (even in the absence of a significant stenosis), resulting in stent failure and a recurrence of symptoms.

Infection
Infection is rare, occurring in less than 1% of cases. Infection is likely to result from bacterial contamination at implantation, although any cause of bacteraemia may potentially infect a stent. It is likely to be more common with stent grafts. The principles of management are the same as an infected prosthetic surgical graft, namely removal of infected synthetic material and revascularization using autologous material via an alternative route if possible.

Intra-arterial thrombolysis

The aim of thrombolysis is to re-establish perfusion by the local infusion of a thrombolytic agent (e.g. recombinant tissue plasminogen activator (rtPA), streptokinase, or urokinase), via a transluminal catheter, into the thrombus. As the volume of thrombus to be lysed is greater than myocardial thrombolysis, direct instillation of the thrombolytic agent is required. Local administration in comparison to systemic use also reduces the risk of haemorrhagic complications by localizing highest doses where they are required. The thrombolytic can be administered by a bolus dose, low-dose infusion, or by pulse–spray techniques where intermittent jets of thrombolytic agent also help to mechanically disrupt the thrombus. Removal of thrombus can also be enhanced by percutaneous thrombus aspiration. Arterial access is usually via a femoral puncture and arteriograms are repeated every 6–12 hours to monitor progress. It may require 24–48 hours of treatment during which the patient must remain supine and be closely monitored, often in a high dependency unit setting. Heparin is administered concurrently and may be continued until definitive treatment to any underlying flow-limiting lesion is performed (i.e. angioplasty, stent, or surgery).

Activation of the fibrinolytic cascade can cause serious bleeding complications and therefore thrombolysis is reserved, in the absence of contraindications, for the treatment of limb-threatening acute ischaemia. This can include *in situ* native-vessel thrombosis, graft thrombosis, and thromboembolism. As lysis requires several hours of treatment, it should not be used to treat severely ischaemic limbs that require more urgent reperfusion. The role of thrombolysis versus surgery remains controversial. Case selection is important and complications are more likely in female patients and those over 80 years old. There is some evidence that thrombolysis is better than surgery for graft thrombosis while surgery is more effective for native vessel occlusions. Overall, limb salvage occurs in 75%, amputation in 12.5%, and death in 12.5%.

Early complications from the administration of local thrombolytic agents

Major haemorrhage

Occurs in 5–10% of patients. This can be pericatheter, retroperitoneal, or gastrointestinal. Particular vigilance should be paid to occult bleeding into the retroperitoneal space following femoral puncture. The classic signs are tachycardia and hypotension, but with no obvious source of external blood loss. Occasionally these patients may present with signs of femoral nerve irritation, and severe groin pain should not be dismissed lightly. Significant bleeding requires resuscitation, stopping the thrombolytic infusion, checking the clotting, and administering fresh frozen plasma and packed red cells as necessary.

Minor haemorrhage

Occurs in 10–30% of patients and is usually puncture-site related. Haematomas and femoral false aneurysms may result. Intramuscular injections are contraindicated and venepuncture should be avoided.

Stroke

Occurs in 2–3% of patients and can be haemorrhagic or embolic. Cerebral hypoperfusion and ischaemic stroke may also result from major haemorrhage.

Distal embolization

Occurs in 4% of patients and is usually managed with continued lysis or suction thrombectomy. In those patients who fail to improve, surgical thromboembolectomy may be required to salvage the limb.

Pain

Results from distal reperfusion, puncture sites, and general musculoskeletal discomfort from lying supine for a prolonged period of time. Compartment syndrome may also occur with successful reperfusion.

Reperfusion sequelae

Reported in 2% of patients and includes the risk of acute compartment syndrome (see Chapter 9, Complications of gastrointestinal surgery, p.159).

Immunological reactions

Immunological reactions occur with streptokinase and may render it ineffective if the patient has been previously exposed, or result in allergic reactions. Streptokinase is less effective than rtPA.

Complications of varicose vein surgery

Introduction

Varicose veins are common. Surveys suggest a prevalence of 40% in men and 32% in women in Western populations, although most clinical series comprise an excess of women (1.5–3.5:1). Surgery is undertaken for symptomatic varicose veins or for complications arising from them. Eighty per cent of procedures are undertaken for primary varicose veins arising from saphenofemoral junction (SFJ) incompetence with long saphenous vein (LSV) reflux or saphenopopliteal junction (SPJ) incompetence with short saphenous vein (SSV) reflux. Surgery is performed under general anaesthesia and consists of a high tie, LSV strip, and multiple stab avulsions (MSAs) for the former and SPJ ligation and MSAs for the latter. Surgical treatment is still most commonly performed but less invasive treatment options such as laser or radiofrequency ablation and foam sclerotherapy are growing in popularity, although their long-term results are not yet clear. Recurrent varicosities may warrant revisional or re-do surgery, which is technically more complex with a higher chance of complications. An honest and frank discussion about what treatment can offer and the potential complications is not only required so your patient can give fully informed consent, it will also reduce complaints and litigation.

Early complications

Bleeding/haematoma

All patients are bruised following venous surgery and this relates to stripping of the LSV and the stab avulsion sites. Intra-operative head-down tilt, evacuation of haematoma in the LSV tunnel, and compression dressings applied immediately post-operatively minimize this. Some advocate the use of a tourniquet to minimize intra-operative blood loss and subsequent bruising. Dressings are left on for between 24 hours and 1 week. About 5% of patients develop a discrete haematoma in the groin, long saphenous tract, or at avulsion sites. Large haematomas may be drained but smaller ones are usually managed conservatively, although the patient should be warned that the 'lump' may persist for several weeks. Occasionally, as bruising or haematomas resolve, an unsightly brown pigmentation may persist due to haemosiderin deposition within the subcutaneous tissues. Many patients, particularly those undergoing re-do surgery or surgery for large varicosities, are left with induration around avulsion sites, which can take many weeks to resolve.

Venous thromboembolism (VTE)

The reported incidence of symptomatic deep venous thrombosis following varicose vein surgery is around 1%. However, if ultrasound surveillance is used post-operatively, DVT has been detected in 5% of legs but the majority of these are confined to the calf and resolve spontaneously. The risk of VTE following primary varicose vein surgery in an otherwise young, fit individual, who mobilizes rapidly and is without other risk factors (e.g. prior or family history of VTE, use of combined oral contraceptive, etc.), is low. Current SIGN (Scottish Intercollegiate Guidelines Network) guidance recommends the use of TED stockings for all patients and the administration of prophylactic low molecular weight heparin (LMWH) for those with additional risk factors. These include prior or family history of VTE, re-do or prolonged surgery, and causes of delayed post-operative mobility (e.g. elderly, obese, etc). Some surgeons recommend prolonged anticoagulation (several weeks) in patients with a history of VTE.

Women on the combined oral contraceptive pill are at increased VTE risk but this must be balanced against the risk of stopping it pre-operatively (risk of pregnancy, effect of anaesthesia on pregnancy, and risk of any termination). These should be discussed pre-operatively and if the balance of risk is in favour of discontinuation this should occur 6 weeks prior to surgery and be accompanied by a documented instruction to use other forms of contraception! If the pill is to be continued, then TED stockings and prophylactic LMWH should be used. Many surgeons also recommend LMWH administration at home for 1 week post-operatively. The pill should be restarted only when the patient is fully mobile.

In the case of women on hormonal replacement therapy, there is little evidence on which to base practice. However, routine prophylaxis (TEDS and LMWH) can easily be justified as age >40 years is an independent risk factor for VTE. A 1-week course of a LMWH may also be offered.

Surgical site infection

Surgical site infection occurs in 2–3% of patients and usually involves the groin wound. This is particularly so in the obese, diabetics, and patients who develop haematomas. Prophylactic antibiotics have been found to reduce this complication.

Nerve injury

Superficial cutaneous nerves

This is the commonest nerve injury and occurs at the site of avulsions. Areas of altered sensation or pain are present in about 25% of limbs at 6 weeks. Medial thigh symptoms can be particularly disabling. Many resolve in time but around 10% may have persistent symptoms and patients should be specifically warned of the possibility of this complication. Inadvertent injury to non-venous structures is particularly common below the level of the ankle joint and for this reason MSA should be avoided here.

Saphenous nerve

The courses of the saphenous nerve and LSV meet just over one-hand's breadth below the knee. Historically, the LSV was stripped to the ankle but this was associated with saphenous nerve injury (saphenous neuritis) in 10% of patients. To minimize this complication, modern practice involves LSV stripping to only just below the knee. Nerve injury presents with pain and paraesthesia affecting the medial aspect of the leg down to and including the first toe. This may take many months to settle or be permanent. The saphenous nerve may also be injured during below-knee MSAs. The neuropathic pain can be very difficult to control and may warrant referral to a chronic pain specialist. A variety of drugs is offered including gabapentin, pregabalin, amitriptyline, carbamazepine, and topical capsaicin.

Sural nerve

The sural nerve accompanies the short saphenous vein (SSV) in the leg. Stripping of the SSV is also associated with sural nerve injury and so not performed by many surgeons. Sural nerve injury presents with pain and paraesthesia over the lateral aspect of the leg and its management is similar to that of saphenous nerve injury.

Femoral nerve

True femoral nerve injury is a rare complication of groin dissection and is more likely during re-do surgery. More commonly, an inadvertent femoral nerve block results from local anaesthetic infiltration to reduce post-operative pain. This results in sensory loss to the anterior thigh and quadriceps weakness. Vigilance to this should be maintained post-operatively as the patient may fall and cases of consequent ankle sprains and fractures are documented!

Common peroneal nerve

The common peroneal nerve is vulnerable to injury during dissection of the popliteal fossa and MSAs around the neck of the fibula. Injury results in sensory loss to the lateral aspect of the leg and foot drop. The use of local anaesthetic in the popliteal fossa may block the peroneal nerve and produce a temporary foot drop. Therefore, care should be taken during infiltration of the popliteal fossa with local anaesthetic, especially in thin patients. Injury at the fibular neck may also occur if the post-operative bandages are applied too tightly.

Lymphocele

Damage to afferent lymph vessels or saphenous lymph nodes in the groin, particularly after redo surgery, can result in a localized collection of lymph (lymphocele). Lymphatic leaks and lymphoceles may also affect MSA sites. Lymphoceles can be easily aspirated although they tend to re-accumulate. Ultimately, 90% resolve spontaneously but this may take many months.

Major venous injury

As access to the SPJ in the popliteal fossa is more difficult, the junction less distinct than the SFJ, and the popliteal vein thin-walled, the risk of major venous injury is more common during SPJ ligation. Damage to the common femoral vein (CFV) can occur during groin dissection, particularly during re-do surgery. Bleeding may obscure the operative field and the blind use of clamps and crude attempts at suturing may damage the CFV. Misidentification of the LSV and CFV can lead to inadvertent ligation or even stripping of the CFV, and so the saphenofemoral junction should be clearly identified before ligation and division. In those rare cases where the common femoral vein is ligated and/or divided, the long saphenous can be used to create a panel or spiral graft to replace the affected segment of the CFV. Following this the patient should be heparinized and warfarinized.

Arterial injury

Division and even stripping of the common and superficial femoral arteries has been reported and causes major complications.

Over-tight bandaging

Ischaemia can result if the compression dressings are applied too tightly; this is a particular risk in patients with pre-existing peripheral vascular disease. Capillary return in the toes should be inspected after bandaging. In the presence of disproportionate post-operative pain all dressings should be removed to allow wound inspection. Bandages that have been applied too tightly may cause a compartment syndrome. Common peroneal nerve injury may also occur as described above.

Intermediate complications

Recurrent varicosities

The incidence of recurrent varicosities 'as bad as before' is 26% at 10 years. The term 'recurrent varicosities' should be distinguished from those patients with persistent varicose veins (those veins simply missed at the original surgery). Truly recurrent varicose veins can result from the following:

Inadequate surgery

Recurrent varicose veins may develop as a result of mid-thigh perforator incompetence following failure to strip the LSV. A small number of recurrences are due to developing incompetence from a duplicated saphenous system unnoticed at previous surgery. Many recurrences originate from the SFJ, which may be inadequately ligated, or from major tributaries that are not ligated, or a combination of both.

Neovascularization

The formation of small vessels between the ligated SFJ and the remnant of the LSV, often across fibrous scar tissue, is known as 'neovascularization'. This can account for up to half of recurrent saphenofemoral junction incompetence if the LSV is not stripped.

The use of prosthetic patches or autologous materials as a barrier to prevent neovascularization has not gained widespread acceptance.

The development of new sites of reflux

This usually involves the development of SPJ incompetence, although in the absence of an initial duplex scan, subclinical SPJ incompetence may have already existed at the time of initial surgery.

Spider veins

Pre-existing spider veins can worsen after superficial venous surgery in around 3% of patients. They tend to develop at the site of stab avulsions.

Complications of sclerotherapy

Venous sclerotherapy can be performed on patients with isolated superficial primary varicose veins, residual veins after surgery, or for spider or thread veins. It involves an intraluminal injection of sclerosant (e.g. 0.5–3% sodium tetradecylsulphate depending upon the size of the vein, polidocanol, or hypertonic saline) followed by compression dressings and can be performed in the outpatient department. A number of complications may occur:

- Brown pigmentation – post-procedure bruising can occur and the extravasation of blood and subsequent haemosiderin deposition can result in pigmentation in around 3% of patients.
- Thrombophlebitis – sclerosants work by chemically inducing a thrombophlebitis that heals with fibrosis resulting in a permanently occluded vein. If inadequate compression is applied allowing a larger volume of blood to thrombose within the vein, a clinically significant thrombophlebitis may result. This resolves with time and analgesia/anti-inflammatory preparations are symptomatically helpful. Deep venous thrombosis complicates less than 1% of cases, but is a particular risk if pain limits mobility post-procedure.
- Ulceration – extravasation of sclerosant can occur if the vein or venule is not cannulated adequately. This can result in skin necrosis with ulceration and unsightly scarring.
- Inadvertent arterial injection – this is a rare but documented complication with dire consequences!
- Allergy – to the sclerosant injection or constituents (e.g. latex) of the dressings may occur.
- Nerve injury – directly from the injection or from incorrectly applied bandages.

Complications of endovenous ablation

Under ultrasound guidance dilute local anaesthetic solution is infiltrated around the LSV or SSV. The vein is then cannulated and a catheter passed along it to the level of the junction with the deep veins. The superficial vein is then ablated with either laser or radiofrequency energy. Treatment of visible varicosities is variable with some surgeons performing immediate MSA under local anaesthesia or sclerotherapy. The number and prominence of varicosities tends to decline after LSV or SSV occlusion so many surgeons wait a period of time before treating residual troublesome veins. Endovenous intervention is less invasive than conventional surgery and so return to normal activities is more rapid. However, the long-term results are awaited.

Complications may occur from the method of ablation or from adjunctive techniques used to treat visible varicosities, namely MSA or sclerotherapy. Specific complications of endovenous laser or radiofrequency ablation include:

- Bleeding/bruising from puncture site.
- Phlebitis.
- Skin burns.
- Skin pigmentation/skin discolouration.
- VTE – generally lower risk as patients rapidly ambulant but more likely following SPJ/SSV closure compared with SFJ/LSV treatment.
- Infection – low risk as small puncture.
- Nerve injury – saphenous, sural, or peroneal nerve injury may occur but is rare.
- Injury from tight dressing.
- Major vessel injury.
- Recurrent varicose veins.

Complications of orthopaedic surgery

Complications of arthroplasty

Arthroplasty can be defined as the operative formation or restoration of a joint. This can involve excision, reconstruction, or replacement of the joint with a prosthesis. In this section replacement arthroplasty will be covered.

Common to all arthroplasties

Infection

Prosthetic joint infection is a devastating complication. This complication is generally classified into early (within 3 weeks), haematogenous, and chronic. For hip arthroplasty the early post-operative incidence should be 0.5% or less, using prophylactic antibiotics and laminar flow theatres. Overall, it is estimated that the incidence of infection is approximately 1% over the lifetime of the prosthesis. Knee arthroplasty has similar infection rates. Risk factors for infection include malnutrition, immunocompromise, diabetes, psoriatic arthropathy, rheumatoid arthritis, and previous peri-articular infection.

The presence of persistent erythema, dusky discolouration, tenderness, poor wound healing, fever, or more-than-expected pain during reha-bilitation should raise the suspicion of an early infection. Elevated inflammatory markers (WCC, ESR, and CRP) are also suggestive of an infection. Aspiration of the joint and evaluation of the Gram stain and microbiological culture of the fluid is diagnostic in 75% of cases. Isotope bone scan is not very helpful in the first 18 months following surgery.

Treatment

Superficial SSIs usually settle with a course of intravenous followed by oral antibiotics. Treatment should be aggressive, with an anti-staphylococcal agent (flucloxacillin 1g every 6hrs). Superficial SSIs usually settle with this regimen within 2 weeks. If infection is not controlled by this regimen or a deep infection is suspected, re-exploration of the wound, arthrotomy, thorough debridement and copious irrigation can salvage the prosthesis. This should be undertaken promptly if a deep infection is suspected. If infection fails to settle in spite of this, management should be more radical. Responsible microorganisms include *Staphylococcus aureus* and *Staphylococcus epidermidis* (the latter typical in late infection).

Thrombosis

Thromboembolism is unfortunately a common complication after ortho-paedic surgery. It has therefore invoked much research and debate over the best form of prophylaxis; however, the subject is still controversial. The National Institute for Health and Clinical Excellence (NICE) have produced guidelines in regards to this, suggesting that all elective surgery and hip fractures should be offered mechanical prophylaxis (calf pump, foot pump) combined with low molecular weight heparin. In the presence of risk factors this treatment should be continued for 4 weeks following operation. Some surgeons still elect to treat patients with a 6-week course of aspirin (150mg od).

Periprosthetic fractures

Periprosthetic fractures are fractures around a joint replacement prosthesis. They can occur any time after implantation, from during the operation (e.g. preparing and manipulating the femur in THR) to more than 10 years after. The incidence of periprosthetic fracture in TKR surgery is 0.6–2.5%. Causes include: surgical error in implanting, stress riser effect of implant, osteolysis, infection, and revision surgery. They present with pain and an inability to weight-bear, usually following injury. Diagnosis is confirmed by X-ray.

Treatment

The treatment of periprosthetic fractures is complicated due to osteoporosis, bone defect and implant presence making fixation difficult.

- Conservative – splintage of periprosthetic fractures is an option for stable aligned fractures with no implant loosening.
- Surgery – this includes implant replacement with an implant that stabilizes the fracture or fixation of the fracture around the implant. If the implant is loose or deformed then the best option is probably to revise the implant and thus remove the complications of non-union, malunion, and fixation problems.

Nerve damage

Nerve damage is a surgical complication that may be minor or major. Around the knee, the infrapatellar branch of the saphenous nerve is often cut, causing a troublesome neuroma or a patch of anaesthesia (this often improves with time). In hip replacement surgery, the nerves at risk during the operation differ depending on approach. The anterolateral approach risks damage to the femoral nerve, usually due to retraction of the anterior structures. The superior gluteal nerve may be damaged in over-exuberant proximal dissection. In the posterior approach the sciatic nerve is at risk.

Aseptic loosening

Aseptic loosening is one of the major causes of late implant failure. Wear particles cause an adverse tissue response over time, contributing to bone loss around the implant. The failure rate can be influenced by many factors, including the prosthesis used and patient factors (such as age, sex, weight). Once infection has been excluded, this can usually be treated with a one stage revision.

Procedure specific

- Total hip replacement.
- Total knee replacement.

Total hip replacement

Dislocation

Dislocation of hip prostheses occurs in 1–5% of patients in the first 3 months following THR performed electively for hip arthritis. The incidence of dislocation is much higher, usually around 10%, if this procedure is performed early for a femoral neck fracture. At least 40% of dislocations occur in the first month after surgery. The direction of dislocation is generally determined by the surgical approach used, thus posterior dislocation is more common with the posterior approach.

Causes

Improper orientation and positioning of the components or inadequate soft-tissue tensioning predispose to hip dislocation post-operatively. Improper compliance of the patient with prescribed post-operative rehabilitation usually precipitates the dislocation. There has been a reduction in rates of dislocation following THR, by use of larger heads on the femoral stem and metal on metal bearings (PMID: 17823033).

Recognition

Sudden onset of severe pain in affected hip with shortening, which is either internally or externally rotated. Confirmation of diagnosis is by X-ray.

Treatment

The hip dislocation should be reduced under a general anaesthetic by closed manipulation as soon as possible. If successful, check for stability in various positions of the limb, and document the findings. Following reduction the hip is maintained in the most stable position, determined by image-intensifier screening (this is usually in abduction). This is accomplished using an abduction brace, which should be continuously worn by the patient for a period of 6–12 weeks. About two-thirds of these cases stabilize with treatment in the brace. If dislocation recurs following removal of the brace, surgical treatment is likely to be essential for either repositioning of the components or re-tensioning of the hip. If closed reduction fails, open reduction of the dislocation should be undertaken and the above regime of bracing followed.

Leg length discrepancy

Limb length discrepancy following THR can adversely affect an otherwise excellent outcome. It has been reported in different case series to occur in 16–27% of cases. However, this seemingly high rate of limb length discrepancy can be attributed to other causes such as lumbosacral scoliosis, pelvic obliquity, periarticular muscular spasm, and residual contracture of the hip. These other causes should improve with time. It is recognized that all but 0.5% of symptomatic leg length discrepancies recover from their initial symptoms.

Hip resurfacing

Avascular necrosis of femoral neck

In hip resurfacing the femoral neck is preserved. This may have its blood supply compromised during surgery, leading to AVN and the need for subsequent revision. Femoral neck fracture is an additional complication as compared to traditional total hip replacements.

Total knee replacement

Arthrofibrosis

This is a rare complication that presents with a painful knee that has a poor range of motion following knee replacement. These patients may never gain a functional range of motion following surgery, or they may lose motion after initially doing well. This condition has to be differentiated from reflex sympathetic dystrophy and, after ruling out infection, can be successfully treated by manipulation and physiotherapy. Rarely, an arthrotomy with removal of intra-articular adhesions and scar tissue may be necessary.

Extensor mechanism problems

Fractures of the patella around the patellar component of the prosthesis may occur and, if undisplaced, can usually be managed conservatively. Immobilization for 4–6 weeks with external cast/splintage, followed by guided active exercises, usually leads to full recovery. Displaced fractures may need to be treated by internal fixation, with or without revision of the patellar component.

Progressive patellar maltracking with lateral subluxation of the patella may occur with continued follow-up. Patellar tendon avulsion is a serious complication for which treatment is frequently unsuccessful. Primary repair, if unsuccessful, leads to a lack of extensor mechanism for the knee, which will have to be treated by a locked knee brace or surgical arthrodesis.

Complications following surgical treatment of fractures

The following complications can occur with any of the various types of internal fixation or external fixation of fractures.

Infection

Iatrogenic infection is now the most common cause of chronic osteomyelitis. Both superficial surgical site infection and deep infection (osteomyelitis) can occur after surgical treatment of fractures, and present with local pain, redness, swelling, warmth, and, in the later stages, abscess formation, wound dehiscence, and discharge. The patient may show systemic features of pyrexia and tachycardia. Tests include ESR/CRP (↑), WCC (↑), and blood culture (positive in 60%). Radiographs of the involved area show soft-tissue swelling in the first 2 weeks, but later osteolysis develops around the implants. MRI and isotope scans can have limitations due to the implant and healing fracture. In the case of external fixators, the pins may become loose due to a surrounding osteolysis.

Treatment

Identification of the offending organism is important, thus a wound swab and blood for culture should be obtained. IV antibiotics should be instituted with activity against *Staphylococcus aureus*. Deep infections require a combination of IV antibiotics and surgical debridement. It is important to completely remove all hardware as it is impossible to eliminate all implant-associated infection due to organisms growing in a biofilm, shielding them from antibiotics. Pin-site infection is very common, even with meticulous care. Antibiotics are required with local pin-site dressings. If pins become loose, the pins need re-siting with reapplication of an external fixator and a course of antibiotics.

Non-union

A non-union is a failure of healing progression on three successive monthly radiographs. Infection needs to be excluded as a cause. Causes of non-union can be divided into local factors (loss of soft tissue or bone, soft tissue interposition, intact fellow bone, local infection, poor blood supply), surgeon factors (distraction, poor splintage or fixation), and patient factors. There are different types of non-union:

- Atrophic – rounded-off bone ends due to the fragments becoming osteoporotic and atrophic. Usually due to poor blood supply.
- Oligotrophic – not hypertrophic and callus is absent. Usually due to significant fracture displacement or distraction.
- Hypertrophic non-union – this is where the bone ends are expanded ('elephant's foot'/'horse hoof') due to large amount of callus. Generally due to inadequate fixation or premature weight-bearing causing excessive fracture movement.
- Pseudoarthrosis – an established non-union with rounding of bone ends and an artificial synovial-type cavity formed around these.

Treatment
- Conservative – if non-symptomatic it can be treated conservatively. Some hypertrophic non-unions may heal with functional bracing and/or low frequency pulsed ultrasound.
- Surgical – in undeformed hypertrophic non-union, rigid internal fixation is usually successful. This may be augmented by freshening of the bone ends and bone grafting. With atrophic non-union, there is fibrous tissue in between sclerotic bone ends. The fibrous tissue and sclerotic bone ends must be excised and the subsequent gap filled with either bone graft or in the case of segmental bone loss, a vascularized bone graft (e.g. fibular graft) or bone transport with a three-dimensional fixator (Ilizarov frame). It is important to eradicate any infection at the non-union site before attempting definitive surgical treatment.

Malunion

This is where the fractured bone unites in an unsatisfactory position (angulated, rotated, or shortened). This is caused by a failure in reduction, failure of holding in a reduced position, or gradual collapse of comminution.

Treatment
This depends on the site and degree of malunion. General rules are: <10–15° in long bone is usually acceptable; angular deformities in children generally remodel over time but rotation will not; and lower limb shortening of >2cm is not well tolerated. If correction is indicated, planned corrective osteotomy with further internal fixation should be carried out. Alternatively, osteotomy with external fixation (Ilizarov frame) can be used.

Avascular necrosis (aseptic necrosis, osteonecrosis)

This is bone necrosis caused by a deficient blood supply. Certain regions have a high propensity to undergo AVN due to their already tenuous blood supply. These are:
- the femoral head
- the proximal pole of the scaphoid
- the lunate
- the body of talus.

It may cause local pain, non-union of fractures, and may lead to disabling arthritis or disorganization of a joint.

AVN can also occur spontaneously in patients on steroid therapy, in sickle-cell disease, and as part of decompression sickness (e.g. deep-sea diving).

The ischaemia that causes AVN occurs only a few hours following the fracture/dislocation. However, the clinical and radiological sequelae may not manifest themselves for 2–3 years. There are no direct symptoms of AVN, only pain from the resulting non-union or collapse. Radiologically, there is an increase in density of the avascular fragment with some relative osteopenia of the surrounding bones from the reactive hyperaemia and disuse of the surrounding area.

Diagnosis

Usually evident with follow-up radiographs. ^{99}Tc-radioisotope bone scanning with high resolution may show the area as a cold spot. A magnetic resonance imaging (MRI) scan can reliably pick up areas of AVN as early as 2 weeks following the injury.

Treatment

Attempts to revascularize the area have been tried with vascularized bone grafts or muscle pedicle grafts, but success is variable. Treatment usually involves surgical removal of the avascular part followed by the salvage procedure for the joint (e.g. arthrodesis or joint replacement/excision arthroplasty).

Growth disturbance

In those of skeletal immaturity, damage to the physis may lead to abnormal or arrested growth. Transverse injuries are seldom problematic if adequate reduction has been achieved. Fractures that transverse the growing portion, however, can lead to complete growth arrest or more commonly partial growth arrest. These can result in angular deformities or progressive limb length discrepancies. Severe growth plate injuries should be monitored closely.

Septic arthritis

This is defined as inflammation of a joint caused by infection. Most cases occur in children and are a result of haematogenous spread. It can, however, arise as a consequence of surgical intervention or penetrating injury. Prompt treatment of this is imperative, as chondrolysis is quickly established. Antibiotics alone do not halt this destruction and surgical drainage or joint lavage is urgently needed.

Clinical features

Pain and swelling of the affected joint are the usual presenting symptoms. On examination the joint is warm and tender to touch with restricted movements. There may be systemic features such as pyrexia, tachycardia, sweating, and rigors.

Microorganisms

The most common offending organism is *Staphylococcus aureus*. Other organisms are possible, e.g. *Haemophilus influenzae* in children (the incidence of this is reducing since the introduction of HiB vaccine), *Gonococcus* in young, sexually active adults, and *Pseudomonas* spp. and other Gram-negative bacteria in IV drug abusers.

Treatment

This is a surgical emergency. Radical treatment by arthrotomy, copious irrigation of the joint, and synovectomy, with systemic intravenous antibiotics (initially flucloxacillin and modified as necessary depending on the results of culture and sensitivity), stands the best chance of eradicating the infection.

Complications following hand surgery

Infection

When thinking of infection in the hand it is important to understand the possible spaces where it may occur.

- Felon – infection of the finger pulp.
- Paronychia/Eponychia – nail fold infection.
- Joint infection – especially 'fight bite' injuries to the MCP joints.
- Flexor sheath infections – this area contains the long flexor tendons to the fingers and thumb. Infection within this compartment leads to adhesions and tendon tethering, and thereby loss of function. It is important to remember that the flexor sheaths of the thumb and little finger extend into the palm.
- Hypothenar space – this encloses the hypothenar muscles but not the long flexor tendons or their sheaths. If infection is confined to this space, it is less problematic than the other areas in the hand.
- Mid-palmar space – this is a space that lies deep to the flexor tendons and the common synovial sheath; it contains the lumbricals and is dorsally bounded by the interossei. Infection may spread from here into the flexor sheath via the lumbrical canal.
- Thenar space – this space encloses the thenar muscles, the flexor tendon of the thumb, and, sometimes, the flexor tendon of the index finger. Infection here causes abnormal function of these fingers.

Infection in the above spaces generally presents with pain in the hand with swelling, which is most marked over the dorsal aspect of the hand. Night pain is a sinister feature. The four cardinal signs of flexor sheath involvement (Kanavel's signs) are intense pain increased on passive extension of the involved digit, flexed posture, uniform swelling, and percussion tenderness over the course of the tendon sheath. There is pain on passive or active movements of the involved fingers, and the finger assumes a flexed posture with any passive stretching/straightening leading to severe pain along the flexor sheath. With an extension of the infection, tenderness and swelling can be noted in Parona's space, just proximal to the carpal tunnel on the volar aspect of the wrist.

Treatment

In the acute stage, IV antibiotics are the mainstay of treatment with elevation. If the signs improve in the first 24 hours surgery may be avoided. Gentle physiotherapy avoids the onset of adhesions and prevents contractures. If infection does not respond or if the patient presents late (after 48 hours of onset), surgical intervention is required. Investigation using ultrasound or MRI to localize the collection may be needed. Incision and drainage is needed for mid-palmar, thenar, and hypothenar infections using both a volar and dorsal approach. If a flexor sheath is involved, it can be opened directly and irrigated or have a window made proximally and distally in the sheath followed by continuous irrigation of the sheath with Ringer's lactate or saline. Physiotherapy is continued post-operatively to maintain hand and finger function.

Tendon adherence

This occurs following any tendon repair or a surgical procedure or injury in the proximity of a tendon. Adherence is most common following flexor-tendon repair in zone 2, and presents with a reduced active range of movement in spite of continued physiotherapy. Diagnosis should always be considered when the passive range of movement exceeds the active range of movement in a finger.

Treatment

This is treated by surgical tenolysis (freeing of the tendon adhesions) but should not be undertaken for >3 months following the repair, when the risk of re-rupture is reduced and full passive motion is obtained. It is important to conserve critical pulleys (especially A2 and A4) on tenolysis. A further course of active rigorous physiotherapy following the tenolysis restores active finger movements.

Scar contracture

This is another complication that can reduce the range of movement in the fingers. Longitudinal incisions forming scars across flexion creases in the fingers usually lead to this complication; such incisions should therefore be avoided. Contractures present with tightness of the scar with an inability to extend the fingers fully. This is treated in the initial stages by scar massage and gentle stretching and, once the scar matures, if there is a significant residual contracture, surgical intervention is required. This can be by incision or excision of the scar. Excision of the scar requires skin grafting, while incision of the scar usually resolves with Z plasty.

Inadvertent neurovascular injury

This complication may occur with injury to digital neurovascular bundles, particularly whilst doing a fasciotomy for Dupuytren's disease. If recognized at the time of surgery, the digital nerve should be repaired by epineural sutures under magnification. If recognized following surgery, there is the risk of neuroma formation and loss of protective sensation in the finger and re-exploration with surgical repair of the nerve should be carried out. The aim of surgery is to restore the protective sensation in the finger and to prevent neuroma formation.

Complications after spinal surgery

The following complications may occur following any form of spinal surgery.

Paralytic ileus

This complication may occur due to reflex inhibition of bowel function. It is more common with anterior approaches to the lumbar spine and is treated in the usual way, with gastrointestinal decompression and IV fluids. This complication is temporary and bowel function returns within a day or two following surgery. If not, a more organic cause should be suspected and investigated (e.g. inadvertent bowel injury).

Infection

Infection occurs in less than 1% of patients after spinal surgery. As illustrated previously in this chapter, infection can be superficial or involve deeper structures. Vertebral osteomyelitis and/or an epidural abscess may occur. The patient presents with an increase in local pain. There may be systemic features and if an epidural abscess or a granulomatous lesion develops in association with this, a corresponding neurological abnormality might develop. It is important to chart neurological signs regularly after any spinal surgery.

Treatment

Treatment is along the usual lines with intravenous antibiotics and close observation. If there is suspicion of an abscess formation, this needs localization and surgical drainage.

Neurological deficit

Usually, there is some neurological dysfunction pre-operatively in most patients and it is important to document this carefully. If any fresh neurological abnormality occurs post-operatively or if there is progressive neurological involvement then prompt investigation and action are indicated. Careful observation, particularly of any post-operative sphincter disturbances, is required.

Causes

Haematomas can cause neurological compression. Residual intervertebral disc fragments, sequestration or prolapse at another level may not be recognized at the time of surgery. Inadvertent neurological injury, particularly with instrumented spinal surgery using pedicle screws and distraction, is another cause.

Management

Determine the level of possible neurological involvement, obtain urgent local imaging (e.g. CT or MRI scanning), and treat the pathology detected. Neurological injury may cause causalgic-type nerve pain and may need the involvement of a chronic pain-management team.

Other complications

Failure of fusion and persistent pain after attempted intervertebral fusions (particularly at multiple levels), instability following extensive laminectomy, and undue stresses adjacent to fused vertebral segments cause persistent low back pain (the Failed Back syndrome). Empyema, persistent pneumothorax, or excessive blood loss from a large haemothorax may occur following a thoracotomy for anterior thoracic spinal operations. It is important to learn to anticipate these complications and institute prompt treatment.

Arthroscopic surgery

The following specific complications can occur following arthroscopic surgery of any joint.

Infection

Septic arthritis of the joint may occur and needs to be treated promptly, as described earlier.

Synovial fistula

Persistent discharge of synovial fluid occurs from a fistulous opening out to the skin surface through an arthroscopy port in 6/1000 patients. This is treated by splintage of the joint and occlusive dressings with non-steroidal anti-inflammatory agents in the early stages. If drainage fails to cease by 8 weeks, surgical excision of the fistula needs consideration with or without a synovectomy of the involved joint.

Compartment syndrome

This is a rare complication, particularly after a knee arthroscopy, and may occur if the irrigation fluid extravasates into the calf through a capsular tear, causing abnormal tension in the muscle compartment of the leg. However, the sequaelae from this are reported to be minimal.

Other complications

Quadriceps inhibition may occur after knee arthroscopy, but this is temporary and can be treated by active physiotherapy. Joint stiffness and florid RSD may occur, particularly in the hand following a wrist arthroscopy. This is managed in the usual fashion. Haemarthrosis is rare, but it can occur after an arthroscopic synovectomy or lateral release in the knee. If bleeding is not controllable arthroscopically, an arthrotomy with drainage of the arthrosis and diathermy haemostasis might be necessary. Treatment is indicated if there is symptomatic joint involvement.

Anterior cruciate ligament reconstruction-related complications

ACL reconstruction is a very common procedure done arthroscopically. The most common methods used are patellar tendon and hamstring tendon grafting. Following ACL repair, graft failure can occur in 1.9% of patellar tendon reconstructions and 4.9% of hamstring reconstructions. The risk of infection following ACL reconstruction is thought to be <2%. A cyclops lesion (fibrous nodule occupying the intracondylar notch) can cause a mechanical block to full extension post-ACL reconstruction, usually occurring 4 months post-operatively. This can be removed arthroscopically. In patellar tendon reconstruction, the harvesting of the graft causes pain on kneeling. Over-zealous harvesting of the patellar tendon graft can result in patellar fracture or patellar tendon rupture, resulting in loss of extension.

Non-specific orthopaedic complications

Post-traumatic ossification (myositis ossificans)

Heterotopic ossification can occur after any injury, most commonly around the elbow, or following muscular injuries to brachialis, deltoid, or quadriceps. Classically the muscle bellies are affected; however, in some cases it may be fixed to underlying bone.

Recognition

Clinically, patients complain about pain, with local swelling and soft tissue tenderness. If the underlying bone is affected, they may present with subjective stiffness and a reduced range of movement. X-rays of the involved part show 'fluffy' calcification, which looks similar to immature callus. Serum alkaline phosphatase is raised and an isotope bone scan may demonstrate a hot spot in this area in the active stages of bone formation.

Treatment

Gentle active exercises in the initial phases, but passive stretching should be avoided altogether. It is necessary to wait for the heterotopic bone to mature (indicated by maturation of the bone with serial radiographs), the serum alkaline phosphatase level to return to normal, and for a negative isotope bone scan (which then indicates that the process has reached an inactive stage). The heterotopic bone can be removed at this stage with improvement of function. There is a risk of recurrence of heterotopic ossification with surgical excision, and prophylactic indomethacin or radiotherapy should be given to prevent this.

Post-traumatic arthritis

This occurs due to damage of a joint surface from a displaced intra-articular fracture. Surgical reconstruction can restore normal joint congruity. Accurate reconstruction of the joint surface minimizes, but does not eliminate, the risk of post-traumatic arthritis. Treatment of this complication should follow the general principles of managing painful arthritis in a joint.

Fat embolism syndrome (FES)

This is a condition characterized by unanticipated respiratory compromise following long-bone fractures.

Pathomechanics

The syndrome follows small-vessel occlusion by fat globules. There are two current theories to explain this phenomenon: the mechanical theory, where fat emboli are released directly into the venous system from the bone marrow of the fractured bone; and the biochemical theory, where hormonal changes, as part of the metabolic response to trauma, cause systemic release of fatty acids as chylomicrons.

Clinical features

These usually follow long-bone fractures in the lower limb (femur, tibia/fibula). The syndrome presents with dyspnoea, tachycardia, anxiety, tachypnoea (sustained respiratory rate >35/min), a petechial rash above the level of the nipples, fever, retinal changes, and, sometimes, jaundice.

There is a 'lucid' symptom-free period of 1–2 days after the fracture before the onset of these symptoms. Gurd and Wilson's criteria for diagnosis are:

- Major signs: respiratory insufficiency, cerebral involvement, and petechial rash.
- Minor signs: fever, tachycardia, retinal changes, jaundice, and renal changes.

FES can be diagnosed when one major and four minor signs are present plus fat microglobinaemia.

Investigations

- Arterial blood gases – PO_2 <9kPa, PCO_2 >8kPa, pH <7.3 breathing room air.
- Fat globules in blood, urine, and sputum.
- ST segment changes on ECG and $S_1Q_3T_3$, suggesting right ventricular strain.
- Thrombocytopenia, anaemia, and hypofibrinogenaemia are suspicious of FES, but are non-specific.
- Chest radiograph – serial radiographs reveal increasing diffuse pulmonary infiltrates.
- Chest CT – may be normal.

Treatment

Supportive, maintaining oxygenation and ventilation whilst awaiting spontaneous resolution. Early surgical stabilization of fractured long bones, especially in polytrauma, within 24 hours of injury. Oxygen administration in the post-injury period reduces the incidence of FES. Corticosteroids in low doses have been shown to reduce the incidence of FES, but their routine use remains controversial.

Osteomyelitis

Osteomyelitis is the infection of bone following a penetrating injury, haematogenous or direct spread from adjacent tissues. Osteomyelitis may be acute, subacute, or chronic depending on the clinical presentation.

Bacteriology

Staphylococcus aureus is the commonest pathogen amongst all age groups. In newborns (up to 4 months), Gram-negative bacilli and group B *Streptococcus* may be implicated. In children, group A *Streptococci* and coliforms are characteristic. Unusual organisms include *Serratia* and *Pseudomonas* spp. (especially amongst IV drug abusers), anaerobes, *Salmonella* (in patients with sickle-cell disease), *Brucella* (in meat handlers), fungi, spirochaetes (*T. Pallidum* following sexual contact), and mycobacteria (TB/leprosy/fishermen). In post-operative osteomyelitis there is usually a mix of pathogenic bacteria: *Staphylococcus aureus, Proteus, E. Coli,* and *Pseudomonas*.

Pathology

The initial stage of osteomyelitis is inflammatory. Polymorphonuclear leucocytes invade the area with an exudation of fluid. The interosseus pressure rises, causing intense pain and obstruction to blood flow. By the second or third day, pus forms and forces its way to the surface of the bone causing a subperiosteal abscess. This is called the 'suppuration phase'. Following this, bony necrosis occurs (third phase) following increasing vascular compromise. The fourth phase is new bone formation, where reactive periosteal bone (involucrum) may form around the infective focus (sequestrum and involucrum). If the infection persists, the pus tracks through holes in the involucrum (cloacae) to the skin, forming discharging sinuses. This heralds the transition to a chronic phase subsequent to uncontrolled acute osteomyelitis. If the infection is controlled and intraosseous pressure relieved at an early stage then this whole process can be controlled.

Clinical features

Manifestation is usually at least a week after fracture treatment or a surgical procedure on bone. In acute osteomyelitis there is local warmth, swelling, skin oedema, and erythema. These signs may be absent if infection occurs deep to the deep fascia, particularly in the femur. The patient is usually febrile. Subacute osteomyelitis presents with pain, but local and systemic features are remarkably absent. There may be percussion tenderness on the affected part of the bone.

Chronic osteomyelitis presents a few months after the inciting event or after an acute osteomyelitis that has been modified in its course by inadequate treatment. There may be some local pain, swelling, and erythema but these are usually not severe. One or more sinuses on the skin may be discharging purulent material, sometimes containing pieces of white necrotic bone. Systemic features are typically absent.

Investigations

Acute osteomyelitis is a clinical diagnosis and treatment should not be delayed. Blood culture and local wound swab is appropriate for culture and sensitivity to confirm the empirical choice of therapy. Laboratory investigations include ESR/CRP (↑), WCC (↑), blood culture (positive in 60%). Radiographs show soft tissue swelling in the first 2 weeks and periosteal reaction.

Chronic and subacute osteomyelitis may be more difficult to diagnose clinically, and may need further investigation. Plain radiographs may demonstrate osteolysis and a periosteal reaction. Haematological investigations are usually normal. Isotope bone scan, using ^{99}Tc-labelled, shows the infective focus as a hot spot, but occasionally can give false-positive and false-negative results. The ^{111}In-labelled leucocyte scan is more specific. Bone biopsy is the definitive confirmatory investigation in doubtful cases. This also helps in identifying the offending organism and its antibiotic sensitivity.

Treatment

Acute osteomyelitis

Splint the affected limb for pain relief. Start intravenous antibiotics after obtaining a blood sample for culture and any local sample from the affected part, if feasible. Use an antibiotic with activity against *Staphylococcus aureus*, e.g. flucloxacillin. Clinical signs should be monitored: leucocyte count, CRP, and ESR (or plasma viscosity) to determine response to treatment. Continue IV antibiotics until CRP returns to normal, and switch to oral antibiotics for a further 4 weeks. Usually a 6-week course of antibiotics (at least) is needed for eradication of infection. If the condition is not settling with IV antibiotics in the first 24 hours, the patient is likely to need surgical drainage.

Subacute and chronic osteomyelitis

Treatment usually requires surgical sequestrectomy and drainage of any abscesses, augmented by local or systemic antibiotics. Multiple surgical procedures may be necessary.

Complications

Local deformity, scarring, and growth disturbance may occur. Sinuses may rarely turn malignant (Marjolin's ulcer) and chronic infection may lead to systemic amyloidosis.

Complex regional pain syndrome (reflex sympathetic dystrophy, shoulder hand syndrome)

This is a clinical entity that causes pain, vasomotor instability, functional impairment, trophic skin changes, and osteoporosis. It can occur after any limb trauma or surgery, splintage, nerve injury (causalgia), or extravasation of thiopental during induction of anaesthesia.

Mechanism

This is unclear. A widely accepted hypothesis is that the condition is mediated and maintained by the autonomic nervous system, and is thought to be due to a sustained efferent sympathetic activity.

Clinical features

The four cardinal features include disproportionate amount of pain, swelling, stiffness, and discolouration.

Three phases are recognized:

- Acute (hyperaemic) phase – pain, hyperaesthesia, increased local warmth, and oedema. Also the skin looks stretched and shiny with loss of normal wrinkles and creases.
- Dystrophic (ischaemic) phase – the oedema spreads further, joints become stiff, and muscle wasting develops. Pain remains the main symptom and is usually burning in nature. The skin becomes moist, cyanotic, and cold. Hair becomes coarse and the nails show ridges and are brittle.
- Atrophic phase – trophic changes become irreversible. Skin becomes pale, smooth, glossy, and tight. Surface temperature falls and thickened hair falls out. There is extreme weakness and limitation of movement of all involved joints (e.g. fingers and wrist). Pain, although less prominent, persists.

Diagnosis

This is usually clinically obvious. X-rays of the involved part show patchy osteoporosis (known as Sudeck's atrophy). Three-phase isotopic bone scans show increased uptake in early and delayed phases with increased activity in a periarticular distribution.

Differential diagnosis

Tenosynovitis, bursitis, myofascial pain, Raynaud's phenomenon, and sometimes peripheral nerve injury without a sympathetic nervous system component.

Treatment
This is difficult. In the early stages, NSAIDs and physiotherapy usually result in a good response. If there is no improvement in the first few weeks, different modalities may have to be tried simultaneously or sequentially. These are: physiotherapy, nerve blocks including regional block using guanethidine, surgical or chemical sympathectomy, and psychotherapy. It is important to maintain function of the involved part and alleviate the stresses produced by the syndrome on the central nervous system.

Compartment syndrome

This is an orthopaedic emergency. It is defined as a pressure within a closed anatomical space that exceeds the perfusion pressure within that compartment. It has the potential to cause irreversible damage to the contents of the closed space. It is usually seen in muscle compartments in the limbs and occurs most commonly in the leg, but can also occur in the forearm, thigh, foot, and hand.

Causes
This can be divided into external pressures (plaster-cast), restriction in the compartment wall (circumferential burns), and causes of intracompartmental swelling (crush injury, fracture, reperfusion injury). The most common fractures that cause compartment syndrome are of the elbow, forearm, and proximal third of the tibia.

Recognition
The diagnosis of compartment syndrome is primarily clinical. Pain, especially on passive extension of the compartment, is the most important sign. The compartment may feel tense to palpation and skin paraesthesia may develop early. Other signs appear later but treatment should be instituted before these have manifested (paralysis, pulselessness).

Investigation
This is unnecessary in an alert and lucid patient and treatment is based on clinical findings. Investigation is only needed if diagnosis is unclear clinically, or in cases of head injury or sedated patient where there is an altered level of consciousness. Compartment pressures are usually measured with a needle manometer. Fasciotomy is indicated if the compartment pressure rises above 30mmHg or is within 30mmHg of the diastolic pressure.

Treatment
Urgent fasciotomy where the skin and enveloping fascia of the involved compartment(s) are incised in their entire length and left open. In the leg, all four compartments (anterior, lateral, superficial posterior, and deep posterior) should be decompressed.

Complications of amputation

Introduction

The major indications for lower limb amputation in vascular surgery are for non-reconstructable critical limb ischaemia, non-viable acute limb ischaemia, trauma, and for diabetic foot infection. Amputation is therefore needed to preserve life, prevent the spread of infection, alleviate pain, and promote mobility. Common amputations performed are digital, ray (digit plus metatarsal), transmetatarsal, below knee (BKA), and above knee (AKA).

Early complications

Within 30 days.

Complications of poor wound healing

The primary aim of any major lower limb amputation is to leave the patient with enough leg to mobilize and rehabilitate, while achieving primary wound healing. The energy required for walking is increased by 60% for unilateral BKA and 120% for unilateral AKA. As a result, following AKA only 40% of patients achieve grade III–V mobility (i.e. unlimited household mobility or better) compared to 80% of those with BKA (note: grade 0 is bedridden and grade V is unlimited mobility). The enhanced mobility associated with a BKA must consequently be balanced against the risk of wound breakdown when choosing the level of amputation. In practice, if the skin of the calf is warm, free from trophic change and infection, and intra-operative tissue bleeding is adequate at the proximal edges of the amputation, then primary healing after BKA is likely to take place. Wound breakdown occurs in around 20% of all BKAs and requires conversion to an above knee level. However, once a BKA has healed the chance of requiring an ipsilateral AKA is only 4%. Poor healing is principally due to ischaemia related to underlying peripheral arterial disease but poor surgical technique, such as excessive suture tension or poor haemostasis, compromises already poor perfusion and predisposes to necrosis and infection. Several techniques have been investigated to predict wound healing after BKA (e.g. angiography, ankle systolic pressures, transcutaneous oxygen partial pressures, isotope blood studies, thermography, and laser Doppler flowmetry) but none have been shown to be sensitive enough for routine clinical practice.

Infection

Operating on bacterially colonized, frankly infected or ischaemic tissues means that the risk of surgical site infection is high. Broad-spectrum antibiotics (e.g. intravenous cefuroxime and metronidazole, unless pre-operative sensitivities dictate otherwise) are thus given prophylactically; in the presence of pre-operative infection a full treatment course (5 days or more) should be given. Infection can lead to oedema, which causes increased tissue tension, and the resultant ischaemia may lead to wound breakdown or skin flap necrosis. Consideration should be given to leaving the skin flaps open in the presence of gross infection or contamination. Osteomyelitis is another potential consequence and generally requires conversion to a higher level of amputation. Bacteraemia may also follow and result in SIRS or even MODS. Common pathogenic organisms include *Staphylococcus aureus*, *Streptococci*, Coliforms (Pseudomonads, *Proteus* spp.), and *Bacteroides* spp. Vigilance should be paid to an increasing prevalence of MRSA-related wound colonization, with the potential risk of post-operative wound infection resistant to 'routine' antibiotics, and systemic disturbance. Clostridial fasciitis and myonecrosis (gas gangrene) is a rare cause of infection. It should be distinguished from anaerobic cellulitis (necrotizing fasciitis), which may be caused by anaerobic *Streptococci* or a synergistic infection. Both are gas-producing infections and cause profound systemic disturbance (SIRS and MODS) with high mortality

(📖 see Chapter 2, Infection, p.29). Some advocate the use of penicillin as prophylaxis for all patients, particularly diabetics or patients who are immunosuppressed.

Bleeding and haematoma
Many surgeons place a small-bore suction drain to avoid this complication. Haematoma formation carries the added risk of infection and wound breakdown. Intra-operatively, meticulous care should be taken to individually ligate all bleeding points.

Stump pain
Wound pain is usually managed in the immediate post-operative period with a patient controlled analgesia system (PCAS) or epidural anaesthetic. In those patients in whom an epidural cannot be used, the surgeon can insert an epidural catheter into either the tibial or sciatic nerve sheath, depending upon the level of the amputation, and a similar local anaesthetic infusion regimen can be administered. Severe and prolonged pre-operative limb pain increases the risk of post-operative phantom limb pain. However, there is conflicting evidence that good pre-operative analgesia by epidural use reduces phantom pain in the long term. Excessive post-operative pain may result in joint contractures, limits ambulation, and increases the risk of the complications of recumbency.

Joint contractures and muscle wasting
Adequate pain control and intensive physiotherapy are required to prevent joint contractures and muscle wasting. In the knee, a fixed flexion deformity of more than 20 degrees necessitates increased hip flexion and lumbar spine extension, which makes mobilization difficult. An angle over 35 degrees makes it impossible to fit even a kneeling prosthesis. To achieve a good functional result for mobility, patients require a minimal fixed-flexion deformity at the knee and certainly less than 20 degrees. Aids such as tricep springs, monkey bars, and rope ladders facilitate early mobilization in bed and promote the development of upper body strength. Patients should have access to their own wheelchair and be referred on to the regional limb-fitting service. Finally, an early comprehensive assessment is essential to facilitate early discharge from hospital. A full nutritional evaluation, with support if intake is inadequate, should be made in the elderly and debilitated to enhance rehabilitation.

The complications of recumbency
Prolonged recumbency particularly affects elderly patients undergoing AKA. It carries an increased risk of thromboembolic events, chest infections, and pressure sores.

Late complications

After 30 days.

Stump neuroma

Stump neuromas may affect the sciatic nerve following AKA. The bulbous nerve end can cause severe pain when compressed against the prosthesis, and for this reason the sciatic nerve is always divided as proximally as possible. They may require excision if they are persistently problematic after failed injection with local anaesthetic and steroids.

Phantom limb pain

Phantom limb sensation is any feeling in the amputated limb except pain and occurs in virtually all patients. When this sensation is uncomfortable or painful it is described as phantom limb pain and may affect as many as 75% of amputees. Phantom limb pain should be distinguished from pain in the residual limb (see below). The cause of phantom limb pain is not fully understood but may be due to the persistence of the sensory cortex and is often more severe in the distal extremities, which have the largest cortical representation. It decreases with time and mild cases may only require explanation and conventional analgesia, but severe cases may require specialist pain team advice. Commonly prescribed medication includes gabapentin, pregabalin, amitriptyline, or carbamazepine. Other techniques to relieve pain include regional nerve blocks, transcutaneous electrical nerve stimulation, dorsal column stimulators, acupuncture, hypnosis, and biofeedback.

Poorly fitting prosthesis

Having achieved primary healing the ideal amputation stump should be conical, have adequate muscle coverage without redundant tissue, and bear minimal pressure through the suture line. If these criteria are not met, because of a technically poor operation, the fitting of limb prostheses is difficult, with an adverse effect on mobilization and the risk of ulceration.

Bone spikes or spurs

These arise if the bone ends are not adequately smoothed at operation. They can cause pain and ulceration. If the amputation stump is required for mobility then revision of the stump should be considered.

Stump ulceration

Ulceration can occur as a result of bone spikes, inadequate muscle coverage of the bone ends (in a muscle-wasted or debilitated patient), infection, ischaemia, or an ill-fitting prosthetic device causing pressure or friction. Ulceration can also allow recurrent infection and the development of osteomyelitis. This usually requires revision of the stump.

False aneurysms and arteriovenous fistulas

Although these are rare, they can involve the superficial femoral or crural vessels. They are usually amenable to interventional radiological techniques but if this fails open surgery may be required.

Pain in the residual limb and complex regional pain syndrome

Stump ischaemia, infection, neuromas, bone spurs, false aneurysms, arteriovenous fistulas, or a poorly fitting prosthesis may cause pain in the residual limb. Persistent pain may still be felt in the absence of these factors and be attributable to complex regional pain syndrome (CRPS), a rather confusingly termed diagnosis that includes causalgia and reflex sympathetic dystrophy. It presents with intractable burning pain in the amputation stump with allodynia and hyperaesthesia and may be accompanied by trophic change to the skin and vasomotor/sudomotor disturbance. The pathogenesis of CRPS remains unclear but following an injury or operation (which may be relatively trivial) afferent nociceptive nerves may become sensitized. Treatment is similar to phantom limb pain and may include sympathectomy. Advice from a specialist chronic pain team is recommended.

Complications of urological surgery

Introduction

Urological surgery is one of the oldest surgical specialties, with recognized pathology of the urinary tract being as old as our *Homo sapiens* species. Five thousand-year-old mummies from ancient Egypt have been found to harbour large bladder stones and circumcision was arguably the first elective operation to ever be performed. It is only in recent times however, that urological surgery has been recognized as a specialty in its own right. With the development of fibre optic equipment the modern day urologist can now visualize the entire urinary tract internally and carry out endoscopic intervention. This is a far cry from the practice of urine tasting, undertaken by Hippocrates in the seventeenth century, to identify genitourinary disease.

Urology is an important specialty. Almost 20% of all surgical emergencies have a urological cause. Despite this, it is a field that few trainees and doctors are exposed to. The field of urology can be broadly divided into six sub-specialties (📖 see Fig. 18.1 below).

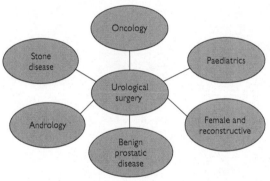

Fig. 18.1 The main urological sub-specialties.

This chapter presents the common urological procedures that fall under each of these sub-specialties. The focus is to give a brief overview of the procedure and its indication, describe the common complications that may arise and their management, and provide a list of alternatives to the initial procedure. With regards to operative complications, the more frequent complications have been listed first.

General principles in urological surgery

Pre-assessment clinic

Ideally all patients undergoing elective urological surgery should be seen in a pre-assessment clinic. This allows potential problems to be identified early and rectified prior to surgery. This should include:

- Full history and examination. In particular the patient's past medical history is of importance in determining their fitness for the proposed procedure. A full drug history must also be taken as, for example, aspirin and other anti-platelets should be stopped prior to the procedure to reduce the risk from bleeding. If the patient is on warfarin this may need to be stopped and the patient brought in for heparinization prior to their procedure.
- Blood tests. As a minimum a FBC, coagulation screen, U&E, and group and save/cross-match should be taken, with other tests as clinically indicated. Anaemia, sepsis, or electrolyte disturbance should be corrected prior to surgery.
- A urine dipstick analysis. This is mandatory and a sample of urine should be sent for culture. Any urinary tract infection must be treated prior to surgery to prevent sepsis.
- A chest X-ray.
- An ECG to identify any cardiac dysfunction.
- An ECHO and lung function test in any patient with significant impairment of cardiac or respiratory function.
- Early anaesthetic review. The anaesthetist should be informed of any potential problems to allow adequate preparation. The cancellation of an operation at the last minute because of anaesthetic issues is frustrating to the patient and entirely avoidable.
- Consent. Taking consent well in advance of the procedure allows the patient to return with any questions they may have after thinking things through.

Cross-matching

Throughout this chapter it is clear that post-operative bleeding is a common complication of urological surgery. For this reason patients should have blood ready, if indicated for certain procedures, prior to entering the operating theatre. A pre-operative group and save or cross-match is advised. Policy varies from Trust to Trust.

TURBT – group and save
TURP – cross-match 2 units
Prostatectomy – cross-match 2 units
Nephrectomy – cross-match 2–4 units
PCNL – cross-match 2 units

Adapted from the Reynard J, Brewster S, and Biers S (2005), *Oxford Handbook of Urology*, Oxford University Press, Oxford.

Prophylactic antibiotics

Another recurrent theme throughout the chapter is the complication of post-operative infection. This risk is reduced by identifying urinary tract infection pre-procedure and treating adequately. Many units also use prophylactic antibiotics peri-operatively. Exact regimens vary according to local microbiological policy, but common antibiotics utilized include ciprofloxacin, nitrofurantoin, cefuroxime, and gentamicin.

The risk of venous thromboembolism

VTE is uncommon following urological surgery. However, its incidence increases with more extensive procedures. The prevention of VTE is far better than its cure. All patients should be considered for TED stockings, a prophylactic dose of LMW heparin, and early mobilization, at a minimum.

Local and general anaesthesia

Many urological procedures are undertaken with sedation, local anaesthetic, general anaesthetic, or sometimes a combination of these. The risks of each should be discussed with the patient as appropriate during the consent process.

Oncological urology

Oncological urology involves malignant and pre-malignant conditions of the urinary tract. Most procedures detailed below are concerned with resection of the affected anatomical site. Common procedures include:
- radical and partial nephrectomy
- nephro-uretectomy
- check cystoscopy
- transurethral resection of bladder tumour (TURBT)
- radical cystectomy and ileal conduit formation
- radical cystectomy and neobladder formation
- prostatectomy (radical perineal or radical retropubic)
- trans-rectal ultrasound (TRUS) prostatic biopsy
- complete and partial amputation of the penis
- radical orchidectomy

Radical and partial nephrectomy and nephrouretectomy

Renal tumours comprise 2% of all malignant conditions. Renal malignancy may be seen in childhood with nephroblastoma, or present later in life, such as renal cell carcinoma. Transitional cell carcinomas occur and can affect any part of the urinary tract from the renal calyces to the urethra. The operation chosen depends on the site and stage of the disease. Small renal tumours may be treated with partial nephrectomy, and more extensive lesions with radical nephrectomy. Both these procedures may involve the removal of the adrenal glands, renal fat, and lymph nodes. Nephrouretectomy is performed for tumours of the ureter and involves the excision of both the kidney and the affected ureter. Frequently pre-operative embolization of the affected kidney is undertaken via percutaneous angiography to reduce the risk of intra-operative bleeding. Nephrectomy may also be performed for transplant purposes.

Indication

The procedures are both diagnostic in obtaining histology of the excised lesion and therapeutic for disease resection (palliation or putative cure).

Post-operative complications

- Infection at the incision site or intra-abdominally, which may require antibiotic therapy or surgical radiological interventions.
- There is a significant risk of haemorrhage, which may require correction with a blood transfusion or warrant interventional surgery.
- Pneumothorax can occur as a result of diaphragmatic injury. This needs chest drain insertion.
- Damage to surrounding structures (such as liver, spleen, or bowel) may occur, needing additional surgical intervention.
- With renal resection, renal impairment and hypertension may result.
- A temporary urinary catheter is inserted post-procedure, which increases the risk of urinary tract infection.
- An abdominal drain is also placed. Resultant complications include prolonged drainage and local wound infection.

- Seroma at the incision site which may require aspiration.
- Adjuvant therapy is often advised for malignancy in addition to the surgical procedure.
- Malignancy may recur at other sites in the urological tract or at distant sites.
- Anaesthetic risks, such as DVT, PE, chest infection, MI, and death, are rare.

Alternatives to surgery include radiotherapy, tumour blood vessel embolization alone, and immunotherapy. Many of these operations are performed via a laparoscopic approach, which reduces the risk of many of the associated complications.

Check cystoscopy

Cystoscopy involves the introduction of a fibro-optical instrument into the bladder via the urethra. It allows the inside of the bladder to be visualized. It is commonly performed to identify bladder neoplasms in patients who present with suspicious symptoms such as that of painless haematuria. The procedure is commonly performed using topical local anaesthesia.

Indication

Diagnostic: to inspect the bladder for suspected pathology and obtain histological samples by biopsy.

Post-operative complications

- Temporary dysuria and haematuria is common post-procedure.
- Gross haematuria may cause clot retention necessitating the insertion of a three-way catheter.
- Urinary tract infection may require antibiotic therapy.
- Biopsies may need to be taken during the cystoscopy if a lesion is identified.
- Bladder perforation rarely occurs but requires treatment with prolonged catheterization or progression to open surgical repair.
- Acute urinary retention.

Transurethral resection of bladder tumour (TURBT)

Most bladder tumours are transitional cell in origin. Fortunately almost 80% of bladder tumours are diagnosed as superficial tumours (with sparing of the bladder musculature). Such tumours are suitable for TURBT – the most conservative bladder tumour surgery. TURBT involves the introduction of a cystoscope into the bladder with resection of the tumour undertaken by thermal or laser ablation. This is frequently performed by EUA.

Indication

The procedure is diagnostic, allowing biopsies of suspicious lesions to be taken. It is also therapeutic as lesions may be treated at the same time by resection.

Post-operative complications

- Urinary tract or systemic infection may require antibiotics.
- Haematuria is common and may cause clot retention. In this instance a three-way catheter needs to be inserted.

- Bladder perforation may occur. This may warrant a prolonged urinary catheter, or in more severe cases, the need for open surgery.
- A temporary urinary catheter is inserted post-procedure. The catheter may also be used to introduce chemotherapy agents (such as mitomycin) into the bladder post-procedure to minimize the risk of recurrence.
- The tumour may be incompletely excised or recur.
- Instrumentation of the urethra may result in stricture formation.

Alternatives include chemotherapy, radiotherapy, or cystectomy.

Radical cystectomy and ileal conduit

Extensive bladder tumours that cross the muscular wall require more radical open surgery to completely remove the bladder and surrounding structures. An ileal conduit is created from an intestinal loop, anastomosed to the ureters and diverted to the abdominal skin where it forms a stoma. In the male radical cystectomy also involves the removal of the prostate and pelvic lymph nodes, whilst in females the ovaries, uterus, upper vagina, and pelvic lymph nodes are removed.

Indication

Diagnostic, by obtaining histology for staging, and also therapeutic in the removal of bulky malignant disease.

Post-operative complications

- A temporary naso-gastric tube may be used post-procedure, carrying a risk of aspiration pneumonia.
- An abdominal drain(s) is also placed. Resultant complications include prolonged drainage and local infection.
- Infection at the incision site may require antibiotic therapy or drainage.
- Seroma at the incision site may require aspiration.
- An incisional hernia may develop.
- Post-operative bleeding may occur requiring transfusion or additional operative procedures.
- Short bowel syndrome may occur leading to diarrhoea and nutritional deficiencies that require treatment.
- Anastomotic dehiscence of bowel may lead to peritonitis and death.
- Stomal problems such as stricturing, herniation, or retraction may occur necessitating a further procedure.
- Rectal perforation may occur during the procedure, needing a temporary colostomy.
- Urinary anastomotic leakage requires a further operative procedure.
- Strictures of the ureter may develop.
- Renal function may decline with time contributing to renal failure.
- In males there is a significant risk of impotence and anorgasmia leading to infertility.
- In females sexual intercourse may become painful due to a shortened vagina.
- Adjuvant therapy is often advised for malignancy in addition to the surgical procedure.
- Malignancy may recur at other sites in urological tract or at distant sites.

- Damage to surrounding structures (such as liver, spleen, bowel, and diaphragm) may occur, mandating additional surgical intervention.
- Anaesthetic risks (such as DVT, PE, chest infection, MI, and death). Admission for intensive or high dependency care is often required.

Alternatives include cystectomy with the creation of a neobladder or radiation therapy.

Radical cystectomy and neobladder

An alternative to ileal conduit formation post-radical cystectomy is the creation of a neobladder. This technically challenging operation creates a new bladder formed out of bowel that is anastomosed to the ureters and urethra, without the need for stoma formation.

The indications and complications of surgery are as for radical cystectomy and ileal conduit formation. In addition patients may need to regularly self-catheterize as the neobladder (which is denervated of all neurological control) empties poorly, leading to hydronephrosis and renal failure.

Alternatives are radical cystectomy with ileal conduit formation or radiotherapy.

Radical prostatectomy (perineal and retropubic)

Prostatic cancer accounts for around 7% of all male cancers. Radical prostatectomy removes the diseased gland and can be performed in one of two ways. Perineal prostatectomy involves excision of the prostate via an incision underneath the scrotum whilst a retropubic approach involves a lower abdominal incision. Both procedures also remove the seminal vesicles with tying off of the vasa deferentia.

Indication

Therapeutic in removing the diseased prostate gland.

Post-operative complications

- Incontinence can follow the procedure, which may require treatment with pelvic floor exercise, catheter insertion, or incontinence pads.
- There is a significant risk of impotence and anorgasmia leading to infertility.
- Rectal perforation may occur during the procedure resulting in colostomy (less than 5%).
- Post-operative bleeding may occur requiring transfusion or additional operative procedures.
- Infection at the operative site may require antibiotic therapy or drainage of pus.
- A temporary urinary catheter is inserted post-procedure, which increases the risk of urinary tract infection.
- An abdominal drain is also placed and resultant complications include prolonged drainage and surgical site infection.
- Seroma at the incision site may require aspiration.
- An incisional hernia may develop.
- Rarely a faeco-urinary fistula develops, requiring further operation.
- Adjuvant therapy is often utilized in addition to the surgical procedure.

- Anaesthetic risks (such as DVT, PE, chest infection, MI, and death). Intensive care admission is often required.

Alternatives include brachytherapy, radiotherapy, and hormonal therapy, which also have specific complications.

Trans-rectal ultrasound prostatic biopsy (TRUS)

TRUS is used to biopsy a prostatic lesion that is suspicious of malignancy. Such suspicion may be alerted on digital rectal examination, an elevated PSA, or a rapidly increasing PSA. A trans-rectal ultrasound probe is introduced. Under ultrasonic guidance needle biopsies of the prostate are obtained across the rectal wall.

Indications

Diagnostic in order to obtain prostatic biopsies to determine if malignancy is present or not.

Post-operative complications

- Temporary haematuria is common.
- Urinary tract infection is anticipated and prophylactic antibiotics should always be given to prevent infection. Patients with post-operative pyrexia should be admitted to hospital as sepsis can occur in up to 1%.
- Haematospermia also occurs and is temporary.
- Rectal bleeding is common. Where bleeding is significant the patient should be admitted to hospital. Transfusion and additional procedures may be necessary.
- Patients may go into acute urinary retention mandating catheterization.

Complete and partial amputation of the penis

Carcinoma of the penis is rare and is usually of squamous cell origin. Partial or complete penile amputation aims to prevent disease progression.

Indication

Therapeutic in removal of the diseased section of penis.

Post-operative complications

- A temporary urinary catheter is inserted post-procedure, which increases the risk of urinary tract infection.
- Surgical site infection is common and may need antibiotic therapy.
- Bleeding may require transfusion or further surgery.
- Penile shortening occurs.
- There may be difficulty in directing the stream of urine. Many men have to sit down to urinate post-operatively.
- The neo-meatus is prone to stricturing, which may require further intervention.
- Erectile dysfunction can occur as a result of penile nerve damage and significant psychological distress.
- A partial procedure may need to be converted to a complete amputation if the resection margins are histologically not clear.
- The malignancy may recur.
- Adjuvant therapy is often necessary.
- Urethral strictures can occur.

- If lymph nodes are involved and these are resected, additional complications include lymphoedema and infection.

Alternatives include topical therapies and radiotherapy.

Radical orchidectomy

Testicular tumours predominantly affect young men and are classified as teratomas or seminomas. Orchidectomy is removal of the affected testicle using a groin incision.

Indication

Therapeutic in removing the diseased testicle.

Post-operative complications

- Reduction in fertility. Many men choose to undertake pre-operative sperm storage if they feel that they have not yet completed their families.
- Infection of the operative site.
- Bleeding.
- Adjuvant therapy is often needed.
- If a silicone testicular implant is used there is an associated risk of infection and cosmetic dissatisfaction. The prosthesis tends to ride high in the scrotum, may feel different to its neighbour, and have a palpable suture at one end.

Benign prostatic disease

Benign prostatic hypertrophy (BPH) is a common condition whereby the cells of the prostate enlarge with age. This results in varying degrees of obstructive uropathy, giving rise to the symptoms of prostatism. It is common, with approximately 80% of men over the age of 80 years affected to some degree. The commonest operation performed for BPH is transurethral resection of the prostate (TURP).

Transurethral resection of the prostate (TURP)

TURP is a very common procedure, performed mostly for benign prostatic hypertrophy, seen frequently in men over the age of 60 years. It can also be used in the resection of prostatic malignancy. The aim of surgery is to remove the obstructing portions of the prostate gland to restore urinary flow. The procedure is performed using a cystoscope with thermal or laser ablation of the prostate. Given the large number of procedures carried out per year it is important to have a grasp of the complications of the operation and their incidence.

Indication

Therapeutic to alleviate urinary obstruction and lower urinary tract symptoms.

Post-operative complications

- Detrusor over-activity is common post-procedure resulting in residual symptoms (30%).
- Impotence commonly occurs (10–20%).
- Re-obstruction occurs in 10% of men within 10 years requiring a repeat procedure.
- Instrumentation of the urinary tract may lead to stricture formation (10%).
- Surgery may not cure all the symptoms of prostatism. Some patients fail to void post-surgery requiring intermittent self-catheterization or a permanent indwelling catheter.
- Urinary tract infection is common (2–5%).
- Significant bleeding may lead to clot retention and necessitate the insertion of a three-way catheter with irrigation. Transfusion may also be necessary (2–5%).
- TURP syndrome results from over-absorption of irrigation fluid leading to hyponatraemia and cardiac overloading (2%).
- Incontinence can follow the procedure, which also warrants the insertion of a catheter or the use of incontinence pads (1%).
- Dysuria and haematuria temporarily follow the operation.
- Anorgasmia can lead to fertility problems.
- Bladder perforation is rare but requires treatment with a prolonged urinary catheter or open surgical correction.

Alternatives to TURP are green light laser prostatic resection, prostatic stents, use of catheters (long-term indwelling or intermittent self-catheterization), and the use of drugs such as alpha blockers and 5-alpha reductase inhibitors.

Stone disease

Around 2% of the UK population has a stone affecting the urinary tract. Most stones are derived from calcium oxalate, calcium phosphate, or magnesium ammonium phosphate. The consequences of stones can range from renal colic to pyelonephritis and renal failure. Different procedures exist depending upon the site and size of the stones. Common procedures undertaken in litho-urology include:
- open nephrolithotomy
- open ureterolithotomy
- percutaneous nephrolithotomy (PCNL)
- ureteroscopic stone removal
- cystolithopaxy
- extracorporeal shockwave lithotripsy (ESWL).

Open nephrolithotomy and ureterolithotomy

Open nephrolithotomy involves the retrieval of a renal stone from within the kidney itself. Pyelolithotomy and ureterolithotomy refer to removal of stones from the renal calyceal system and ureter respectively. These open techniques are usually reserved for very large or complex stones that cause ongoing symptoms such as infection or pain. The procedures involve a 10–15cm flank incision to allow stone retrieval.

Indication
Therapeutic in removing the obstructing calculus.

Post-operative complications
- The abdominal incision is prone to infection and herniation.
- A temporary urinary catheter is inserted post-procedure, which increases the risk of urinary tract infection.
- Significant renal haemorrhage may require transfusion, embolization, or nephrectomy.
- An abdominal drain is frequently inserted. Prolonged drainage and surgical site infections are potential complications.
- Temporary ureteric stenting or a nephrostomy tube may become necessary as part of the procedure with associated risks and need for removal at a later date.
- A urinary fistula may develop from the renal tract to the open abdominal wound necessitating additional procedures.
- Strictures of the urinary tract may develop.
- Damage to surrounding structures (such as liver, spleen, bowel, and diaphragm) may occur, mandating additional surgical intervention.
- The procedure may fail to remove the stone.
- Stones can re-accumulate.
- Anaesthetic risks (such as DVT, PE, chest infection, MI, and death).

Alternatives include ureteroscopic removal and ESWL.

Percutaneous nephrolithotomy (PCNL)

With improvements in technology open procedures are becoming increasingly rare. PCNL is a good alternative to open procedures, which carry a relatively higher risk of post-operative complications. The recovery time following PCNL is also much quicker. The procedure involves a small posterior incision to allow a nephrostomy tube to be introduced into the kidney. With the nephrostomy in place an ultrasonic lithoclast or laser with copious irrigation can be introduced into the urinary tract to fragment stones.

Indication

Therapeutic in alleviation of the stone burden.

Post-operative complications

- Infection of the urinary tract (including pyelonephritis) and wound site occurs in 10% of patients, which may progress to systemic sepsis. Antibiotics may be needed.
- A temporary urinary catheter is inserted post-procedure, which increases the risk of urinary tract infection.
- Significant bleeding occurs in 10% of patients requiring transfusion, embolization, or nephrectomy. However, haematuria almost always occurs temporarily post-operatively.
- Failure to gain access to the urinary tract via the nephrostomy occurs in 10% of patients. Multiple puncture sites are sometimes necessary or occasionally an open procedure must be resorted to.
- Damage to surrounding structures occurs in 5% (such as liver, spleen, bowel, and diaphragm) needing additional surgical intervention.
- In less than 1% of patients, the kidney may be severely damaged by attempted nephrostomy insertion. Should this happen, nephrectomy might be necessary.
- The procedure may fail to remove the stone and sometimes a ureteric stent is inserted to bypass the obstructing stone.
- Stones may recur.
- A transient pyrexia is common post-PCNL.
- Over-absorption of irrigating fluid can cause hyponatraemia and cardiac overloading.

Alternatives are open procedures, ureteroscopy, and ESWL.

Ureteroscopic stone removal

This procedure is useful for stones confined to the ureter. Ureteroscopy involves instrumentation of the ureter by introducing a ureteroscope externally via the urethra and bladder. Under direct vision using the ureteroscope, stone extraction may be undertaken by a lithoclast or basket retrieval. The placement of a ureteric stent is common during this procedure, facilitating the passage of stone fragments generated by the lithoclast.

Indications

Therapeutic in the removal of ureteric stones.

Post-operative complications
- Infection of the urinary tract (including pyelonephritis) occurs in 10% of patients, which may progress to systemic sepsis. Antibiotics may be needed.
- A temporary urinary catheter is inserted post-procedure, which increases the risk of urinary tract infection.
- Significant bleeding occurs in 10% of cases, requiring transfusion, embolization, or nephrectomy. However, haematuria almost always occurs temporarily post-procedure.
- There is a 1% risk of ureteric injury: perforation, stricture, or avulsion.
- If a ureteric stent is inserted an additional procedure is required to remove it at a later date. Stents tend to cause post-operative dysuria.
- The procedure may fail, especially if the ureter is too narrow to allow instrumentation.
- Instrumentation may push the stone backwards into the kidney, rendering it irretrievable. This requires alternative procedures to remove the stone.
- Ureteric colic may occur on stone fragmentation resulting in prolonged hospitalization.
- Stones may recur.

Alternatives are open procedures, PCNL, and ESWL.

Cystolithopaxy

Cystolithopaxy is the telescopic removal of bladder stones. A cystoscope is introduced externally via the urethra into the bladder. Stone extraction is undertaken with a lithoclast or laser.

Indication
Therapeutic in removal of bladder stones.

Post-operative complications
- A temporary urinary catheter is inserted post-procedure, which increases the risk of urinary tract infection.
- Temporary dysuria and haematuria are common.
- More significant bleeding may result in clot retention and may require the introduction of a three-way catheter with irrigation.
- Stone fragments may persist.
- Stones may recur.
- 'Stones' seen on imaging of the renal tract may actually turn out to be neoplasms on cystoscopy. A biopsy might become necessary as part of the procedure.
- Urethral strictures can occur as a result of instrumentation.
- Rarely, bladder perforation occurs, which requires a temporary urinary catheter to allow healing, or in more severe cases progression to an open surgical repair.

Alternatives are to observe or proceed to open surgery.

Extracorporeal shockwave lithotripsy (ESWL)

ESWL is a non-invasive procedure that uses a lithotripter to generate ultrasonic shockwaves that fragment renal stones into smaller fragments allowing spontaneous passage. ESWL works best for larger stones between 4mm and 2cm that are situated in the upper urinary tract.

Indication

Therapeutic in fragmenting upper renal tract stones, thereby allowing spontaneous passage.

Post-operative complications

- Renal and ureteric colic are common complications as stone fragments descend into the urinary tract. This may result in prolonged hospital admission. On occasion fragmented stones may cause obstruction lower down the urinary tract.
- Haematuria for a short period post-procedure is also common.
- Stone fragmentation leads to the release of bacteria. This predisposes to local urinary and systemic sepsis. This may require oral or intravenous antibiotics. Percutaneous nephrostomy and drainage is occasionally required in overwhelming renal infection.
- Failure of fragmentation or large stone fragments that fail to pass may require repeat ESWL treatments or alternative procedures such as ureteroscopy.
- For stones in the range of 1–2cm in diameter, prior stent insertion under ureteroscopy may first be desirable to aid fragment passage.
- Stone recurrence.

Alternatives to ESWL are those outlined previously: open or endoscopic surgery or simple observation.

Andrology

Andrology is the study of the male reproductive and genito-urinary system. The urologist is frequently involved in procedures in this anatomical region, be it for cosmesis, family planning, or to improve functional impairment. The common procedures undertaken are:
- penile straightening (Nesbitt's procedure)
- vasectomy and its reversal
- varicocele repair
- epididymal cyst removal
- cystoscopy and urethral dilatation
- cystoscopy and optical internal urethrotomy
- catheterization (urethral and supra-pubic).

Penile straightening

Curvature of the penis, or Peyronie's disease, is a condition that affects approximately 0.5% of men. The underlying aetiology is the development of fibrosis within the tunica albuginea of the penis. Curvature is most prominent on erection, which is often painful and makes intercourse difficult. Nesbitt's procedure aims to correct the curvature by incising the penis. The development of additional scar tissue post-operatively helps to correct the original deformity.

Indication

Cosmetic and functional in correction of penile curvature.

Post-operative complications

- Cosmetic dissatisfaction with degree of correction.
- Recurrence of curvature.
- Penile shortening always follows this procedure.
- Wound infection and incisional skin separation may occur. It is important to try and avoid erections and intercourse until the wound is fully healed.
- Bruising and swelling of the penis and scrotum is common post-procedure.
- Damage to penile nerves during the procedure may lead to impotence and occurs in around 15–20% of patients.
- Damage to penile nerves may also result in temporary or permanent parasthesiae of the penis.

Given the risk of impotence, the Nesbitt's procedure is usually reserved for men who are experiencing severe difficulty with sexual intercourse. There are different surgical approaches available such as a penile suture technique and excision of fibrotic tissue with graft replacement. ESWL and drugs such as tamoxifen have also been used to some (but limited) effect.

Vasectomy

Vasectomy is performed for male sterilization. It involves small incisions bilaterally in the scrotum. Each vas deferens is located and divided. The ligated ends are sutured preventing spermatozoa entering the ejaculate. It is a permanent method of birth control and should be considered to be irreversible.

Indication

For males who have completed their families and who wish to be sterile.

Post-operative complications

- Two separate semen samples (both of which must be negative for spermatozoa) are required before unprotected intercourse should commence. This may take up to 12 ejaculations to occur. Alternative contraceptive measures should be utilized in the interim.
- A testicular lump or sperm granuloma occurs in 10% of men.
- Chronic testicular pain may develop in up to 5% of men.
- Infection of the urinary tract, orchitis, and epididymitis may occur, necessitating antibiotic therapy (2.5%).
- Scrotal bruising is common post-procedure. More significant bleeding occurs in 2.5% of patients and may require an additional procedure to achieve haemostasis.
- Short-term failure (surgical failure) occurs in 1%.
- Long-term failure (caused by recannulization of the vas deferens) occurs in 1 in 800.

Many other forms of contraception are available as an alternative to vasectomy. Vasectomy should be considered as an irreversible procedure. Although the vas deferens can be surgically re-anastomosed, stricture formation may result, impeding fertility and preventing pregnancy.

Varicocele repair

Varicosities of the testis can be an uncomfortable condition associated with sub-fertility. Incompetent testicular veins lead to dilated, tortuous vessels within the scrotum, collectively known as a varicocele. They are usually left sided and may be associated with renal pathology. Varicocele repair is usually performed laparoscopically. A small incision is made in the abdomen. Abnormal vessels are ligated or clipped.

Indication

Therapeutic in alleviating the discomfort that varicoceles cause, and may improve male fertility.

Post-operative complications

- Shoulder tip pain is common following the procedure and is short lived.
- Wound infection and sepsis may occur.
- The procedure may fail to rectify the varicosities.
- Significant bleeding from damaged blood vessels may need transfusion or conversion to open surgery.
- Testicular atrophy may occur should the blood supply to the testicle be compromised. This may lead to reduced fertility.
- Damage to surrounding structures (such as liver, spleen, diaphragm, bowel, and blood vessels) may need open surgery.

Epididymal cyst removal

Epididymal cysts are very common benign lesions that increase in prevalence with age. They are sometimes mistaken for testicular malignancies. The collecting tubes of the epididymis dilate causing the resultant swelling, which can cause testicular discomfort. The procedure to correct the cyst involves a small incision over the epididymis and removal of the dilated sac.

Indication
Therapeutic in removal of the cyst.

Post-operative complications
- Scrotal bruising is common.
- Haematocele requiring surgical intervention.
- Orchitis and epididymitis requiring antibiotic therapy.
- Recurrence of the epididymal cyst (may be ipsilateral or contralateral).
- Epididymal scarring can result in sub-optimal fertility.

As there is a small risk of impaired fertility, operative intervention is best avoided until a man has completed his family. Simple observation or needle aspiration are alternatives.

Cystoscopy and urethral dilatation/optical urethrotomy

These procedures are performed to alleviate urethral strictures that cause bladder outflow obstruction. They may be benign or malignant in aetiology. Both techniques involve the use of a cystoscope to allow internal inspection of the urethra and bladder. With urethral dilatation, balloon devices are utilized to increase the luminal diameter. With optical urethrotomy a telescopic knife or laser is used to resect the stricture. During the procedure biopsies may be taken.

Indication
Therapeutic in alleviating the stricture and its resultant urinary tract obstruction.

Post-operative complications
- A temporary urinary catheter is inserted post-procedure, which increases the risk of urinary tract infection.
- Temporary dysuria and haematuria are common.
- Post-procedure patients are required to intermittently self-catheterize to prevent secondary stricture formation.
- Stricture recurrence may follow any instrumentation of the urinary tract.
- Rarely impotence can occur post-surgery.

Observation is an alternative. Insertion of a permanent catheter may also be used; urethral or supra-pubic.

The same procedure can be carried out in females with a similar spectrum of complications.

A word on urinary catheterization

Urinary catheterization is one of the commonest procedures undertaken in urology. It is considered in this section because of the large number of male patients who require catheterization predominantly as a result of urinary retention secondary to prostatic pathology.

Urethral catheters

A urethral catheter is passed externally via the urethra into the bladder. There are numerous types and sizes. Although a simple procedure to carry out, it can have serious complications if poorly performed.

Indication

The indications for catheterization are numerous and include retention, incontinence management, and monitoring fluid balance in the critically ill patient.

Post-procedural complications

- Dysuria is common post-procedure and may respond to topical local anaesthetic.
- Urinary tract infection is common and is related to the duration of catheterization.
- Paraphimosis may occur in men if the foreskin is not retracted following the procedure. This causes great discomfort to the patient and although it can usually be rectified on the ward, it may require operative intervention.
- Failure to catheterize. This may be a result of urethral strictures, prostatic obstruction, or a tight bladder neck. Asking the patient to cough or 'bear down' is useful in overcoming prostatic and bladder neck resistance. If catheterization is difficult, a useful technique is to use a more rigid intermittent self-catheter, which may allow the bladder to be reached and facilitate catheterization with a standard urinary catheter. However, multiple attempts at catheterization must be avoided and should be left to more experienced individuals.
- Urethral strictures may occur secondary to multiple, over-zealous attempts at catheterization.

Supra-pubic catheters

A supra-pubic catheter is a percutaneous catheter that traverses the abdominal wall to enter the bladder. It should only be performed by trained medical staff to minimize extra-vesicular organ damage.

Indication

Supra-pubic catheters are often used in patients in whom urethral catheterization has failed or in patients who require long-term catheterization.

Post-procedural complications

- Dysuria and haematuria may occur post-procedure.
- Urinary tract infection is common and may require antibiotic therapy.
- Bladder irritation from the catheter can cause pain.
- The catheter may frequently block, requiring flushing or replacement.
- Long-term supra-pubic catheters need to be changed every 12 weeks – this is a simple procedure that can be carried out by a district nurse.

• There is a risk of damage to surrounding structures in less than 1% of patients (most notably bowel, which results in faecal peritonitis). The risk of injury is increased when supra-pubic catheterization is attempted 'blind' and it is for this reason that it is preferable to insert the catheter during cystoscopy.

Problems with catheter management

The main problems encountered with catheter management are blockage, failure to catheterize, and an inability to remove the catheter.

Catheter blockage

Catheter blockage is caused either by debris from the bladder or more commonly from clots in the patient with haematuria. The 'eye' of the catheter is very small and is hence easily blocked. The patient will fail to pass urine and will complain of increasing supra-pubic pain.

If the blockage is thought to be due to debris or a small clot then a catheter flush may be undertaken with strict aseptic precautions. This is performed by disconnecting the urinary catheter from the leg bag. A 50ml syringe is taken and normal saline flushed quickly via the port into the bladder. Rapid fluid injection aims to dislodge the obstruction. By aspirating back, the offending debris or small clot is often retrieved into the syringe. The catheter is then reconnected to the leg bag.

If the patient is experiencing gross haematuria there is little to be gained in flushing a standard catheter. It will quickly re-obstruct with the accumulation of further clots. In this instance a three-way catheter is required. The three-way catheter has three ports: one to inflate the catheter's balloon, one to allow free drainage of urine from the bladder, and one to allow rapid infusion of fluids into the bladder. Via this third port large volumes of normal saline are instilled into the bladder. This dilutes any haematuria and prevents clot formation and hence catheter obstruction. The patient remains comfortable as the instilled fluid and urine passes out quickly into the leg bag via the large diameter exit port.

Failure to catheterize

Failure to catheterize is a common occurrence and amongst others can be due to phimosis, tight urethral strictures, and prostatic obstruction.

If difficulty is being experienced, call for assistance — two pairs of hands makes things much easier. If resistance is felt after a significant proportion of the catheter has been introduced, a tight urethral sphincter or prostatic obstruction may be the cause. Asking the patient to 'bear down' or cough at this point often allows progress to be made. Using additional lubricating local anaesthetic is another useful technique. If difficulty is still arising, the insertion of an intermittent self-catheter (ISC) may be helpful. ISCs are more rigid catheters used by patients for self-catheterization. The extra rigidity that they offer may allow successful catheterization. The ISC may then be removed and immediately followed with the introduction of a regular catheter, which is usually successful.

However, multiple traumatic attempts at catheterization must be avoided. Seek speciality help early — a supra-pubic catheter may be indicated.

Inability to remove the catheter

Inability to remove a catheter can be an embarrassing experience for the healthcare professional and a worry for the patient. The cause is usually failure of the intra-vesicular balloon holding the catheter in place to deflate, and is easily rectified. One method used is to over-inflate the balloon with saline. The balloon eventually bursts, allowing removal of the catheter. The amount of fluid to be insufflated is surprisingly high to cause balloon rupture and the energy of the burst may cause local damage to the bladder lining. Retained portions of the balloon within the bladder may cause urinary tract infection or bladder outlet obstruction. For this reason this method should be avoided. Preferably the input tubing should be cut above the one-way valve. This allows the balloon to deflate quickly and facilitate removal.

Female and reconstructive surgery

The urologist generally undertakes procedures on the female genito-urinary system as a result of continence issues. Surgical intervention outside of this domain falls to the realm of the gynaecologist. The common procedures undertaken are:

- colposuspension
- sling procedure for urinary stress incontinence
- cystoscopy and injection of peri-urethral bulking agents.

Colposuspension and sling procedure

Both of these procedures are used for urinary incontinence, which is common in ageing multiparous females. With colposuspension a lower abdominal incision is made. Through this incision the bladder neck is elevated with the placement of strategic sutures to improve continence. With the sling repair a vaginal incision is used to place surgical tape in a sling-like fashion to support the proximal urethra.

Indication

Therapeutic in attempting to alleviate urinary incontinence.

Post-operative complications

- 30% of patients suffer from detrusor over-activity and symptoms of frequency, which may require medical therapy.
- Around 10% of patients will be over-corrected leading to acute urinary retention, which necessitates a long-term or intermittent self-catheter.
- In 2% of patients sling erosion occurs, leading to recurrence of incontinence.
- A temporary urinary catheter is inserted post-procedure, which increases the risk of urinary tract infection.
- An abdominal drain is also placed. Resultant complications may include prolonged drainage and local infection.
- Infection at the incision site, which may require antibiotic therapy.
- Seroma at the incision site (colposuspension), which may require aspiration.
- An incisional hernia (with colposuspension) may develop.
- Rectoceles may develop.
- Post-operative bleeding may occur, requiring transfusion or additional operative procedures.
- Failure to improve continence.
- Pain on sexual intercourse.
- Reaction to the sling can cause adhesion formation.
- Rarely bladder perforation occurs, which requires a temporary urinary catheter to allow healing, or in more severe cases progression to an open surgical repair.

Alternatives are catheterization, incontinence pads, and peri-urethral bulking agents.

Peri-urethral bulking agents

To improve continence the injection of bulking material around the urethral outlet aids sphincter function. Injection takes place during cystoscopy.

Indication

Therapeutic in improving urethral bulk and thereby reducing incontinence.

Post-operative complications

- Temporary dysuria and haematuria are common.
- Urinary tract infection requiring antibiotic therapy.
- Failure to improve symptoms or recurrence of incontinence.
- Over-correction leading to urinary retention.

Alternatives include colposuspension, slings, catheters, and incontinence pads.

Paediatrics

Common procedures in paediatric urology include:
- circumcision
- scrotal exploration for suspected testicular torsion
- hydrocele repair
- orchidopexy
- hypospadias repair
- posterior urethral valve resection.

Circumcision

Circumcision (removal of the foreskin) is one of the earliest recorded elective surgical procedures.

Indication

The indications for circumcision are few, but include: phimosis, recurrent balanoposthitis, and recurrent urinary tract infections. Many surgeons worldwide continue to operate for religious purposes.

Post-operative complications

- Psychological distress to the patient.
- Cosmetic dissatisfaction.
- Surgical site infection, which may need antibiotics, occurs in 2%.
- Prolonged bleeding necessitating a further procedure occurs in 2%.
- Acute urinary retention occurs in 1%.
- Suture retention (despite absorbable suture use) necessitating removal in clinic.

Circumcision is not a trivial procedure. The alternative is to treat infective aetiologies with broad spectrum antibiotics.

Scrotal exploration for suspected testicular torsion

Testicular torsion is one of the emergency conditions seen in urology. Although torsion can occur at any age, the peak incidence is in early adolescence. Suspicion of torsion requires urgent surgical exploration as testicular viability diminishes after 6–12 hours of impeded blood flow. A scar in the testicle is better than an empty hemiscrotum.

Indication

Should there be any suspicion of testicular torsion, a diagnostic testicular exploration is required. If the operation demonstrates torsion, then therapeutic correction may be undertaken simultaneously.

Post-operative complications

- Bilateral fixation of both testicles may be necessary if torsion is identified.
- Testicular atrophy may still ensue despite operation, resulting in potential fertility issues.
- Need for unilateral orchidectomy if testicular necrosis has commenced.
- Bleeding post-procedure may result in a haematocele necessitating drainage or a further surgical procedure.

- Wound and testicular infection may occur, warranting antibiotic therapy.

Doppler ultrasound to assess testicular vascularity is an alternative to immediate surgery but such delay jeopardizes potential testicular viability.

Hydrocele repair

The underlying defect is a patent processus vaginalis. This allows the tracking of peritoneal fluid into the testicle forming a hydrocele. If the processus vaginalis is sufficiently large a scrotal inguinal hernia may also develop. Hydrocele repair involves ligation of the processus vaginalis through a groin incision.

Indication

Therapeutic correction of the hydrocele.

Post-operative complications

- A coincidental inguinal hernia may also be present, necessitating repair at the same time (and needs pre-operative recognition).
- Haematocele formation requiring surgical drainage.
- Surgical site or testicular infection warranting antibiotic therapy.
- Re-accumulation of the hydrocele requiring additional procedures.

Observation is a valid alternative to surgical intervention. Most hydroceles spontaneously resolve with obliteration of the processus vaginalis. However, persistence of fluid past 18 months of age usually requires operation. Needle aspiration is also an alternative.

Orchidopexy

At birth approximately 5% of all full-term male babies have either a unilateral or bilateral undescended testis. However, testicular descent continues for the first 3 months leaving only a small proportion of male babies with problems thereafter. Operative intervention aims to preserve future fertility and reduce the risk of malignancy with cosmetic improvement. An inguinal incision is used to mobilize the undescended testicle and place it into the scrotum, whilst taking care to preserve the vas deferens and testicular vessels. Orchidopexy is usually carried out by the age of 2 years.

Indication

To move the undescended testicle into the scrotum to preserve future fertility and reduce the risk of malignancy.

Post-operative complications

- Testicular atrophy as a result of testicular vessel damage is seen in 5% of patients. This may actually compromise future fertility.
- Surgical site and testicular infection warranting antibiotic therapy occurs in 2%.
- Significant bleeding and haematocele formation necessitating surgical drainage or an additional procedure again occurs in 2% of patients.
- The testicles may re-ascend (failed procedure), which happens in less than 1% of cases.

- Cosmetic dissatisfaction: some patients are left with a 'high riding' testicle within the scrotal sac.
- There is no guarantee that this procedure will prevent infertility or malignancy.

Observation of the undescended testicle is the only other approach, but the risks of infertility and malignancy increase rapidly the longer the testicle remains outside of the scrotal sac.

Hypospadias repair

Hypospadias is a congenital condition affecting approximately 1 in 300 males. The underlying aetiology is a failure of urethral tubularization. The triad of symptoms consists of a ventral urethral meatus, chordee, and a dorsal hooded foreskin. Correction is undertaken by the age of 2 years and aims to create a terminal urethral meatus and a straight erection. As part of the procedure the foreskin is often utilized to reconstruct the shortened urethra.

Indication
Therapeutic in correction of the congenital defect.

Post-operative complications
- Psychological distress to the patient.
- Cosmetic dissatisfaction: the penis appears as if it has been circumcised and may not straighten adequately (persistent chordee).
- A urethral fistula may develop in 10–15% of patients, mandating further procedures.
- Urethral stricture and meatal stenosis may occur in later life, necessitating repair.
- The urethral graft may leak urine or develop into a urethrocele, mandating further procedures.
- Wound and urinary tract infection warranting antibiotic therapy.
- A urinary catheter is inserted post-operatively to aid urethral graft take. This is associated with a risk of urinary tract infection.
- Bruising is common. Prolonged bleeding may require surgical intervention.

The alternative is to leave the hypospadias uncorrected. This often causes great distress to the patient, particularly as they approach adulthood.

Posterior urethral valve resection

Posterior urethral valves are a rare condition affecting male infants with an incidence of 0.5 per 10 000 births. The abnormal urethral valve, thought to be a remnant of the cloacal membrane, causes bladder outlet obstruction with resulting bilateral hydronephrosis. The condition is usually detected on antenatal ultrasound scanning. The urethral valve is thermally ablated under cystoscopic vision.

Indication
Therapeutic in removing the posterior urethral valves that cause hydronephrosis and resulting renal damage.

Post-operative complications
- Renal insufficiency may develop in up to 30% of all treated survivors in later life.
- Paternity may also be impaired in 30% of patients in later life.
- Failure of procedure mandating further attempts.
- Urinary catheter insertion to promote healing increases the risk of urinary tract infection.
- Temporary dysuria and haematuria.
- Urethral stricture development in later life.

An alternative to an endoscopic procedure is to carry out an open procedure or one can simply observe the patient.

Pelviureteric and vesicoureteric junctional obstruction are similar conditions found predominantly in female infants. Corrective procedures are similar and carry corresponding risks.

The impact of other surgical procedures on urology

The work of many other surgical specialties can involve urologists. The main complications that urologists see as a result of other surgical procedures are:
• ureteric injury following gynaecological surgery
• acute urinary retention following abdominal and pelvic surgery.

Ureteric injury following gynaecological surgery

Ureteric injury is one of the most serious complications following gynaecological surgery. The close anatomical relationship between the ureter and the female reproductive organs results in ureteric injury in approximately 1% of all gynaecological surgical cases.

The common aetiologies of ureteric injury include: crush injuries from surgical clamp application, ligation as a result of suturing, complete and partial transection, and ischaemia as a result of electocautery. The consequences of ureteric injury are varied depending on the underlying aetiology. Minor injuries may spontaneously resolve. A tight ligature causes hydronephrosis and renal impairment. Stricture formation may also be seen. With ureteral necrosis or transection, urinary extravasation occurs resulting in urinomas and urinary ascites.

Over 70% of ureteric injuries are detected during the post-operative period, when classically patients complain of flank pain, with pyrexia and a prolonged ileus. On suspicion of such injury renal tract imaging is required. Intra-venous and CT urograms are sensitive modalities for detecting ureteric injuries, whereas ultrasound scanning clearly shows the complications such as hydronephrosis.

Operative treatment is usually necessary and depends on the aetiology. Clamped or ligated ureters simply require release of the constricting article. Partial transections respond well to ureteric stenting, which allows for ureteric moulding and prevents stricture formation. More serious transections and necrosis may require ureteral resection and anastomosis. Other procedures include ureteroureterostomy and transureteroureterostomy.

Acute urinary retention following non-urological surgery

Acute urinary retention is a common post-operative complication. It may occur following any surgical procedure but is particularly common following surgery to the abdomen and pelvis. The incidence of urinary retention following colorectal surgery is quoted as being as high as 15%.

There are several mechanisms thought to be responsible for post-operative retention. Post-operative pain is thought to be a major factor. Pain prevents the patient from activating musculature to increase intra-abdominal pressure to aid micturition. This, coupled with aggressive fluid resuscitation post-procedure, seems to account for most cases of retention. The innervation of bladder function is complex consisting of both sympathetic and parasympathetic fibres. It is the parasympathetic fibres that are responsible for activating detrusor contraction. Handling of such fibres during surgery temporarily diminishes parasympathetic innervation and may also contribute to urinary retention.

Treatment of post-operative retention is aimed at appropriate analgesia, sensible fluid administration, and the use of urinary catheters on a temporary basis until the patient is able to void.

Complications of ENT and head and neck surgery

Introduction

When dealing with any specific complication of ENT surgery, consideration needs to be given to the safety of the airway and integrity of the neurovascular system. An appropriately experienced anaesthetist and an adequately equipped operating theatre are essential.

For the purposes of this chapter, the definitions of complication timings are:

- Immediate: 0–6hrs.
- Early: 6–72hrs.
- Intermediate: >72hrs but <1 week.
- Late: >1 week.

Complications of ear surgery

Immediate complications

Myringotomy and ventilation tube (grommet) insertion

Complications are rare. The ear canal can be so narrow that even a small grommet cannot be inserted safely. Bleeding secondary to damaging a dehiscent internal carotid artery or internal jugular vein has also been described. In the event of such a problem, the ear should be packed immediately with bismuth iodoform paraffin paste (BIPP) gauze until bleeding has settled.

In the event that the grommet immediately falls into the middle ear cleft, consideration needs to be given to undertake a tympanotomy to retrieve it.

Myringoplasty/tympanoplasty/ossiculoplasty

Ossicular dislocation

Dislocation of the bones that form the ossicular chain can be corrected at the time of surgery or delayed to a later date.

Tearing of the tympanomeatal flap

Raising a flap in the meatal canal to access the middle ear occasionally causes trauma or perforation to the tissues from suction or drill trauma. Protect the flap by reflecting it out of harm's way.

Damage to the chorda tympani

This nerve is usually encountered when raising the tympanic membrane off the annulus. Damage or transection is noticed by the patient as a loss of taste sensation or a metallic taste localized to the ipsilateral side of the tongue. The nerve should be preserved if possible. However, taste disturbances generally settle within a short time if the nerve is sacrificed.

Mastoid surgery

Facial nerve palsy

This should be looked for immediately post-operatively and is normally the result of blunt nerve damage in a dehiscent facial nerve canal. However, if there is any chance that surgical disruption has occurred, then immediate re-exploration of the ear is mandatory. A physically disrupted nerve requires either primary re-anastomosis or cable grafting.

Local anaesthetic infiltration in the region of the facial nerve may cause a transient post-operative facial nerve palsy, particularly if the nerve is dehiscent in the middle ear. Assuming the surgeon is confident that there has been no trauma to the nerve, then re-exploration is not necessary. If the palsy is profound and longer lasting, eye care is required to avert corneal ulceration.

Cerebro-spinal fluid (CSF) leak
(See Chapter 22, Neurosurgical complications, p.425.)

Confirm with B2 transferrin assay. Commence antibiotics, nurse the patient in a semi-upright position, and inform the operating surgeon. Medical options include diuretics (furosemide) and carbonic anhydrase inhibitors (acetazolemide). Surgical repair, required in about 15% of cases, is best undertaken via a trans-mastoid approach with a fascial graft and tissue glue used to close the defect.

Cochlear implant
As with a stapedectomy, a perilymph 'gusher' is sometimes encountered when the footplate is perforated. The defect should be closed immediately and no further procedure undertaken.

Early complications
Myringoplasty/tympanoplasty/ossiculoplasty
Sensory neural hearing loss (SNHL)
From direct or indirect damage to the adjacent cochlear or labyrinth.

Conductive loss
This is due to tympanic membrane or ossicular disruption. Comparison of Weber's and Rinne's tests before and after operation helps to determine whether iatrogenic loss has occurred and its nature. Pure tone audiometry should be performed routinely before surgery and after if indicated. Under exceptional circumstances, re-exploration should be considered.

Vertigo
Acute onset of vertigo may similarly result from vestibular damage, perilymph fistula, or an overly long ossicular prosthesis pushing on the oval window (displacement of prosthesis is sometimes a late complication). Exploration is required in the second two examples. An untreated perilymph fistula ends with a dead ear. Vestibular sedatives (e.g. prochlorperazine) may be required for a short time if vertigo is severe.

Skin hypersensitivity
Occurs after packing of the ear post-operatively with impregnated wick and is more often seen with BIPP dressings.

Cochlear implant
Routine post-operative radiological assessment of the position of the implant is necessary. Incorrect position necessitates relocation.

Intermediate complications

Meningitis

Rarely complicates cochlear implantation, and vaccination (pneumovax) should be administered pre-operatively to reduce the risk. Treat with high-dose antibiotics.

Late complications

Myringotomy and ventilation tube (grommet) insertion

Infection

Often causes early extrusion. Treat with aural toilet, topical antibiotics, and water avoidance.

Persistent perforation of the tympanic membrane

This may occur after ventilation tube extrusion. It is more common with larger diameter grommets and T-tubes. If the perforation persists for more than one year then grafting of the defect should be considered.

Myringoplasty/tympanoplasty/ossiculoplasty

Failure of tympanic membrane graft

Graft reconstruction of the eardrum fails in approximately 20% of cases. If infection is present, non-ototoxic topical antibiotics should be administered for at least 10–14 days and aural toilet performed.

Mastoidectomy and its variants

A recurrently discharging mastoid cavity requires aural toilet, and topical antibiotics. Surgical revision of the cavity may be indicated if there is an anatomical reason, e.g. high facial ridge or rough cavity walls. However, this should only be considered after failure of prolonged medical treatment.

Recurrent cholesteatoma occasionally occurs and may necessitate revision surgery.

Bone-anchored hearing aid (BAHA) implantation

Failure of osseointegration/excessive bone growth

Removal and revision is required if a sleeper fixture is not already in place.

Cochlear implant

Scalp flap failure

This is more likely in those with KID syndrome (keratitis-ichthyosis-deafness) due to systemic skin factors.

Device failure

This is fortunately a rare problem as technology improves. Refer to implantation team if suspected.

Complications of nasal surgery

Nasal surgery involving the anterior ethmoid sinuses and the adjacent nasal cavity is relatively safe. Minor intra-operative bleeding is frequent. Post-operative packing for 4–12 hours is usually all that is required if it occurs. Posterior ethmoid and skull-base surgery are associated with more significant complications.

Immediate complications

Septoplasty/septorhinoplasty

Haemorrhage

Consider re-packing the nose with an additional post-nasal space pack. ITU transfer is rarely necessary in a haemodynamically stable patient.

CSF leak

(📖 See Chapter 22, Neurosurgical complications, p.425.)

A complication of FESS/intra-nasal polypectomy or rhinoplasty. It usually settles spontaneously. Nurse semi-upright, give antibiotics, and advise the patient not to blow their nose. Non-healing leaks are surgically explored and repaired using fascia, perichondrium, or a local transposition flap closure using septal mucosa.

Altered sensation to incisors, upper lip, and gingivae

The nasopalatine nerve supplies these and is at risk when raising the mucoperichondrial flap in nasal surgery. Symptoms are usually transient.

Intra-nasal polypectomy/functional endoscopic sinus surgery

Ophthalmic complications

In the immediate post-operative phase, eye observations should be performed every 15 minutes when the lamina papyracea has been or is suspected to have been breached. Examination for diplopia, loss of red colour perception, proptosis, and signs of ophthalmoplegia is required. Intervention should not be delayed if intra-orbital bleeding is suspected. Blindness may result if these early signs are ignored. Treatment is immediate surgical decompression, intra-nasally or externally via an external ethmoid approach.

Early complications

Septoplasty/septorhinoplasty

Septal haematoma

A septal haematoma is classically cherry red and unilateral, causes pain, and should be drained under local or general anaesthetic as a matter of urgency. Intravenous antibiotics should prevent septal abscess formation.

Skull base procedures
Meningitis
A particular risk if the skull base and dura have been disrupted with an ensuing CSF leak. Treat with high-dose antibiotics and consider surgical closure.

Intermediate complications
Septoplasty/septorhinoplasty
Septal abscess formation
An unrecognized septal haematoma often leads to an abscess. Intravenous antibiotics and drainage under general anaesthetic are required to halt potential cartilage destruction. Place a non-suction drain or leave a drainage hole in the flap.

Late complications
Septoplasty/septorhinoplasty
Septal perforation
This can be the result of a poorly managed septal abscess or insufficient blood supply to the septum when bilateral mucosal perforations have occurred and have not been repaired. Treatment options include reduction of nasal crusting with saline douches, local rotational or advancement mucosal flap repair, or septal button placement in larger perforations.

Supra-tip nasal deformity
May result from loss of septal cartilage support (poor surgical technique or septal necrosis). Surgical reconstruction may be required.

Adhesions
These occur between septum and the lateral nasal wall. May cause problems with nasal breathing and require surgical division.

Complications of airways endoscopy

Immediate complications

Microlaryngoscopy, laryngo-pharyngoscopy

Dental injury

Instrumentation of the oral cavity or oropharynx always risks damage to the teeth and adjacent mucosa. Patients with bad dentition should be warned of possible post-op problems. Appropriate protection should always be used.

Airway fire

An airway fire can result from laser use, particularly if an inappropriate anaesthetic tube is employed. If fire occurs, remove the endo-tracheal tube immediately as this removes the source of concentrated oxygen and the fire extinguishes itself. Re-intubate as soon as it is safe to do so and treat burnt areas as appropriate. Beware of potential for airway oedema and safeguard airway.

Laryngospasm

The vocal cords are particularly sensitive to irritants such as blood. Adduction of the vocal cords results in inspiratory stridor. The period immediately after surgery is most dangerous, when the patient has just been extubated. Although spontaneous resolution within 30–60 seconds is the norm, high flow oxygen should be administered and consideration given to re-intubation.

Rigid oesophagoscopy with or without dilatation

Oesophageal perforation

Must always be considered during and after the procedure. If there is any question that perforation has occurred then placement of a naso-gastric tube and commencement of antibiotics is required. A contrast swallow at 24hrs will confirm or refute the diagnosis. Consider an external approach to surgically close a high, large perforation.

Early complications

Rigid oesophagoscopy with or without dilatation

Missed oesophageal perforation

Observations of pulse, temperature, and for chest pain should be undertaken. Cervical oesophageal perforations are generally treated conservatively; lower perforations should prompt referral to a cardiothoracic or specialist oesophageal surgeon. Failure to make the diagnosis early can result in mediastinitis, which is associated with a significant mortality rate, particularly in the elderly. A contrast swallow is advisable when deciding to commence feeding orally.

Late complications

Direct microlaryngoscopy with biopsy

Vocal cord adhesions

This can occur when two opposing epithelial surfaces are left raw, resulting in the formation of anterior glottic web. Consider surgical division.

Complications of oro-pharyngeal surgery

Immediate complications

Tonsillectomy/uvulopalatopharyngoplasty

Primary haemorrhage

This may be controlled with ligatures, suturing the anterior to the posterior pillar, or packing. Sedation on ITU for 24 hours may be required in extreme cases. An underlying clotting problem should be considered.

Adenoidectomy

Post-nasal space packing is indicated until haemostasis has been achieved. 1 in 10 000 adrenaline-soaked packs may help achieve this, though the use of adrenaline requires care.

Early complications

Tonsillectomy/uvulopalatopharyngoplasty/adenoidectomy

Reactionary haemorrhage

This is potentially insidious. The first indication of continuing blood loss is often the vomiting of blood and/or tachycardia and hypotension. Very young children only have to lose 100ml of blood before they become surgically shocked. Management of reactionary haemorrhage is focused on maintenance of the airway, breathing, and circulation.

Patients with minor haemorrhage require removal of any clot and close observation. Application of an adrenaline-soaked swab to the affected side and subsequent regular gargling of dilute hydrogen peroxide solution may suffice. If not, place the patient in the recovery position with a Trendelenburg tilt, establish intravenous access, fluid resuscitation, and return to theatre. The patient should also be placed on antibiotics.

Intermediate complications

Tonsillectomy/uvulopalatopharyngoplasty/adenoidectomy

Secondary haemorrhage

This is usually associated with local infection, which allows premature separation of the protective slough covering the tonsillar/adenoidal bed. Management is with broad spectrum intravenous antibiotics and analgesia. Re-exploration is unlikely to be required.

Late complications

Tonsillectomy/uvulopalatopharyngoplasty

Velopharyngeal incompetence

Over-zealous soft-palate surgery or those with a submucosal cleft palate run the risk of velopharyngeal incompetence resulting in hyper-nasal speech and food regurgitation into the nasal cavity. In severe cases a pharyngoplasty may be required.

Adenoidectomy

Hyper-nasal speech

Excision of grossly hypertrophied adenoids, especially if the soft palate is short, can result in palatal incompetence and pronounced hyper-nasal speech.

Complications of tracheostomy

Tracheostome formation after laryngectomy is far less likely to be associated with any of the complications listed below, which primarily relate to formal tracheostomy formation.

Tube displacement

The tube may become displaced at any time after insertion. Displacement can be complete or partial. Partial displacement, commonly into the pretracheal space, is particularly dangerous if unrecognized. This can be avoided by using an appropriately sized tube and secure fixation with tapes and/or sutures.

Re-introduction of a misplaced tube is sometimes facilitated by railroading it over a bougie introduced into the tracheal lumen. Local surgical emphysema in the neck tissues is a tell-tale indication of tube displacement.

Immediate complications

Haemorrhage

Bleeding may be from an anterior jugular vein, thyroid isthmus, terminal branches of the superior thyroid artery, or skin edges. Reactionary haemorrhage may occur due to poor haemostasis at the time of surgery or a slipped ligature.

Trauma to adjacent structures

Injury to paratracheal structures should be avoided by ensuring that a midline approach is maintained. Trauma to the recurrent laryngeal nerve, oesophagus, pleura, and left brachiocephalic vein (particularly in children, in whom it is high) can all occur.

Hypoxia

In some patients, chronic airway obstruction results in hypercapnia; with the formation of a tracheostomy the obstruction is overcome and the pCO_2 immediately falls, with a loss of respiratory drive and the potential for respiratory arrest. Anticipation of such problems and close cooperation with anaesthetic colleagues is required.

Intermediate complications

Tube obstruction

Crusting or retained tenacious secretions can occlude the tube lumen. This can be avoided by attentive nursing care, adequate humidification, the warming of inspired gases, and regular physiotherapy. The tube should be changed regularly. Many modern tubes have removable inner tubes, which makes tube clearance much easier.

Lower respiratory infection

Acting as an infected foreign body, a tracheostomy tube forms a source of infection for the lower airway. Regular physiotherapy, early mobilization, and tracheobronchial toilet reduce this risk.

Dysphagia

This can be due to compression of the oesophagus by the inflated tube cuff or stenting of the larynx, preventing it from moving vertically during deglutition.

Late complications

Tracheal stenosis

This is usually the result of circumferential stenosis of the trachea due to mucosal ischaemia secondary to too high a cuff pressure being maintained for too long a period of time. Modern low-pressure cuffs have largely led to the disappearance of this problem.

Tracheo-oesophageal fistula

This can lead to aspiration pneumonia. Its incidence has been significantly reduced with low-pressure cuffs.

Major haemorrhage

A rare complication, usually related to poor placement or sizing of the tube and erosion of the innominate artery. Warning bleeds usually pre-empt major haemorrhage. If not taken seriously, this has a high mortality.

Complications of routine neck surgery

Certain procedures are associated with specific complications. Particular care should be taken to avoid damage to the accessory nerve when operating in the posterior triangle.

Immediate complications

Sistrunk's procedure

Recurrence

The risk of cyst recurrence can be reduced by good surgical technique. Very rarely, hypothyroidism can result if the cyst represents the only viable thyroid tissue in the neck.

Branchial cyst excision

Nerve damage

Meticulous surgical technique minimizes subsequent damage to adjacent nerves, e.g. accessory nerve, hypoglossal nerve.

Submandibular gland excision

Haemorrhage and nerve damage

The main post-operative complications relate to poor haemostasis and nerve injury to either the marginal mandibular, lingual, or hypoglossal nerves.

External pharyngeal surgery

This particularly relates to pharyngeal pouch excision.

Immediate complications

Pharyngeal/oesophageal perforation

As for direct oesophagoscopy. If there is any chance of a perforation, or one has been closed, a drain should be left in the wound.

Early complications

Recurrent laryngeal nerve damage

Damage to both the recurrent laryngeal nerve and the superior branch of the laryngeal nerve is possible. The risk of nerve damage is less when treatment of the pouch is undertaken endoscopically.

Intermediate complications

Fistulas

Careful repair of the pharyngotomy following pouch excision is important if a fistula is to be avoided. If the neck has been adequately drained, fistulas usually close in 7–10 days. A naso-gastric tube should be left in place and the patient given intravenous antibiotics.

Late complications

Stricture

An iatrogenic post-cricoid stricture can develop at the site of closure. Symptoms may present later following exacerbation by scarring and fibrosis. Aspiration may also result. Repeated dilatations may help although management is very difficult for a persisting stricture.

Complications of laryngectomy (with or without partial pharyngectomy)

Immediate complications

Primary haemorrhage

The most common cause is bleeding following slippage of a ligature from, for example, the superior thyroid artery. Locate the source, apply clips, and re-ligate.

Early complications

Reactionary bleeding

Blockage of large-bore suction drains can turn a troublesome small bleed into a life-threatening problem with subsequent haematoma formation, infection, and wound breakdown, so must be avoided.

Wound breakdown

This is more likely to occur in patients in a poor nutritional state and those who have undergone previous radiotherapy or synchronous flap reconstruction of a skin or mucosal defect. Every effort should be made to encourage healing by primary intention. Naso-gastric feeding should continue and the patient should be placed on antibiotics. Significant breakdown may require a flap reconstruction if a prolonged period of conservative management fails.

Intermediate complications

Pharyngocutaneous fistulas

These are related to pre-operative factors (prior radiotherapy, poorly controlled diabetes, anaemia, poor nutrition), peri-operative factors (inadequate suturing), and post-operative factors (untreated infection, seroma, or haematoma). Radiotherapy is the most significant of these factors. Infected skin with areas of necrosis requires debridement and control of local infection by dressings and antibiotics. Nutrition is provided by naso-gastric tube or gastrostomy until the fistula closes. Fistulas do not close in the presence of residual disease. Any suspicious-looking granulations need to be biopsied to rule out residual disease. Hyperbaric oxygen therapy is used in some centres in an attempt to promote healing.

Surgical closure of fistulas that persist beyond 4 weeks should be considered. A number of options are available; a pectoralis major myocutaneous flap is a commonly employed choice.

Late complications

Pharyngeal stenosis

This is caused by excessive resection of mucosa with inappropriate primary closure. It can be avoided in large pharyngeal resections by undertaking immediate surgical reconstruction of the pharynx to maintain a good lumen. Repeated serial dilatations may be required if stenosis does occur.

Stenosis of the tracheostome

A stoma button may help prevent stenosis. Stomaplasty or small rotational flaps are options designed to address this problem.

Aspiration and dysphagia

These are a risk in partial laryngectomy. Dysphagia is common with supraglottic resections and is difficult to overcome.

Aspiration usually presents with cough, poor voice and/or right basal pneumonia. Strategies available are thyroplasty, PEG feeding, or 'completion laryngectomy'.

Complications of neck dissection

This operation can be radical, functional, or selective. For the purpose of this chapter, a radical neck dissection is considered.

Immediate complications

Venous air embolism
The patient is commonly operated on in the reverse Trendelenburg position. Should a low-cut stump of the internal jugular vein be lost into the superior mediastinum prior to ligation, for example, the negative pressure in the vein draws air into the venous circulation and carries a significant mortality. The patient should be placed in the head down position and the root of the neck explored appropriately.

Pneumothorax
This is caused by damage to the cervical pleura when operating low in the neck. This may be overlooked in the ventilated patient. A plain chest radiograph should be taken if indicated post-operatively.

Nerve damage
The phrenic, hypoglossal, lingual, vagus, accessory, brachial plexus, and lower branches of the facial nerve are all at risk during a radical neck dissection. Injury to the sympathetic trunk produces a post-operative Horner's syndrome. The latter has no functional significance but may be cosmetically unacceptable.

Early complications

Haemorrhage
Likely causes are bleeding from the superior or inferior ends of the divided jugular veins, superior or inferior thyroid pedicles, or the external carotid artery. Drain volume is normally reliable for assessing blood loss but a blocked drain is potentially falsely reassuring. Management is the same as that after any operation: ensure maintenance of the airway prior to identifying and ligating the bleeding vessel.

Airway obstruction
A neck dissection rarely causes upper airway oedema with compromise of the airway. This is more likely, however, after bilateral radical neck dissections with ligation of both internal jugular veins. Loss of one vein results in an acute three-fold rise in intracranial pressure. Resection of both veins results in an eight-fold rise and this is much more likely to be associated with upper airway venous congestion and oedema. Symptoms include headache and agitation. Examine for facial swelling and congestion, which can be minimized by recovering the patient in an upright position, avoiding constricting neck dressings, and preventing neck hyperextension. Medical treatment traditionally involves the use of intravenous 20–25% mannitol with or without concurrent dexamethasone administration.

It is also occasionally seen after a unilateral radical neck dissection in an irradiated patient. Anticipation of the risk should be followed by an elective tracheostomy.

Intermediate complications

Chylous fistula

Thoracic duct damage is estimated to occur in 2% of radical neck dissections. More commonly left-sided, 25% occur on the right side. Most fistulas close spontaneously, although prolonged drainage has significant biochemical and nutritional implications; protein loss leading to hypoproteinaemia can be troublesome. It can also result in local wound breakdown.

The decision about whether to treat conservatively or re-explore the neck is based largely on the amount of chyle being collected over a 24-hour period. If the fistula continues to drain in excess of 600ml of chyle per day after the first post-op week, then consideration needs to be given to surgical intervention.

Seroma

Suction drainage reduces this risk. Failure to recognize seroma compromises the viability of the overlying skin and leads to delayed wound healing. Seromas can be managed by regular aspiration under aseptic technique and pressure dressings until dry.

Late complications

Carotid artery rupture

This can occur after a culmination of a number of factors: infection, a salivary leak, radiotherapy, and recurrent disease. There is nearly always a preceeding herald bleed 48 hours before rupture. At this stage rupture can be avoided by returning the patient to theatre, resecting any necrotic tissue (including a section of carotid artery) and covering the exposed vessel ends with a vascular muscle flap, e.g. pectoralis major.

Massive rupture should be controlled with finger pressure, the airway secured by re-inflating the tracheostomy tube (if still in place), and fluid replacement (ideally with blood). Cerebral blood flow is maintained by head-down tilt. The artery should be isolated, clamped, transfixed, and divided. No attempts should be made to suture or graft the defect; a further rupture is almost inevitable if this is attempted.

Neurological complications are more likely if a period of prolonged hypotension precedes surgical intervention. If anticipated and the patient makes it to theatre, the prospect for survival is reasonably good.

Scar contracture

Skin crease incisions are cosmetically most desirable. Trifurcations are less aesthetic and prone to contracture.

Incisions perpendicular to the normal skin crease lines result in the greatest degree of scar contracture. Conventional Z-plasty techniques redistribute the resulting skin tension.

Parotidectomy – superficial/total

The parotid gland is frequently operated on for benign disease – neoplasms, chronic sialadenitis, and sialolithiasis. Fortunately, the most common tumours (pleomorphic salivary adenomas and adenolymphomas) tend to occur in the superficial lobe of the parotid.

Immediate complications

Haemorrhage

If a large wound haematoma forms, the patient must be returned to theatre for evacuation and haemostasis.

Facial nerve damage

Malignancy may necessitate sacrifice of the main trunk or branches of the nerve. The chance of inadvertent damage is reduced by a meticulous technique that exposes the nerve throughout its intraglandular course. Consideration should be given to the use of intra-operative nerve monitoring. Complete nerve section requires immediate repair. Microneural anastomosis or grafting using the greater auricular, sural, or medial cutaneous nerves should be undertaken.

Simple neuropraxia, more severe after 24 hours than in the immediate post-operative period, recovers fully provided all branches are anatomically intact at the end of the operation. If eye closure is compromised, corneal ulceration may be avoided with Hypromellose eye drops and taping the eye shut at night until resolution. Lateral tarsorrhaphy or botulinum toxin injection is advised in a severe or prolonged palsy.

Intermediate complications

Salivary fistulas

Spontaneous resolution occurs commonly after 7–10 days so conservative management and/or sterile aspirations of any accumulated secretions should be all that is required. Anti-sialagogues are of little benefit.

Formal re-exploration is reserved for non-healing fistulas. Post-operative low dose radiotherapy to the affected gland may be considered in older patients.

Late complications

Frey's syndrome

This presents approximately 6 months post-operatively with gustatory sweating accompanied by vasodilatation of the skin innervated by the auriculotemporal nerve.

Treatment options in those cases that persist include intracutaneous injection of botulinum toxin, re-raising the skin flap, and vestibular neuronectomy.

Thyroid surgery/parathyroid surgery

Some of the most significant complications relate to endocrine function. Meticulous attention to haemostasis is required during thyroid and parathyroid surgery due to the highly vascular nature of the area. Patients who have tertiary hyperparathyroidism are altogether less well and need close monitoring by renal physicians and early transfer to their care post-op.

Immediate complications

Haemorrhage

Airway compromise results if a large haematoma forms. Oxygen should be administered and a clip remover used to open the wound immediately. Stitches in the platysma layer should also be cut and the haematoma evacuated. Only then should the patient be returned to theatre for definitive haemostasis and re-closure. Airway oedema may take longer to settle and may require provision of a temporary alternative airway.

Thyrotoxic storm

Patients with inadequately controlled hyperthyroidism are at risk. Symptoms include tachycardia, hyperpyrexia, and agitation. Operating on these patients can result in arrhythmias, heart failure, and malignant hyperthermia, with significant mortality. Consider administration of cool intravenous fluids, propranolol, thiouracil, potassium iodide, and dexamethasone in doses appropriate to the severity of the condition.

Tracheomalacia

Long-standing tracheal compression from a large multinodular goitre can produce softening and collapse of tracheal rings. This is a rare cause of immediate post-operative respiratory obstruction. It may show on pre-operative CT scanning and should be anticipated.

Recurrent laryngeal nerve injury

Damage can be caused by intra-operative traction, haematoma formation, ligation, diathermy, or sectioning at the time of surgery. Unilateral nerve damage results in a weak, hoarse voice. Reassure the patient if the symptoms are mild; if they are severe, consider a thyroplasty or cord injection at a later date. Bilateral incomplete nerve injury produces respiratory distress and airway obstruction, necessitating re-intubation and tracheostomy. In bilateral complete injuries, the cords adopt the cadaveric position; the voice is very poor, but dyspnoea is not pronounced. Aspiration is likely and may necessitate the use of a cuffed tracheostomy tube.

Superior laryngeal nerve injury

This nerve is at risk during dissection of the superior pole of the thyroid and causes a subtle change in voice quality and projection. This is of great importance to those who rely on the quality of their voice for work or recreation.

Early complications

Hypocalcaemia

This may result from devascularization or inadvertent removal of all or most of the functioning parathyroid tissue. Ask about peri-oral and digital tingling sensations, and examine for latent carpal-pedal spasm and a positive Chvostek's sign. Mild hypocalcaemia (adjusted ionized calcium <2.2mmol/l but >2mmol/l) is usually transient but may require oral calcium supplements if symptomatic. Adjusted calcium levels >1.8mmol/l but <2mmol/l require oral calcium supplements (for example 1–2µg of 1-alpha-hydroxycholecalciferol given daily), but if severe (<1.8mmol/l or symptomatic) require intravenous calcium gluconate. Levels should be monitored regularly until stable.

Hypocalcaemia after partial parathyroidectomy

This is usually transient, but if severe, temporary oral calcium supplements are required. Monitor calcium regularly.

Late complications

Hypothyroidism

After total thyroidectomy patients develop hypothyroidism if not treated. Start levothyroxine supplementation day 1 post-operatively (triiodothyronine 20mg 8 hourly if likely to have future radio-abalative treatment). Arrange for thyroid stimulating hormone levels to be monitored.

Persistent hyperparathyroidism after parathyroidectomy

Other causes of hypercalcaemia should be excluded. Radioisotope or magnetic resonance imaging (MRI) localization studies can identify ectopic glands – the commonest reason for failure. Referral to an experienced surgeon is advised because the risk of permanent recurrent laryngeal nerve injury and hypoparathyroidism after re-operation is considerable.

General miscellaneous complications associated with head and neck surgery

Regarding head and neck cancer patients, they are often long-term smokers and heavy drinkers and are consequently at risk of alcohol and nicotine withdrawal.

In spite of counselling pre-operatively, the psychological trauma of surgery can have a major effect on them over the immediate and early post-operative period. This can be alleviated by appropriate clinical and psychological support. In addition, antidepressants are sometimes required.

Chapter 20

Complications after breast surgery

Introduction

Surgery of the breast may be performed for various reasons, namely for oncological diagnosis or clearance, removal of benign lumps to exclude cancer or for reassurance, and for aesthetic or reconstructive purposes. Breast surgeons are increasingly employing oncoplastic techniques during tumour clearance and there needs to be awareness of the potential complications of such techniques in addition to those that may follow 'traditional' breast surgery.

Aesthetic and reconstructive surgery of the breast may involve the use of tissue expanders, implants, and flaps. Complications following aesthetic or reconstructive breast surgery can occur within breast tissue, implant material, flap tissue, or in flap donor sites.

Complications

Complications that follow oncological investigations of the breast, i.e. fine needle aspiration or Core (Trucut) biopsy, include haematoma, infection, and (rarely) pneumothorax. Complications that occur after local excision, mastectomy, axillary surgery, or reconstruction are as follows:

Immediate

- haemorrhage
- injury to axillary structures
- pneumothorax.

Intermediate

Breast

- seroma
- haematoma
- wound infection
- wound dehiscence
- skin/skin flap necrosis
- fat necrosis
- nipple necrosis (partial or complete)
- flap failure/necrosis
- implant extrusion/infection/contracture/failure.

Axilla

- lymphocele or lymphoedema of arm
- paraesthesia
- reduced shoulder movement.

Late

Breast

- tumour recurrence
- deformity/asymmetry
- hypertrophic or keloid scarring.

Axilla

- frozen shoulder
- scar contracture.

Specific complications

Seroma
Collections of lymphatic fluid are often seen following large volume breast excisions, mastectomies, axillary clearance, and in flap donor wounds, e.g. latissimus dorsi. Drainage via surgical drains in the immediate post-operative period followed by repeated aspiration may be necessary if symptomatic. Topical antibiotics (tetracycline, bleomycin), quilting of raw surfaces, and fibrin glue have all demonstrated varied success in reducing seroma rates.

Haematoma
Meticulous haemostasis is the key to avoiding haematomas. Small haematomas often resolve with conservative treatment. Large haematomas require evacuation because of late sequelae of calcification, fat necrosis, and breast asymmetry.

Wound infection
Significant surgical site infection rates of up to 5% are quoted with even higher rates of minor SSI if close post-discharge surveillance is undertaken. There is little evidence that antibiotic prophylaxis reduces the risk of breast infections.

Skin/skin flap necrosis
Necrosis of wound edges or skin flaps is the result of wounds being closed under tension, following poor tissue handling, or when excessively thin flaps are used. Wound complications are more prevalent in smokers, diabetics, and particularly in post-radiotherapy patients. Non-viable tissue requires debridement. Clean wounds may be left to heal by secondary intention when they are small, but if defects are large they need closure with skin grafts or flaps.

Fat necrosis
Excessive use of deep breast sutures that strangulate fat, haematomas, or infection may result in areas of fat necrosis within the breast. These may present as a palpable lump, with or without skin dimpling, and diagnosis is by exclusion, reached after a triple assessment.

Nipple necrosis
This is an uncommon but disastrous complication that may follow peri-areolar incisions for duct ectasia, surgical access (for removal of gynaecomastia, for example), or mammoplasties.

Flap failure/necrosis
Partial or complete flap failure of the deeper tissues in a flap, as in a myocutaneous flap, may follow breast reconstruction. Small areas of flap necrosis may present as palpable thickening or lumps. They may resolve or need surgical correction.

Lymphoedema
The risk of lymphoedema increases with the level of axillary dissection and use of radiotherapy. Level III axillary dissection is associated with a 10% risk of symptomatic lymphoedema. The addition of radiotherapy increases this to more than 30%. Early recognition and treatment in specialized lymphoedema clinics is essential. Compression garments and physiotherapy help control the condition. Long-standing lymphoedema may be rarely complicated by angiosarcoma (Stewart-Treves syndrome).

Paraesthesia
Damage to the intercosto-brachial, thoracodorsal, or long thoracic nerves may occur during an axillary dissection. Rarely there may be direct axonal damage to the brachial plexus. More commonly neuropraxia of the brachial plexus may arise due to traction of the arm during surgery.

Tumour recurrence
Local recurrence may present as areas of thickening, skin changes, or palpable lumps around the surgical site or in areas of lymphatic drainage, particularly the axilla. It is important that changes that present in a patient who has undergone reconstruction are investigated to exclude recurrence.

Deformity/asymmetry
Post-surgical breast deformity can be reduced by the use of appropriately placed incisions and oncoplastic mammoplasty techniques. Incisions in the upper half of the breast can be avoided via a peri-areolar approach. Distortion of the level of the nipple areolar complex is a major determining factor in the patient's perception of her breast asymmetry.

Hypertrophic/keloid scarring
These are more common in wounds closed under tension, darker skinned individuals, and where there is a family history. Massage therapy, silicone gel, and topical and intra-lesional steroids are forms of treatment available but none is entirely satisfactory.

Frozen shoulder
Reduced shoulder movements can be resolved by early physiotherapy. If neglected, frozen shoulder is a late and difficult complication to manage.

Complications of plastic surgery

Introduction

Plastic surgery is one of the oldest surgical specialities, dating back to Sushruta's reconstruction of amputated noses in 600 BC, but the general public and medical profession may both misunderstand the scope of modern day plastic and reconstructive surgery. The number of plastic surgery units in the United Kingdom is comparatively small, and few surgical trainees have exposure to this speciality, in which procedures are varied and often cross the anatomic boundaries that define and limit other specialities.

Complications occur in all branches of surgery; however, these may be minimized by meticulous attention to a strict set of plastic surgical principles (see Box 21.1) and being aware of the pathophysiology of wound healing.

Box 21.1 Surgical principles

- **Tissue handling** – crushing of tissue should be strictly avoided. Use skin hooks or fine-toothed forceps wherever possible.
- **Incisions** – skin incisions should be made at right angles to the skin surface, to avoid shelving and 'undercutting'. In hair-bearing areas, the incision must be made parallel to the hair follicles.
- **Direction** – scars placed within natural wrinkles and parallel to relaxed skin tension lines are often less noticeable. Secondary procedures such as Z- or W-plasty techniques can re-orientate and 'break up' the scar if necessary.
- **Haemostasis** – meticulous haemostasis prior to wound closure reduces the risk of haematomas post-operatively. Haematomas can become the source of wound infection, discomfort, and increased wound tension.
- **Wound evaluation and debridement** – this is often overlooked, especially in traumatic wounds, but has important long-term results. Dirty, devitalized tissue or foreign bodies must be excised, and thorough irrigation should be performed. Foreign material acts as a nidus for infection and may become permanent 'tattoos' or increase the scarring process.
- **Wound tension** – tension should be minimized as much as possible to reduce scar stretch and the risk of wound dehiscence. Dermal sutures should be considered. Wound support such as Steri-strips may be used to prevent wound edges shearing during healing.
- **Wound closure** – sutures should be placed in order to 'evert' the skin edges. Make sure the wound edges are apposed with minimal tension as post-operative oedema may further appose and strangulate the edges.
- **Tissue perfusion** – ensure optimal correction of shock, and correct any metabolic disturbances such as diabetes. Educate the patient with regard to the risks of smoking, and encourage them to stop.
- **Wound care** – sutures on the face should generally not be left in for more than 5 days to reduce the chance of 'hatch mark' scars. Sutures on the trunk and extremities are usually removed after 10–14 days.

General plastic surgery complications

Scarring

Scars are the normal and inevitable result of mammalian connective tissue repair. Each year in the developed world 100 million patients develop scars, as a natural part of the healing process, following elective operations and traumatic events. Scars are comprised of the fibrous replacement of normal skin after injury, although the epithelial component is regenerated, and can occur to varying degrees of aesthetic acceptability.

Scarring covers a wide spectrum of clinical phenotypes (📖 see Box 21.2) and determining the mode of scarring is important in guiding management, both of the current scarring and for planning future surgery. Abnormal scars may cause unpleasant symptoms and be psychologically and functionally disabling. Recent advances in the understanding of embryonic skin healing, and novel scar assessment tools, are leading to the development of new drugs and techniques to prevent scarring.

Box 21.2 Scarring

- **'Normal' scars** – it may be argued that no scar is truly 'normal'; however, a fine white line scar is the most satisfactory outcome.
- **Stretched scars** – these develop in the weeks following surgery as the tissue is stretched and widened due to external forces and increased tension. These scars are typically flat, pale, soft, and asymptomatic. Commonly seen on the trunk and following joint replacement surgery.
- **Atrophic scars** – these scars are depressed below the surrounding skin. They are generally small and often rounded with an indented centre. Common following acne or chicken pox.
- **Scar contractures** – scars crossing joints or skin creases at right angles are prone to shortening and causing contracture. This type of scar is often disabling. They are common following burn injuries. Surgical correction is often needed.
- **Hypertrophic scars** – these are raised scars that develop *within the boundaries of the original incision*. Common in young children, they can occur at any site and may be red, itchy, and painful. They are also common following burn injury.
- **Keloid scars** – these were first described by Egyptian surgeons around 1700 BC. Alibert first recognized them to be a clinical entity in 1806, naming them Cheloide (Greek: *chele* – crab's claw; *oid* – like). Keloid scars are raised scars that have developed *beyond the boundaries of the original incision*. Those from pigmented races are particularly prone to developing keloid scars, which predominate in areas such as the earlobe, sternum, and deltoid regions. A keloid scar does not regress over time, and invariably recurs after excision. Histologically keloids have a swirling nodular pattern of type III collagen fibres. They are often pigmented but in white skin become avascular and white during maturation.

Box 21.3 Management options (in a multi-disciplinary setting)

Non-invasive
- Compression therapy (such as pressure garments with or without gel sheeting).
- Silicone gels and pads.
- Static and dynamic splints.
- Acrylic casts, masks, and clips.
- Psychosocial counselling and advice.

Invasive
- Intra-lesional corticosteroid injection (beware fat atrophy, dermal thinning, and pigment changes).
- Intra-lesional 5-FU injection.
- Radiotherapy.
- Laser therapy.
- Intra-lesional excision and re-suture.
- Intra-lesional excision combined with corticosteroid injection.
- Scar excision with local transposition flap reconstruction (Z-plasty, W-plasty, M-plasty).
- Scar excision and reconstruction (loco-regional flap, free flap).

Management
The severity of scars is often judged by eye; however, they may be assessed quantitatively with a scar assessment guide, such as the Vancouver Scale.

The decision about whether to treat a scar depends upon site, symptoms, functional impairment, timing, and patient wishes. A range of surgical and non-surgical options are available (📕 see Box 21.3).

Surgical scar revision is specialized, and a plastic surgeon may base scar revision on:
- a period of at least 6–12 months for the active process of scarring to have minimized
- the relationship to other anatomical landmarks and relaxed skin tension lines
- the likelihood of hypertrophic or keloid scarring.

Techniques such as Z-plasty, W-plasty, and M-plasty are often employed.

Skin incisions

The ideal scar is flat, fine, lies within or parallel to the natural skin line (relaxed skin tension lines, RSTL), and does not affect function or appearance.

Surgical principles

- Skin incision – incisions are normally made at right angles to the skin. Avoid shelving or undercut incisions on the skin, as they heal leaving thick, unsightly scars. However, in special areas, e.g. eyebrows and scalp, the incision is made parallel to the hair follicles.
- Direction – scars placed within natural wrinkles or parallel to RSTL are less conspicuous. They may require Z-plasty or W-plasty techniques to re-orientate or break up the direction of the scar.
- Tissue handling – gentle handling and avoiding crushing of soft tissues is basic to all aspects of surgery. Consider using skin hooks or fine-toothed forceps to hold deeper tissues and avoid damaging the dermal and epidermal layers of the skin.
- Haemostasis – careful haemostasis prior to wound closure reduces the risk of haematomas post-operatively. These may become sites of wound infection, discomfort, scar distortion, and increased wound tension.
- Wound evaluation – dirty, devitalized tissue or foreign matter must be excised, otherwise these will be a nidus for future wound infection and unsightly scars. Wounds that contain foreign material may become permanent 'tattoos'. This unsightly complication can be minimized by thorough wound cleansing at the time of injury and may need scrubbing debridement with copious irrigation.
- Wound tension – excessive tension results in a widespread scar. Consider deep dermal sutures to reduce tissue tension and review scar alignment.
- Tissue perfusion – areas of the body with a good blood supply heal better than those areas with a poor blood supply. Ensure good perfusion (including optimal correction of shock and avoidance of hypothermia) and nutrition to patients following surgery to reduce risks of delayed wound healing and infection.
- Age/co-morbid factors – older patients produce less conspicuous scars, although their healing rates are slower. Co-morbid factors may affect wound healing due to nutritional, vascular insufficiency, or iatrogenic causes, e.g. chemotherapy.
- Closure – sutures should be placed so that the skin edges are everted and just touching. Post-operative oedema apposes the edges; excessive tension in the area surrounded by the suture may cause tissue necrosis or visible suture marks.
- Wound care – wounds heal better in a moist environment; occlusive dressings allow rapid epithelialization of an incision. After 48–72 hours the incision may be gently cleaned without disrupting wound integrity. Prolonged occlusion under opaque dressings does not allow identification of potential deterioration of the wound. Wound support, e.g. Steri-strips, may be used to prevent wound edges shearing and gaping during healing, and for a limited period following suture removal.

Unsightly scars
Scars are disfiguring. However, in some societies intentional scarring has been used for decorative purposes.

Hypertrophic scar
Raised red scar limited to the area of the incision. These are more common in young children and may occur at any site; they tend to resolve with time. They are possibly due to wound-edge shearing, subclinical infection, excessive tissue tension, or prolonged inflammation.

Treatment
Expectant, silicone gel, pressure, steroid injection. Remember the complications of steroid injections: local hypopigmentation, dermal atrophy, widening of the scar, and telangectasia. Intralesional calcium antagonists may be tried. Vascular specific lasers (585nm pulse-tuneable dye or 532nm) have shown beneficial effects on erythematous hypertrophic scars.

Keloid scars
Raised scar extending beyond the initial incision often shows a progressive increase in size. They are commonly associated with darker skin pigmentation, particularly in those of Afro-Caribbean descent, with family history, or of Celtic ancestry. They tend to occur at high-risk sites, e.g. earlobe and chest. Histology reveals an abnormally high concentration of type III collagen with a disorganized collagen pattern.

Treatment
This is difficult as surgery can make the condition worse. Use combined therapy with surgical excision and non-surgical options, e.g. steroid injections, pressure, radiotherapy, and/or calcium antagonists.

Widespread scars
Flat or recessed scar. These are usually caused by tissue tension pulling the wound edges apart (e.g. removal of sutures too early or not using buried sutures to support the wound) and are seen in areas of increased tissue tension, e.g. limbs. The scar does not contain excessive collagen.

Treatment
Either accept the scar or consider revisional surgery with prolonged wound support or a 'plasty' procedure.

'Morse code' (l — l) scar ('stitch marks')
Seen when skin sutures are left in place for longer than 5–6 days, or if the initial wound closure is so tight that tissue oedema causes dermal necrosis under the suture. Suture abscesses occur at each point of skin entry.

Treatment
Avoid the cause and consider using buried dermal suture technique, e.g. subcuticular closure.

Erythematous scars
Flat pink or red scar in the incision line. Note that all scars are erythematous during the initial stages of wound healing, and particularly following curettage or dermal shaving. They are caused by prolonged angiogenesis and decreased capillary regression and tend to resolve with time. Persistence beyond 12 months indicates a lack of resolution.

Treatment
They respond well to vascular specific lasers, which can be used early to hasten resolution or in later stages to lighten colour.

Pigmented scars
Flat tan/dark scar in the incision line. They are associated with darker skin tones and are due to increased melanogenesis or post-inflammatory hyperpigmentation with deposition of pigment into the dermis.

Treatment
These tend to resolve with time. Prolonged hyperpigmentation may be treated with topical hydroquinone.

Contractures
Wound contraction is a normal part of wound healing; however, a short, thick scar results in a scar contracture. This causes functional effects if the contraction crosses joints or is near the eyelids, and it may also have cosmetic effects by distorting soft tissues.

Treatment
Using techniques to lengthen or break up the contracture, e.g. Z-plasty or Y–V-plasty.

Skin grafts
A graft is a tissue that lacks its own intravascular blood supply and is dependent on the blood supply at the recipient site for its survival. A split-thickness skin graft (SSG) contains epidermis and a variable thickness of dermis; a full-thickness skin graft (FTSG) contains the whole dermis and adnexal structures, e.g. hair follicles. The graft bed must be vascularized, clean, and free of necrotic tissue. Skin grafts will not take on bone, cartilage, or tendon without the presence of periosteum, perichondrium, or paratenon. They are used to repair areas of skin loss or close wounds that cannot be closed by primary suture.

Initial graft adherence to a wound bed is affected by fibrin deposition, which lasts for 72 hours. This is followed by graft revascularization ('take'): the process of serum inhibition (24–48 hours), inosculation (alignment of graft and donor capillaries), and capillary ingrowth and revascularization.

Complications
These are mainly failure of skin grafts and late complications. The partial loss of a skin graft may require re-grafting or leaving the wound to heal by secondary intention; total loss may require re-grafting or another surgical approach, e.g. flaps.

Failure of skin grafts
Haematoma – this is the most common reason for skin graft failure. Careful haemostasis of the graft bed and removal of any residual clot prior to skin graft application with close contact between graft and bed is essential. Firm dressings, fenestrating the graft, and quilting sutures will allow close contact and the escape of any accumulated fluid. If detected early, incise the skin graft over the haematoma and evacuate, and re-dress with firm pressure.

Infection – infection is the second most common reason for skin graft failure. Avoid by attention to the preparation of the wound bed. Early signs of infection (cellulitis or suppuration) should be treated with systemic antibiotics and frequent antiseptic dressing changes.

Graft movement – shearing forces between the graft bed and graft may dislodge the graft from the bed. Grafts should be firmly fixed to the recipient site bed and, if dressed, use a non-shearing dressing technique with relative immobilization of the grafted area. Prolonged immobilization of the patient is not recommended.

Seroma – collections under the skin graft may result in skin graft necrosis. Using firm dressings, fenestrating the graft, and quilting sutures allows close contact and the escape of any fluid. If detected early, incise the skin graft over the seroma and evacuate, then re-dress with firm pressure.

Congestion – venous congestion or lymphatic stasis by prolonged early dependency or proximal constricting dressings results in localized oedema, preventing perfusion of the graft and causing failure. FTSG may show superficial desquamation and may manage to survive if congestion is relieved.

Pressure – excessive pressure (>30mmHg) on the surface of a skin graft causes necrosis.

Late complications

Contraction – primary contraction is the immediate shrinkage of a graft as it is harvested, due to recoil of the elastic fibres within the dermis. Therefore, a FTSG loses approximately 40% of its original area, and a SSG contracts by about 10–20%.

Secondary contraction is clinically more significant and occurs as the graft wound heals. SSGs exhibit secondary contracture more than FTSGs. After wound healing, FTSGs continue growing with the surrounding tissues. SSGs remain in a fixed state and grow minimally compared to the surrounding tissues, and therefore may cause future contractures. This may result in a functional problem, e.g. across flexor or extensor areas, or aesthetic problems due to soft tissue distortion, which may require revisional surgical procedures.

Aesthetic appearance

- Pigmentation – initially a graft appears erythematous, but this gradually fades. Hyperpigmentation may occur in SSGs.
- Elasticity – SSG lacks elasticity of normal skin, appearing thin, shiny, and darker; FTSG gives a better colour match and preserves skin elasticity. FTSGs harvested from above the clavicular areas are a good colour match for the face; SSGs are best avoided in the face.
- Aesthetic units – must be considered when using skin grafts, particularly in the face, avoiding a 'patch' appearance of graft.
- Skin function – as FTSGs contain adnexal structures they take on the characteristics of the recipient area, e.g. sweating. SSGs lack these structures and remain dry, so requiring long-term moisturization to prevent them drying out and becoming keratotic.

- Re-innervation – FTSGs have a greater chance of re-innervation compared to SSGs, with a slow recovery starting after 4–5 weeks and completed by 12–24 months. Sensory recovery of pain, light touch, cold, warm, and heat occur in that order. Patients need to be aware of thermal insensitivity to avoid injury.

Flaps

A flap is a unit of tissue containing its own intravascular blood supply transferred from a donor site to a recipient site.

Classification of flaps

Type (vascularity)
- random (cutaneous)
- pedicled/axial.

Technique (movement)
- advancement
- V–Y, Y–V
- single pedicle
- bi-pedicle
- pivot
- rotation
- transposition
- interpolation/island
- distant
- direct
- tubed
- free (microvascular anastomosis).

Tissue (composition)
- cutaneous
- fasciocutaneous
- musculocutaneous
- muscle
- osseocutaneous
- sensory.

Complications

Flap loss

Survival of a flap is dependent on the blood supply incorporated in its design. Clinical monitoring of flaps enables the early detection of problems; sophisticated monitors (laser Doppler) are available. Ensure patient is physiologically stable at all times post-operatively: well hydrated, warm, and pain-free. Reasons for flap loss are mainly:

- Flap design – partial (distal) flap loss is the most common complication with flaps. The flap designed may be too large for the intrinsic blood supply. Other causes of vascular pedicle compromise are due to extrinsic compression from dressings, sutures, or adjacent haematoma. Mechanical trauma may lead to more extensive total flap loss. A delay procedure to divide part of the vascular supply to a flap, prior to transfer, allows an increase in the surviving length of the flap.
Proper flap design, avoiding pedicle compression, tight wound closure,

and venous congestion, reduces the incidence of pedicled flap loss. Early stages of distal ischaemia may be reversed by correcting the underlying cause, e.g. evacuation of a haematoma or the release of a tight suture.

- Arterial insufficiency – clinical examination of free flaps in particular reveals pale, mottled skin. Capillary refill is sluggish (>2 seconds), which can be demonstrated by pressing a scissors' handle on skin. Pricking the dermis with a sterile needle reveals scant dark blood or serum. Ensure adequate perfusion, circulatory blood-volume replacement, and core temperature. Explore pedicle or anastomosis for intrinsic or extrinsic occlusion, which may be easily relieved.
- Venous occlusion – skin appears cyanotic or dusky. Capillary refill is brisker than normal and dermal blood is dark with rapid bleeding on pricking. Relieve venous occlusion, reduce congestion by elevation, and reduce tissue tension by releasing tight sutures. Venous engorgement may be relieved by the use of medicinal leeches – ask for help in their use.
- Ischaemia – reperfusion injury. Following ischaemia and the establishment of vascular perfusion, direct cytotoxic injury may result from free radicals. This is greater than the damage from the ischaemia itself. Hence, it is important to limit the period of ischaemia to the flap.
- No re-flow phenomenon – following prolonged ischaemia, vascular obstruction within the microcirculation becomes irreversible and it is not possible to re-establish perfusion; this precedes flap death.

Infection

Although flaps are generally resistant to infection, deep infection can devastate flaps. In addition, infection can contribute to flap necrosis. Treat with systemic antibiotics, antiseptic washouts, and wound excision as needed.

Tissue contour

Following flap inset and healing, tissue contour irregularities may require flap debulking/thinning to match the surrounding tissue.

Donor site

Donor site morbidity can occur due to a range of causes:
- loss of, or damage to, donor site muscle
- damage to motor nerves
- inadequate fascial closure
- skin and soft tissue wound and closure problems.

Regional plastic surgery complications

Breast

Operation: breast augmentation
General anaesthetic

Specific risks: haematoma, seroma, infection around implant, capsular contracture, implant rupture, asymmetry of breasts, rippling of implant surface, skin numbness, need for exchange/removal of implants, problems with breastfeeding, special radiological view (Eklund) needed for future mammography.

General risks: wound infection, hypertrophic scarring.

Operation: breast reduction (reduction mammoplasty)
General anaesthetic

Specific risks: haematoma, seroma, abscess, dehiscence, wound breakdown, fat necrosis, reduced/increased/altered skin or nipple sensation, skin/nipple necrosis, dissatisfaction with breast size, inability to breast feed, asymmetry of breast size/breast shape/nipple position, 'dog ears'.

General risks: wound infection, hypertrophic scarring.

Operation: mastopexy
General anaesthetic

Specific risks: changes in nipple sensation, asymmetry of shape and position of nipples, haematoma, recurrent ptosis.

General risks: wound infection, hypertrophic scarring.

Operation: latissimus dorsi flap for breast reconstruction
General anaesthetic

Specific risks: haematoma, seroma, dehiscence, wound breakdown, flap necrosis, asymmetry, shoulder stiffness or reduced shoulder movement, need for implant or expander, implant complications (infection, contracture, rupture, removal, replacement).

General risks: infection (of wound or deeper tissues), hypertrophic or stretched scars.

Operation: free TRAM (transverse rectus abdominis myocutaneous) flap for breast reconstruction
General anaesthetic

Specific risks: haematoma, seroma, dehiscence, wound breakdown, fat necrosis, flap necrosis, asymmetry, anastomotic problems, abdominal hernia/weakness/laxity, necrosis of umbilicus.

General risks: wound infection, abscess, hypertrophic scarring.

Operation: DIEP (deep inferior epigastric artery perforator) flap for breast reconstruction
General anaesthetic
Specific risks: haematoma, seroma, dehiscence, wound breakdown, fat necrosis, flap necrosis, asymmetry, anastomotic problems, abdominal hernia/weakness/laxity, necrosis of umbilicus.

General risks: wound infection, abscess, hypertrophic scarring.

Operation: nipple reconstruction (e.g. skate flap, nipple sharing)
Local or general anaesthetic
Specific risks: haematoma, asymmetry of nipple size/shape/colour, nipple necrosis, reduced skin/nipple sensation, need for tattooing.

General risks: wound infection, hypertrophic scarring.

Operation: correction of gynaecomastia
General anaesthetic
Specific risks: haematoma, seroma, abscess, nipple necrosis, reduced or altered nipple sensation, asymmetry, irregular appearance of breast, rippled, bruising, or indented appearance, inadequate or excess breast tissue excision, skin excess.

General risks: scar, hypertrophic scar, wound infection.

Nodal dissections/malignancy
Operation: groin dissection
General anaesthetic
Specific risks: haematoma, skin flap necrosis, seroma, wound infection, abscess, dehiscence, wound breakdown, lymphoedema, nerve or vessel damage.

General risks: scar, hypertrophic scar.

Operation: neck dissection
General anaesthetic
Specific risks: bleeding/haematoma, skin flap necrosis, wound breakdown, nerve damage causing difficulty swallowing (glossopharyngeal – CN IX), shoulder pain (spinal accessory – CN XI), difficulty breathing (phrenic), and tongue weakness (hypoglossal – CN XII), salivary fistula, lymphatic leakage, air embolus from vessel damage, dehiscence and vessel exposure, seroma, damage to sympathetic chain leading to Horner's syndrome, trigger point sensitivity from division of branches of cervical nerves.

General risks: scars, wound infection.

Operation: parotidectomy
General anaesthetic
Specific risks: haematoma, skin flap necrosis, seroma, sialocoele or parotid fistula, facial nerve palsy, Frey's syndrome.

General risks: scar, infection.

Congenital

Congenital (clefts)
Operation: cleft lip repair
General anaesthetic
Specific risks: bleeding, dehiscence, flap necrosis, scar contracture, hypertrophic scar, fistula formation.

General risks: scars, infection.

Operation: cleft palate repair
General anaesthetic
Specific risks: bleeding, dehiscence, flap necrosis, hypertrophic scar, fistula formation, retarded maxillary growth, nasal/airway obstruction.

General risks: scars, wound infection.

Congenital (urogenital)
Operation: hypospadias repair
General anaesthetic
Specific risks: urethro-cutaneous fistula, meatal stenosis, urethral stricture, recurrent chordee, and urethral diverticula, further operations, bladder spasm due to catheter post-op.

General risks: scars, infection, bleeding.

Lower limb

Operation: fasciocutaneous or muscle flap for lower limb reconstruction
General anaesthetic
Specific risks: haematoma, partial or total loss of flap, need for skin grafts, reduced or altered sensation, bulky flap.

General risks: scars, infection.

Operation: fasciotomy
General anaesthetic
Specific risks: bleeding/haematoma, nerve or vessel damage, need for future skin grafting.

General risks: scars, infection.

Aesthetic

Operation: abdominoplasty
General anaesthetic
Specific risks: haematoma, seroma, abscess, dehiscence, wound breakdown, numbness or reduced skin sensation, dog ears, asymmetry, flap/umbilical necrosis, recurrence of abdominal excess after weight gain.

General risks: scars, hypertrophic scar.

Operation: liposuction
General anaesthetic
Specific risks: haematoma, seroma, fat necrosis, contour irregularity, hypovolaemia, abscess, bruising, reduced or altered sensation, damage to skin,

skin necrosis, lignocaine toxicity, damage to deeper structures (e.g. intra-abdominal perforations), pulmonary fat embolism.

General risks: scars, wound infection, hypertrophic/keloid scarring.

Operation: rhinoplasty
General anaesthetic
Specific risks: haemorrhage, asymmetry, irregularity, over-/under-correction, nasal obstruction, septal perforation, post-operative deformity requiring further surgery, bruising around nose/eyes, implant complications (infection, migration, extrusion), nasal tip oedema, palpable step at maxillary osteotomy sites.

General risks: visible scars, hypertrophic scar, wound infection.

Operation: blepharoplasty
Local or general anaesthetic
Specific risks: blindness from retrobulbar haematoma, dry eyes, asymmetry, orbital cellulitis, ptosis, diplopia, enophthalmos, over-correction and lagophthalmos, ectropion, lash atrophy, epiphora.

General risks: scars, wound infection.

Operation: brow lift
General anaesthetic
Specific risks: haematoma, alopecia, frontalis paralysis, forehead numbness secondary to sensory nerve damage.

General risks: scars, infection.

Operation: face lift (rhytidectomy)
General anaesthetic
Specific risks: haematoma (men > women), flap necrosis, wound breakdown, infection, asymmetry, recurrence, nerve damage to great auricular nerve or facial nerve branches, temporal alopecia, ear deformity, salivary fistula.

General risks: scar, hypertrophic scarring.

Operation: pinnaplasty
Local or general anaesthetic
Specific risks: haematoma, skin necrosis, hypertrophic/keloid scars, suture extrusion, suture failure, recurrence of prominent ears, asymmetry, over-/under-correction, cauliflower ear.

General risks: scars, wound infection.

Operation: botulinum toxin injection
None or local anaesthetic
Specific risks: bruising, temporary unwanted muscle paralysis (leading to ptosis, for example), transient headache/flu-like symptoms, need for further injection, failure of treatment, resistance to toxin due to antibodies.

General risks: bleeding, infection.

Neurological complications after surgery

General complications

Intracranial pressure

cerebral perfusion pressure (CPP) =
mean arterial pressure (MAP) − intracranial pressure (ICP)

Therefore a rise in ICP lowers the CPP. There are significant autoregulatory mechanisms in place, and CPP would have to drop below 40mmHg before perfusion would be impaired. However, high CPPs are not protective against raised ICP. Raised ICP is a common complication of both head injury and surgical procedures. The Monro-Kellie hypothesis states that the contents of the skull (blood, brain, CSF, or space-occupying lesions) are of a constant volume and that in an inelastic box (the skull), an increase in one component necessitates a decrease in another or the pressure will rise.

An ICP greater than 25–30mmHg is likely to be fatal if uncontrolled, and the aim is to keep the ICP <20mmHg.

Causes of raised ICP

- cerebral oedema
- hyperaemia (the normal response to head injury)
- induced masses – haematoma following extradural (EDH), subdural (SDH), or intracranial bleeding (ICB) after a foreign object (such as a bullet) or a depressed skull fracture
- hydrocephalus, due to obstructed CSF flow or decreased absorption
- hypoventilation → raised CO_2 → vasodilatation
- raised BP exceeding autoregulation

Delayed raised ICP usually occurs 3–10 hours after an after initial insult and is associated with a worse prognosis. It may be caused by a delayed haematoma formation, by the onset of ARDS, or developing hyponatraemia.

Treatment

Treat the underlying cause.

Routine measures

Elevate the head to 30–45°, avoid sedation, avoid hypotension, control BP, control blood sugar, intubate if Glasgow Coma Scale (GCS) is <8, avoid hypoventilation, ensure adequate oxygenation.

Extended measures

Heavy sedation and paralysis, CSF drainage (via EVC), osmotic agents (mannitol: maximum permissible serum osmolality is 320mosm/l), hyperventilation, steroids (controversial in head injury and not currently recommended), hypothermia.

Final measures
- high dose barbiturate therapy
- decompressive craniectomy. Removal of a portion of the skull immediately increases the space. This may be coupled with removing portions of haemorrhagic parenchyma and more controversially temporal tip lobectomy (4–5cm on dominant side, 7cm on non-dominant).

Infection

Meningitis

Community acquired meningitis (CAM) is usually more fulminant than post-neurosurgical meningitis. Focal neurological signs are rare, and lumbar puncture (LP) is the investigation of choice (see below).

- In CAM the usual organisms are *Streptococcus pneumoniae* (pneumococcus) or *Neisseria meningitidis* (meningococcus) and should be treated empirically with cefotaxime 2g IV, although with increasing drug resistant strains in the community, vancomycin 1g IV is recommended.
- Post-surgical or post-traumatic meningitis is usually caused by *Staphylococcus aureus*, *Streptococci*, or *Pseudomonas*, and should be treated with vancomycin, and cefotaxime with gentamicin if *Pseudomonas* is the infecting organism.

Osteomyelitis of the skull

Haematogenous spread of infection is rare, and osteomyelitis usually follows a penetrating wound, or overlying scalp abscess. Commonly *Staph. aureus*, *Staph. epidermidis*, or *E. coli* in neonates are the offending organisms.

Treatment

Usually requires surgical debridement, rongeuring back to healthy bone. An infected cranioplasty flap needs to be removed and the skin closed without bony cover. Surgery is followed by an extended course of antibiotics (>4 weeks). Cranioplasty may be performed after 6 months of being infection free.

Surgical site infection

Incidence

0.9–5% of neurosurgical operations. *Staph. aureus* is the commonest infecting organism.

Treatment

- culture the wound
- empirically give IV vancomycin ± third generation cephalosporin
- wound debridement
- re-suture (tension must be avoided), or let wound heal by secondary intention, or consider plastic surgical reconstruction (especially if dura is exposed).

CSF leakage requires re-exploration with a watertight dural closure.

Spinal epidural abscess

Suspicion should be aroused after spinal surgery by the clinical triad of back pain, fever, and excruciating spinal tenderness. There may be a rapidly progressive myelopathy. The classically reported furuncle occurs only in approximately 15%. Abscesses commonly affect thoracic vertebrae (50%), the lumbar (35%), and cervical (15%).

Haematogenous spread is the commonest cause of an epidural abscess from an underlying infected focus (especially IV drug abuse, skin infections, or bacterial endocarditis). Post-surgical infection is rare (0.67% of lumbar discectomy patients) but can be from direct local invasion from psoas abscesses or pressure sores.

By far the commonest organism is *Staph. aureus* followed by *Streptococcus* and *E. coli*. In chronic infections, TB should be excluded, as it is usually associated with vertebral body osteomyelitis (Pott's disease).

Diagnosis

Cultures may be sterile (especially with concomitant antibiotic therapy). Imaging of choice is MRI (gadolinium-enhanced T2 weighted imagery), which shows a high intensity homogenous epidural mass with thin peripheral enhancement.

Treatment

A non-operative approach is only used in those too frail to tolerate surgical treatment. Otherwise, surgical debridement, culture specific antibiotics, plus post-surgery stabilization if necessary (with a TLSO brace) would be indicated.

CSF fistula

There are two types:
- Post-traumatic or after surgery, and these may be immediate or delayed.
- Spontaneous, which is rare.

This condition should be suspected in patients with rhinorrhea or otorrhea following head injury or surgery, or in patients with recurrent meningitis.

Traumatic fistulas occur after 2–3% of head injuries. Anosmia is a common finding in traumatic rhinorrhea (78%) but rare in spontaneous.

Common sites of leaks are percutaneously through the wound, the cribriform plate, sphenoid air cells, petrous ridge, or internal auditory canal; rarely from a lumbar drain site.

Diagnosis

Is this fluid CSF?

Fluid is clear (unless infected or mixed with blood). It tastes salty (to the patient). Quantitative glucose strips often register the glucose in mucus. CSF glucose >30mg%, mucus <5mg%.
- **Ring sign** – used in blood-tinged CSF: drip fluid onto linen, which forms a ring of blood, with a larger concentric ring – double ring or halo sign. An old, simple but unreliable sign.
- **B$_2$-transferrin** – present in CSF, absent in tears and mucus (except neonates and liver disease). It can be measured using electrophoresis in specialist laboratories.
- **Imaging** – CT with thin coronal cuts, and may require water-soluble contrast cisternography if multiple bony defects are seen on plain CT, or if a bony defect does not have associated soft tissue enhancement.

Treatment

Seventy per cent of CSF rhinorrheas stop within 1 week, 85% of otorrheas stop within 5–10 days. There is no proven benefit of prophylactic antibiotics.

Non-operative management

Observe, lower intracranial pressure with bed rest, avoid straining, give acetazolamide (to decrease CSF production), fluid restriction (caution in possible diabetes insipidus). If there is no obstructive hydrocephalus, consider LP or a lumbar drain, but beware of the possibility of causing a tension pneumocephalus.

Operative management

This should be undertaken if CSF drainage continues for >2/52 or is complicated by infection.

Air embolus

This is a potentially fatal complication of any surgery when an opening to air occurs in a non-collapsible vein (e.g. diploic vein or a dural sinus) and when there is negative pressure in the vein (for example when the head is elevated above the heart).

Operations at significant risk of air embolus (e.g. where the patient is in a sitting position) require the use of a pre-cordial Doppler, which will pick up machinery-like sounds, and this coupled with an increase in end-tidal CO_2 is an indication that immediate treatment should be instituted.

Treatment

Find and occlude the site of air entry, or pack the wound with soaking-wet sterile gauze. If possible lower the patient's head. Consider bilateral jugular venous compression. Rotate the patient left-side down (to trap air in right atrium), and then aspirate the right atrium using a CVP line. Give 100% O_2, and discontinue nitrous oxide if being used.

Metabolic post-neurosurgical complications

SIADH (Schwartz-Bartler syndrome)

Symptoms

Mainly related to low sodium – confusion, lethargy, coma, seizure, paradoxical thirst.

Findings

Increased urine osmolality and extracellular fluid, which lead to dilutional hyponatraemia.

Causes

- Malignant tumours.
- Trauma (4.6% in head injury patients).
- Raised ICP.
- Other tumours.
- Meningitis.
- Post-craniotomy.
- Sub-arachnoid haemorrhage (exclude cerebral salt wasting).
- Others – pulmonary, porphyria, drugs (chlorpropramide, oxytocin, thiazides).

Diagnosis

- Plasma sodium <135 mmol/l.
- Serum osmolality <280 mosm/l.
- Increased urinary sodium.
- A high urine osmolality to serum osmolality ratio.
- Normal thyroid, renal, and adrenal function.
- **Not** dehydrated (in which case increased ADH would be appropriate).

Treatment

- Exclude cerebral salt wasting (CSW).
- If due to low haemoglobin then transfuse.
- If mild and asymptomatic then fluid restrict 1l/day (in a child 1l/m^2/day).
- If severe then give hypertonic saline ± furosemide.

Beware central pontine myelinosis.

Cerebral salt wasting

In this complication there is renal loss of sodium due to intracranial disease, leading to a fall in plasma sodium and extracellular fluid volume (especially after subarachnoid haemorrhage).

Findings

↓Extracellular fluid volume and ↑serum osmolality and ↑urinary sodium.

Treatment

Fluid restriction can exacerbate CSW. Replace volume and sodium balance using 0.9% saline, 3% saline, or oral replacement.

Beware central pontine myelinosis.

Fludrocortisone 0.2mg IV can help sodium absorption but may cause pulmonary oedema, potassium loss, and raised BP.

Diabetes insipidus (DI)

This follows a lack of ADH (antidiuretic hormone), which leads to an increased output of dilute urine causing thirst with an increased or normal serum osmolality.

There are two main forms:
- central/neurogenic DI (due to hypothalamic pituitary axis dysfunction)
- nephrogenic DI (due to renal resistance to ADH).

Causes

Familial, idiopathic, post-traumatic, tumour, granuloma, infection, autoimmune, vascular (Sheehan's syndrome), hypokalaemia, hypercalcaemia, drugs (lithium, colchicine).

Diagnosis

A urine osmolality of 50–150mosm/l or a urinary specific gravity (SG) of 1.001 to 1.005 (mannitol can cause both high urine osmolality and SG). Urine output >250ml/hr with a normal or raised serum sodium.

Treatment

If the DI is mild (in a conscious patient), instruct the patient to drink **only** when thirsty. If severe, the patient may not tolerate increased oral intake and urine output. In this case use desmopressin 2.5µg intranasally up to 20 µg twice daily or 0.5–2µg IM/SC.

Seizures

Post-traumatic seizures may be divided into early or late (<7 or >7 days following head injury). There is a 30% incidence after severe head injury (severe being LOC >24hrs, amnesia >24hrs, focal deficit, intracranial haematoma) of early post-traumatic seizures. In high-risk patients (those with acute SDH, EDH, or ICH, open skull fracture, GCS <10, seizure within first 24hrs) anticonvulsants reduce the risk of post-traumatic seizures, and once epilepsy has developed continued therapy reduces the recurrence of seizures.

Treatment

Controversial. Give a phenytoin load 18mg/kg and maintain high therapeutic levels (or carbamazepine), which can be weaned after 1 week in absence of penetrating brain injury, prior seizure history, or development of late post-traumatic seizures.

Thromboembolic disease

Neurosurgical patients are particularly prone to thromboembolic disease due to prolonged operating times, long-term bed rest, paralysed limbs, and predisposing conditions (brain tumour patients have a prevalence of 28% at post-mortem).

The best form of treatment is prevention, and all neurosurgical patients should be considered for commencement of prophylactic low molecular weight heparin and TED stockings, with pneumatic compression boots in theatre. However, in some patients with a significant risk of bleeding or in whom post-op bleeding would be disastrous (e.g. spinal canal surgery), low molecular weight heparin may be omitted pre-op.

Specific complications

Craniotomy

Post-operative haemorrhage is a risk after all operations, and craniotomies have an overall risk of 0.8–11%. However, haemorrhage in the skull carries a significant risk of mortality of 32%.

Craniotomies for brain tumours carry an increased risk of anaesthetic complications of 0.2%, an increased neurological deficit in approximately 10%, and a risk of surgical site infection.

Any neurosurgical patient who deteriorates, especially after initially doing well, requires emergency evaluation and prompt treatment.

Causes of deterioration

- Haematoma: intra-cerebral, subdural, epidural.
- Cerebral infarction: arterial or venous.
- Post-operative seizure (may require intubation if not protecting own airway, CT scan, and a bolus of anticonvulsants).
- Acute hydrocephalus.
- Pneumocephalus (simple or tension). Simple pneumocephalus does not usually require evacuation, but tension pneumocephalus requires prompt evacuation with an urgency similar to an intracranial haematoma.
- Oedema – worsening of oedema is to some extent expected post-operatively, but reversible causes must be ruled out
- Neurological deficit – traction injuries to cranial nerves can cause temporary or permanent dysfunction.
- Systemic – hypoxia, electrolyte imbalance, infection.

Lumbar laminectomy

The overall risk of mortality is 6 in 10 000; usually due to septicaemia, MI, or PE.

Common complications
- Infection – superficial SSI 0.9–5%, deep SSI <1%.
- Increased motor deficit of 1–8%; some are transient.
- CSF fistula.
- Recurrence 4% at 10-year follow-up.

Uncommon complications
- Direct injury to neural structures.
- Injury to structures anterior to anterior longitudinal ligament:
  - great vessels (37–67% mortality)
  - ureters
  - bowel
  - sympathetic trunk.
- Post-operative spinal epidural haematoma leading to cauda equina syndrome (0.21%).
- DVT, PE, reflex sympathetic dystrophy, pseudo-obstruction of colon (Ogilvie's syndrome).
- Failed back syndrome. The failure rate of lumbar discectomy to provide long-term pain relief is 8–25%. Ongoing compensation and legal proceedings are associated with poor prognosis.

Anterior cervical decompression

Exposure injuries
- Perforation of oesophagus, trachea, or pharynx.
- Vocal cord paresis, due to damage to recurrent laryngeal nerve, often a neuropraxia from prolonged retraction. Causes hoarseness, cough, dysphagia, aspiration, or voice weakness. Commoner on right than left.
- Arterial injury, vertebral or carotid, may require surgical repair; just packing may lead to fistula or pseudoaneurysm.
- CSF fistula.
- Horner's syndrome – damage to sympathetic plexus.
- Thoracic duct injury – in exposing lower cervical spine.

Others
- Spinal cord injury – especially with pre-existing canal narrowing.
- Failure of fusion, pseudarthrosis, kyphotic deformity.
- Surgical site infection <1%.
- Haematoma.
- RSD.

Shunts

Categorized by position: ventriculo-peritoneal, ventriculo-atrial, Torkildsen (ventriculo-cisternal space), ventriculo-pleural, and lumboperitoneal.

Many of the post-operative complications of shunts are due to the longevity of their placement. Complications include infection, erosion (particularly in the debilitated), disconnection or damage to the shunt, obstruction (at distal end or at the valve), seizures, or seeding of metastases (theoretical risk).

Other complications are due to their anatomical location. These include blockage (by omentum in VP shunts), need for lengthening (all shunts, but especially VA), inguinal hernia, CSF ascites, peritonitis, and retrograde blood flow into ventricles (VA shunts only, rare).

The settings of the shunt valves themselves can lead to complications of 'undershunting' or 'overshunting' causing raised intracranial pressure or intracranial hypotension respectively.

Shunt infection

This is commonly due to *Staph. epidermidis*, *Staph. aureus*, or Gram-negative *bacilli* (from intestinal perforation). History should be sought for an ectopic infective locus. The vast majority are iatrogenic. A shunt tap should be sent to assess presence of Gram-negative bacteria requiring different antimicrobials.

Treatment

Leaving a shunt *in situ* is only recommended when the patient is terminally ill, a poor anaesthetic candidate, or where slit ventricles make re-cannulation difficult. If a shunt is removed an alternate CSF pathway needs to be instituted, such as an extraventricular drain.

Antibiotics

These need to be given empirically (IV vancomycin ± oral rifampicin), followed by culture-specific antibiotics. Intra-ventricular antibiotics may be used through EVD, but intra-thecal antibiotics are not recommended.

Transsphenoidal hypophysectomy

There are many different indications and approaches for hypophysectomy. The complications are related to both the condition and the surgical approach.

• Hormonal imbalance:
  • deficient ADH, including diabetes insipidus
  • deficient cortisol can lead to an Addisonian crisis if severe
  • hypothyroidism can lead to myxoedematous coma
  • deficient sex hormones leading to hypogonadotrophic hypogonadism.
• Secondary empty sella syndrome – chiasm drops into empty sella turcica causing visual impairment.
• Hydrocephalus.
• Infection, including pituitary abscess.
• CSF rhinorrhea, 3.5% incidence. This may be treated with an intra-sella fat graft and lumbar drainage.
• Carotid artery rupture.
• Damage to cavernous sinus and structures therein.
• Perforation of nasal septum.

Lumbar puncture

The overall risk of serious complications (persistent headache, worsening neurological condition, nerve root injury) is approximately 0.1–0.5%.

Possible complications

- tonsillar herniation
- infection (spinal meningitis)
- 'spinal headache' – usually positional
- spinal epidural haematoma, usually only seen in the presence of a coagulopathy
- nerve root radiculopathy.

The debate about whether to undertake a scan before an LP for safety, at the cost of time delay, is controversial. The cases of LP causing herniation are all pre-1950s and pre-CT scan, were all performed with a large-gauge cannula, and led to therapeutic drainage of large quantities of CSF. The presence of CT scanners in almost all A&E departments means that scans can be obtained promptly, and thus do not delay the administration of antibiotics. However, should the scan take longer than a few minutes to obtain, the risk of taking a few droplets of CSF is minimal. The anecdotal recommendation, if the patient deteriorates suddenly, is to re-inject the CSF through the LP needle.

Head injuries

Head injuries may be divided into penetrating, crush injuries, deceleration injuries, and projectile injuries (e.g. GSW). Each type of injury carries its own complications, and of course many of these overlap.

The most obvious early complication is death, with approximately 0.5% of patients with head injuries dying, either at the scene or soon after reaching hospital (the 'talk and die' cohort). Intracranial bleeding is the commonest mechanism behind this and it is common to all types of head injury, and often requires prompt diagnosis and surgical intervention.

Penetrating and projectile injuries are commonly associated with dural damage and hence CSF leak and its concomitant infective risks.

Crush and deceleration injuries may be more associated with widespread parenchymal damage causing raised intracranial pressure and increased risk of epileptogenesis.

Any injury that affects the base of the skull, as well as risking CSF leak, has the potential to damage cranial nerves as they egress from the skull.

Other risks include:

• Fat embolus, which has the symptoms of drowsiness, confusion, seizures, and cerebral irritation, along with pulmonary symptoms. These often occur 1–3 days following injury and the diagnosis may be confirmed by the presence of a petechial rash.

• Caroticocavernous fistula can occur with minor trauma or with no recollection of trauma at all. It is commonest in middle-aged women. The patient becomes aware of a to-and-fro murmur in their head, in time with their pulse. It is readily auscultated over the eyeball. Look for proptosis and chemosis. Approximately 50% of low-flow fistulas resolve spontaneously and can be safely observed as long as the vision is stable and intra-ocular pressure is <25mmHg. Otherwise, balloon embolization is the treatment of choice.

Complications of hand surgery

Introduction

The most common complication of any hand injury is stiffness, due to a combination of the primary pathology, the effect of surgery, and immobility following surgery. The collaborative effects of inflammation, swelling, and immobility all contribute. Early mobilization is therefore the key to success.

The other most common complications of hand surgery are:
- infection
- poor healing
- deep venous thrombosis
- anaesthetic reactions.

Hand surgery complications in general

While hand surgery comprises a diverse range of pathologies and surgical procedures, there are some aspects to the surgery that are shared by many of the procedures, and that share complications related to them. Prevention is the key (□ see Box 23.1).

Use of a tourniquet

Tourniquet palsy is an infrequent complication of tourniquet use that occurs in 1 in 5000 cases. This is more common after microsurgical than other procedures. While ischaemia and pressure necrosis are largely the postulated underlying aetiologies, risk factors include patients with coagulation disorders, pre-existing neuropathy, thin, malnourished patients, those with systemic lupus erythematosis, and where high tourniquet pressures are encountered due to gauge failure. While all nerves are usually affected to some degree, the radial nerve is the most often affected.

Bandaging and/or plastering

Tight dressings can contribute to pain, stiffness, and distal swelling if mild, or frank ischaemia if severe. While some degree of pressure can be beneficial to prevent swelling or haematoma formation and immobility, dressings should always be loose enough to facilitate vascular supply and drainage. Minimally tight dressings (even gauze or other elastic dressings) if applied circumferentially may lead to distal swelling. Progressive swelling can further contribute to the occlusive effects of the dressing and venous return from the distal parts may become progressively impaired. Swelling may mask progressive problems by hindering assessment and may delay surgery until a reduction in swelling is achieved by elevation and change to a non-compressive dressing.

Tight plaster-casts may also result in local pressure sores, discomfort, and at worst, vascular compromise and compartment syndrome.

Management

- Prevention is the key. If applied with care and non-circumferentially, complications of elastic dressings are much less likely. Multiple layers of gauze applied non-circumferentially deep to the bandage ensures that the deepest layer of bandage cannot provide circumferential pressure.
- When plaster-casts are used, loose application is essential. In the setting of immediate plastering after injury (with further swelling likely to ensue), prospective splitting of the cast immediately after application is suggested.
- Where vascular compromise is suggested, immediate splitting of all occlusive dressings is essential, including plaster-cast, bandage, and gauze.
- Measurement of compartment pressures and compartment fasciotomies may need consideration earlier rather than later.

Inadequate positioning

The hand should be immobilized in a position that aids healing while minimizing the risk of joint stiffness. Splints and other supportive dressings maintain a posture that may thus be both helpful and detrimental. Ensuring the best position is essential. If there is any doubt as to the adequacy of positioning, an X-ray may be useful.

Wound care

Inadequate wound care, in terms of both choice of dressing and frequency of dressing changes, can discourage healing and permit excessive bacterial growth. This bacterial growth occurs in moist, undisturbed conditions, and can be commonly seen beneath occlusive bandages in the crevices and the interdigital web spaces of the immobilized hand. Uncontrolled surface growth can produce direct skin invasion, causing maceration dermatitis, which may progress to cellulitis.

Management
- frequent dressing changes
- ensuring a dry environment
- antibiotics where indicated.

Infection

Infections in hand surgery are uncommon as the hand has an abundant blood supply, with infection rates reported frequently at less than 10%. Predisposing factors for infection include gross contamination, crush injury (both soft tissue and bony crush), systemic illnesses or immunocompromise, smoking, or delay in treatment.

Box 23.1 General preventative principles

- Stop smoking.
- Optimize co-morbid conditions, e.g. diabetes mellitis, renal function.
- Adequate debridement prior to definitive treatment.
- Minimize tourniquet time and pressure.
- Dressings – loose, carefully applied.
- Wound care – keep wounds dry, frequent dressing changes.
- Early mobilization.
- Hand physiotherapy.

Specific hand surgery complications

Trauma hand surgery

Operation: nail bed repair
- Benefits: improve growth of nail plate.
- Anaesthetic: LA.
- Specific risks: abnormal nail growth, nail ridges.
- General risks: bleeding, infection.

Operation: terminalization
- Benefits: improve healing and function of finger.
- Anaesthetic: LA.
- Specific risks: wound dehiscence, sensitive tip, reduced or altered sensation, abnormal nail growth (depending on level).
- General risks: scars, infection, bleeding.

Operation: flexor tendon repair
- Benefits: improve hand function.
- Anaesthetic: GA.
- Specific risks: re-rupture of tendon, scar contracture, adhesions, stiffness with reduced function, bowstringing if pulleys are significantly damaged, need for further operation.
- General risks: scars, infection, bleeding.

Operation: extensor tendon repair
- Benefits: improve extensor/hand function.
- Anaesthetic: LA or GA (depending on level of injury and number of digits affected).
- Specific risks: re-rupture of tendon, stiffness, adhesions restricting movement and function.
- General risks: scars, infection, bleeding.

Operation: washout of infective flexor tenosynovitis
- Benefits: improve symptoms and retain flexor tendon function.
- Anaesthetic: GA.
- Specific risks: damage to pulley or flexor sheath, need for further washout.
- General risks: scars, bleeding.

Operation: nerve repair
- Benefits: improve sensation.
- Anaesthetic: LA or GA (depending on level).
- Specific risks: increased, reduced, or altered sensation, scar contracture.
- General risks: scars, infection, bleeding.

Operation: re-implantation of digit or limb
- Benefits: reattachment of amputated digit or limb.
- Anaesthetic: GA.
- Specific risks: prolonged operative time with long recovery and rehabilitation, failure of re-implantation, need for grafts (vein, nerve, skin), use of skin or muscle flaps, infection, non-union of bone, decreased sensation and range of movement, chronic pain, cold intolerance, further operation.
- General risks: scars, bleeding.

Operation: open reduction and internal fixation of fracture
- Benefits: aid union of fracture and improve hand function.
- Anaesthetic: GA.
- Specific risks: infection (of wound, deep tissues, or osteomyelitis), nerve or vessel damage, skin necrosis, malunion or non-union, palpable or painful hardware, stiffness, arthritic joint (if intra-articular fracture).
- General risks: scars, bleeding.

Operation: closed reduction and Kirschner-wire fixation of fracture
- Benefits: aid union of fracture and improve hand function.
- Anaesthetic: GA or LA.
- Specific risks: infection (of wound, pin-site, deep tissues, or osteomyelitis), nerve or vessel damage, skin necrosis, malunion or non-union, loosening, migration, tendon transfixation, skin irritation, stiffness, arthritic joint (if intra-articular fracture).
- General risks: scars, bleeding.

Elective hand surgery

Operation: open carpal tunnel release
- Benefits: relieve symptoms of numbness, paraesthesia, and pain secondary to median nerve compression.
- Anaesthetic: LA.
- Specific risks: sensitive scar, damage to median nerve, damage to palmar cutaneous branch of median nerve, pillar pain, flexion weakness, pisotriquetral syndrome, chronic regional pain syndrome, recurrence of symptoms.
- General risks: infection, haematoma, dehiscence.

Operation: trigger finger release (stenosing tenosynovitis)
- Benefits: relieve symptoms of locking finger and discomfort and improve function.
- Anaesthetic: LA.
- Specific risks: nerve or vessel damage, recurrence of symptoms, incomplete release of pulley, further operation.
- General risks: scar, infection, bleeding.

Operation: excision of ganglion
- Benefits: excision of cyst, improve symptoms of pain and wrist weakness, cosmesis.
- Anaesthetic: GA or regional block.
- Specific risks: nerve or vessel damage, recurrence, joint (wrist) stiffness.
- General risks: scar, infection, bleeding.

Operation: arthrodesis
- Benefits: fusion of a joint to relieve symptoms and improve hand function.
- Anaesthetic: depends on level – LA (if DIPJ or PIPJ) or GA/regional block if more proximal.
- Specific risks: nerve or vessel damage, nail bed injury (DIPJ joint), infection (pin tract and deep), non-union or malunion of bone, stiffness, skin necrosis, extensor adhesions, painful or prominent hardware, cold intolerance.
- General risks: scars, bleeding.

Operation: Dupuytren's fasciectomy
- Benefits: excision of abnormal fibrous tissue to improve symptoms and hand function.
- Anaesthetic: GA or regional block.
- Specific risks: bleeding/haematoma, nerve or vessel damage, scar contracture, stiffness, continued joint contracture, recurrence, chronic regional pain syndrome, graft loss (in dermofasciectomy).
- General risks: scars, infection.

Consent and other medico-legal issues

Introduction

In relation to post-operative complications, two main legal issues stand out: consent and negligence. Patients need to understand the risks of any surgical intervention, but at the same time be confident that their treatment will be undertaken in a safe and competent manner.

A summary of important aspects of consent, negligence, and other medico-legal factors is provided in the following chapter. Brief summaries are provided in relation to confidentiality, data protection, expert witnesses, medico-legal reports, and record-keeping.

Consent

Has my patient agreed to treatment, having understood the treatment and risks involved? If you can answer 'yes' to this question, then you have probably obtained consent that is legally valid from your patient. However, it is good practice to gain such consent in writing, and indeed it is difficult not to obtain written consent for an operation due to the various guidelines and protocols in hospitals today (📖 see Box 24.1). Written consent provides a useful infrastructure around which to base consent, but its role is purely evidentiary, and a signature on the form does not in itself constitute consent:

'I regard the consent form immediately before operation as pure window dressing ... and designed to avoid the suggestion that a patient has not been told' – Lord Popwell in Taylor v. Shropshire HA *[1998].*

Historical perspective

In 1767, the importance of consent was acknowledged by the courts for the first time in the legal case of *Slater v. Baker & Stapleton*, where surgery had been performed against the wishes of the patient. Consent has taken on greater importance with the development of tolerable and safe treatments, particularly surgical intervention. Prior to anaesthesia and asepsis, many procedures were undertaken *in extremis*, often forced upon restrained patients. Even so, written consent forms date back as early as the Ottoman Empire.

Consent also has an important bearing in relation to experimentation. The development of modern consent law has undoubtedly been shaped by scandals in history, especially in relation to human experimentation. Examples include Nazi experiments highlighted in the Nuremberg trials, those conducted under the Manhattan project involving radioactive exposure of hospital patients without their knowledge, the feeding of radioactive cereal to learning-disabled children at Fernald School in the 1950s, and the Tuskegee Syphilis studies, which ran into the 1970s. Various regulatory agreements including the Declaration of Helsinki were developed to deal with these sorts of issues.

Why is consent important?

Consent is not only important for upholding patient autonomy – the 'right to self-determination' – but it also leads to improved clinical outcomes through better cooperation from patients. Although we as doctors may think we know what is 'best' for patients in terms of medical treatments and likely outcomes, we are less qualified to judge when it comes to what is 'best' for patients within the context of their lives and taking into account their priorities and beliefs. Doctors should therefore guide patients into making decisions by providing them with adequate explanation and information in this context. Consent also remains a moral, ethical, and professional duty – as well as a legal one. Philosophically it is a concept, whereas practically it is a system implemented in the workplace to provide an infrastructure to obtain and document patient acceptance of treatment.

Obtaining consent within the UK National Health Service tends to revolve around the consent form. This is filled in by clinicians and details the relevant procedure along with risks and benefits, and is signed by patients. But it is worth noting that there is no legal obligation to obtain written consent – simply to obtain consent that is valid. Furthermore, a request-based method of consent has recently been described (✍ www.rft.org.uk). The only circumstances in which written consent is mandatory relate to treatments carried out under the jurisdiction of the Mental Health Act 1983 and the Human Fertilisation and Embryology Act 1990.

Nevertheless, many of the procedural aspects of consent are derived through the stipulations of third parties, not the courts. These include the General Medical Council (GMC) and British Medical Association (BMA) guidelines, as well as policies set out by individual Hospital Trusts. It is worth pointing out that consent for anaesthesia has not been adopted in the UK. This is despite the fact that the anaesthetic may pose greater risks than the procedure itself – for example, a nail bed repair or other minor procedure in a small child.

Box 24.1 Types of consent

- No consent ('best interests'). However, subsequent to the Mental Capacity Act 2005, an Independent Mental Healthcare Advocate (IMHA) may be required.
- Implied consent.
- Verbal consent.
- Written consent.
- Advance directive (consenting to or refusing treatment at some future date if capacity is lost).

Refusing treatment

Anyone with an adequate mental capacity can refuse treatment – even if this might lead to the demise of that individual. Hence the result in *Malette v. Shulman* [1990]: a life-saving blood transfusion was not justified in a Jehovah's Witness who had specifically refused this treatment.

Consent law

The law does not, as one might expect, have a single 'rule-book' with which to deal with issues of consent. There exists a two-tier system whereby doctors can be held accountable for undertaking treatment without consent, and this is determined by the 'degree of absence' of consent. Therefore, if there is no consent whatsoever, such as when treatment has been explicitly refused or the patient is treated entirely without their prior knowledge, then this is '*trespass* to the person' (assault/battery). In these circumstances, merely the act of undertaking treatment – even with a perfect outcome and absence of any harm – results in the award of damages if a legal challenge is undertaken on this basis. Such claims are uncommon, and occur in circumstances such as giving blood transfusions to a Jehovah's Witness, or undertaking an additional procedure whilst under anaesthetic that has not been discussed with the patient (unless the need was emergent/life-saving, e.g. *Devi v. West Midlands HA* [1981]).

If some attempt at consent is undertaken, and this is shown to be inadequate, the legal jurisdiction of a claim will be in *negligence*. Most commonly, patients seek compensation due to a lack of awareness of specific risks of surgery, which then materialize as a complication. However, proving negligence is more of a challenge for a claimant. One obstacle has traditionally been a burden of proof from a claimant that had the consent been undertaken appropriately (e.g. adequate explanation of a specific risk), they would have declined treatment on that basis; an onerous task.

The cornerstone of negligence law is based around the Bolam principle, whereby: 'A doctor is not guilty of negligence if he/she has acted in accordance with a practice accepted as proper by a responsible body of medical professionals.' However, the controversial case of *Chester v. Afshar* [2004] has to some extent changed matters, and it is debated that we are closer now to the 'informed consent' position in the USA than ever. What used to be 'the prudent doctor test' (risk disclosure that a prudent doctor would have provided) is now 'the prudent patient test' (risks that a prudent patient would want to know about).

Box 24.2 Common misconceptions regarding consent

- Written consent is mandatory in law (No – but it is good practice and part of NHS guidelines).
- Written consent must be undertaken using specific forms to be valid (No).
- Informed consent means 'really good consent' (No – it has a quite specific legal meaning and is often used inappropriately).
- There is a cut-off of 1%, and risks that are lower than this need not be imparted (No – specific risks are imparted either on the basis of the 'prudent doctor' test or the 'prudent patient' test).

Box 24.3 Essential constituents of consent

- Capacity: adult (over 16 for consent), conscious, and 'of sound mind'.
- Sufficient provision of information.
- Understanding of information provided.
- Absence of duress.

As per *Chatterton v. Gerson*, and Mental Capacity Act 2005.

Children

A person over 16 years of age may give consent to medical treatment as though he/she was an adult. For those under 16, the principle laid down in Gillick applies (*Gillick v. West Norfolk and Wisbech Area Health Authority* [1986]). The parental right to determine whether a child under 16 receives or refuses medical treatment ends when the child achieves a significant understanding and intelligence to enable him/her to fully comprehend what is proposed. Where an apparently competent child refuses treatment, case law suggests that it may still be possible to treat the child provided that someone else with the capacity to consent consents on the child's behalf (in *Re R.* [1991] and *Re W.* [1992]). The position is different in Scotland where those with parental responsibilities cannot authorize procedures a competent child has refused. Sometimes the matter may need to be referred to the courts.

Capacity and advance directives

'Competent patients' decisions about accepting or rejecting proposed treatment are respected. Incompetent patients' choices … are put to one side …. Thus, enjoyment of one of the most fundamental rights of a free society – the right to determine what shall be done to one's body – turns on the possession of those characteristics that we view as decision-making competence.' (Grisso and Appelbaum, 1998: 1.)

This quotation highlights the importance of mental capacity and competence (synonymous). The Mental Capacity Act (MCA) 2005 has formalized many aspects of the law pertaining to competence of patients to consent to treatment. Nobody can consent on behalf of a patient, and so treatment has until recently either progressed in the best interest of the patient (decided by doctors, and documented appropriately, for example using the UK National Health Service 'consent form 4'), or simply not been undertaken (or postponed if incapacity is temporary and treatment non-urgent). However, new procedures have now been introduced since the MCA 2005, whereby patients without capacity may need to be assigned an independent mental health advocate (IMCA) who will become involved in the decision-making and consent process. This is a significant change to the previous situation and readers are urged to refer to the Department of Health website. Of course it is still important to communicate with and involve relatives in such decisions. The GMC has produced guidance on this issue.

If a patient has lost the capacity to consent to or refuse treatment, the doctor should attempt to ascertain whether the patient has previously indicated preferences in an advance statement. The GMC guidance states that the doctor must respect any refusal of treatment given when the patient was competent, provided that the decision given in the advance statement is clearly applicable to the circumstances, and there is no reason to believe that the patient has changed his or her mind. If there is no advance statement then the patient's known wishes should be taken into account.

Negligence

Negligence law aims to protect the public and maintain standards. Without accountability, standards inevitably slip, and almost everyone at some stage requires medical care and should be entitled to expect that care be delivered with due diligence. Negligence does not deal with unavoidable risks of a procedure, which is covered by consent law, unless that consent has itself been undertaken negligently (i.e. the appropriate risks were not disclosed and the patient suffered the consequences of such a specific risk).

In order to determine that a doctor is negligent the claimant must establish three things:
- the doctor owed him/her a duty of care
- there has been a breach of that duty
- the plaintiff has suffered damage as a breach of that duty.

The standard of care required by law is expressed in the Bolam test (*Bolam v. Friern Hospital Management Committee* [1957]). This states:

'... it is the standard of the ordinary skilled man exercising and professing to have that special skill. A man need not possess the highest expert skill; it is well-established law that it is sufficient if he exercises the ordinary skill of an ordinary competent man exercising that art.'

The standard of care relates to the specialty in which the doctor practises. A lack of experience is no defence against an allegation of negligence, but a trainee surgeon may discharge his/her duty by seeking the help of a superior (*Wilsher v. Essex Health Authority*). The prudent trainee will not step beyond his/her capabilities but will always seek advice when in doubt.

The Bolam test has established that a doctor will not be held negligent simply because they hold a different view from other members of their specialty, provided that they can prove that there is a reasonable body of opinion that supports their view. Every doctor has a duty to keep themselves abreast of developments in their field. It is, however, probably reasonable not to be aware of a single paper that might have prevented the negligent act. On the other hand, it is likely that not being aware of practice that has become widespread would be unacceptable to a judge (*Crawford v. Board of Governors of Charing Cross Hospital*).

Proof of medical negligence

It is not sufficient for a plaintiff to show that a surgeon's actions were below an acceptable standard; they must also prove that the damage suffered was a result of the surgeon's poor performance. In *Barnett v. Chelsea and Kensington Hospital* [1968], the casualty officer failed to examine a patient who attended with signs of poisoning. Yet the case was successfully defended when it was established that the poison had no antidote.

The claimant has to show that his/her version of events with expert analysis is, on the balance of probabilities, more likely to be true than that of the defence. Where the issues are equally balanced, the claimant will fail.

An apparent reversal can occur when res ipsa loquitor is pleaded. This literally means 'the facts speak for themselves'. Good examples of this would be a retained swab following surgery or amputation of the wrong leg. In these circumstances, the onus is on the defence to provide an adequate explanation of how the injury occurred that is consistent with an acceptable standard of care.

Box 24.4 Essential record-keeping
- Date and time all entries in the notes.
- Make yourself identifiable in three ways – print your name as the first line of your entry. This is the most important step. Make your entry legible. Sign your entry and provide a contact (e.g. bleep number).
- Document who was present including chaperone(s) if relevant.
- Make sure what is written is an adequate reflection of the encounter, and clarify if need be.
- If notes are written in on your behalf, you should take responsibility for educating and enforcing good record-keeping practice.
- A regular audit of department note-keeping can ensure high standards, and 'name and shame' for poor record-keepers can be positive in these circumstances.

Box 24.5 Dealing with confidential data
- Confidential data should be made available only to those with a valid right to see or use them.
- They should be stored in a protected environment.
- Encryption and password protection are important for electronic storage.
- Data transfer should be minimized, and when undertaken should be done securely.
- Limit sending identifiable data using methods that could lead to loss or interception.
- Register with the Data Controller if you are storing clinical data and/or images.
- Obtain consent for use or disclosure.

Expert witness
In cases of medical negligence and personal injury the court may require assistance to resolve the issues from a medical expert. From 26 April 1999 the Civil Procedure Rules 1999 replaced all previous rules governing the conduct of civil litigation in both the High Court and the County Court in England and Wales. Part 35 of these Rules set out obligations of Experts and Assessors.

The expert has an overriding duty to the court to help on the matters within his/her expertise.

In the case of the Ikarian Reefer, Cresswell laid down guidance on the duties and responsibilities of the expert. This is a key case, and any expert witness should read it.

- Expert evidence presented to the court should be, and should be seen to be, the independent product of the expert, uninfluenced as to form or content by the exigencies of litigation. (See *Whitehouse v. Jordan* [1981] 1 WLR 246. 256.)
- Independent assistance should be provided to the court by way of objective, unbiased opinion regarding matters within the expertise of the expert witness. (See *Polivitre Ltd v. Commercial Union Assurance Co. plc.* [1987] 1 Lloyds Rep. 379. 386. and Re J. [1990] ECR 193. An expert witness in the High Court should never assume the role of advocate.)
- Facts or assumptions upon which the opinion was based should be stated together with material facts that could detract from the concluded opinion.
- An expert witness should make it clear when a question or issue fell outside his/her expertise.
- If the opinion was not properly researched because it was considered that insufficient data were available, then that had to be stated with an indication that the opinion was provisional (see Re J.) If the witness could not assert that the report contained the truth, the whole truth, and nothing but the truth, then the qualification should be stated on the report. (See *Derby & Co Ltd. and Others v. Weldon and Others* [No. 9] *The Times*, 9 November 1990.)
- If after exchange of reports an expert witness changed his/her mind on a material matter, then the change of view should be communicated to the other side through legal representatives without delay and when appropriate to the court.
- Photographs, plans, survey reports, and other documents referred to in the expert evidence had to be provided to the other side at the same time as exchange of reports.

Medico-legal reports and statements

The Civil Procedure Rules lay down certain rules that must be complied with in preparing a report. These are:

- The report must be addressed to the Court stating which party, or parties, have instructed the expert.
- The report must state the substance of all material instructions, whether written or oral, on the basis of which the report is written. It must summarize the material facts of the case.
- Where there is a range of opinion on matters dealt with in the report the range must be summarized and you must make clear the reasons for your own opinion.
- Your conclusions must be summarized.
- The report must conclude with a statement of truth in the following form: '*I believe that the facts I have stated in the report are true and the opinions I have expressed are correct.*'
- There must be a statement that the expert understands his/her duty to the court and has complied with that duty.

- The expert must set out details of his/her qualifications, details of any literature or other material relied on in making the report, and identify any person who carried out any test or experiment that the expert has used, giving the qualifications of such a person.

In preparing a report for the court the expert should be clear on what the court requires. If necessary, guidance can be obtained from the instructing parties or directly from the court. Reports usually refer to one or more of the following six areas:

- an initial statement on the possible merits of an allegation for a plaintiff before notes and other evidence are obtained
- liability
- causation
- current condition
- prognosis
- expert opinion on an area of medicine.

A quote should be given on the cost of a report in advance. It is also advisable to quote an hourly rate for work. This should include travel to meetings with counsel and a rate for attending court.

The report should be typed on A4-size paper. Each sheet should have the name of the claimant and the expert's name in the top left-hand corner. Each paragraph and each page should be numbered. It is useful to enclose a short curriculum vitae for use of counsel and the court. It is inadvisable to use the word 'negligent' in a report. The finding of negligence is the province of the judge. However, phrases such as 'fell below a reasonable standard of care' or 'followed a course of action that could not be supported by any body of medical opinion' are useful to imply serious criticism. Phrases such as 'flagrant disregard' or 'reckless course of action' should be avoided as they may carry criminal connotations.

The court or any party can put written questions to the expert, who has to reply within 28 days. If the expert does not reply within the 28 days, then the party who instructed the expert in the first place will be unable to rely on his/her evidence or will be unable to recover the expert's fee.

Those undertaking significant amounts of expert witness or medico-legal report work will benefit from attending a specialist course, of which there are a number.

Actions after a medical accident

Appropriate action after an accident may avoid litigation or, if litigation does arise, lead to a speedy conclusion of the action.

- Keep good records of the event. Do not alter any previous records, but if previous records have been inadequate, write up your memory of the events and findings leading up to the mishap. Date and sign all entries.
- Fill out an Incident Form or write a full description of the events to your hospital's legal department. Consider informing your defence organization, particularly if the patient has died.
- Give a truthful explanation to the patient. However, be sure of your facts lest you give incorrect information. If the patient is dead or unconscious it is reasonable to inform the next of kin of the situation, unless the patient had expressly forbade the disclosure prior to

losing consciousness. In most circumstances of a medical accident, the consultant in charge of the case should give the explanation; however, if the consultant is unavailable then relatives or the patient should not be left waiting for an inordinate length of time.

• An apology and expression of regret concerning the outcome is not an admission of guilt and so should not be withheld. Every attempt should be made to maintain the patient's confidence in the doctor and not to build up a feeling in the patient that the doctor has become self-centred and defensive. On no account be arrogant. Where appropriate, offer the reassurance of a second opinion or even transfer of the patient to a separate team or hospital if that is what the patient wishes.

Medico-legal protection

It would be unwise for any medical practitioner not to be insured by one of the main medical insurers (MPS, MDU, MDDUS). Whilst most aspects of practice within the NHS are covered by the NHS 'Crown' indemnity, there are many areas for which you are not covered. Furthermore, if there are other issues such as legal action or suspension initiated by the hospital in which you work, GMC proceedings, and issues surrounding harassment at work in which you may be embroiled, then you may find you have no advocate and no cover. The British Medical Association is limited in the areas in which it will provide support and it will always be discretionary.

Acknowledgement

Many thanks to Maurice Hawthorne for the excellent paragraphs on expert witness and reports that were retained from the first edition.

References

Grisso, T. and Appelbaum, P. S. (1998) *Assessing Competence to Consent to Treatment*. Oxford University Press, Oxford.

　　ℬ http://www.gmc-uk.org/guidance/ethical_guidance/consent_guidance/index.asp.

　　ℬ http://www.gmc-uk.org/guidance/current/library/confidentiality.asp.

　　ℬ www.rft.org.uk

Mental Capacity Act 2005:

　　ℬ http://www.opsi.gov.uk/ACTS/acts2005/ukpga_20050009_en_1

Independent Mental Capacity Advocate (IMCA) service:

　　ℬ http://www.dh.gov.uk/en/SocialCare/Deliveringadultsocialcare/MentalCapacity/IMCA/index.htm

Index

Printed and bound by CPI Group (UK) Ltd, Croydon, CR0 4YY